ress Cataloging-in-Publication Data

quivalence/edited by Andre J. Jackson.

ographical references and index.
-6930-4
herapeutic equivalency. 2. Drugs —Bioavailability.
. I. Jackson, Andre J.
1994

93-44588
CIP

d Book Number 0-8493-6930-4
Card Number 93-44588
States of America 2 3 4 5 6 7 8 9 0
aper

GENER
AN
BIOEQUIV

Edite

André J. Jac
Office of Ge
Center for Drug Eval
Food and Drug
Rockville

C
Boca Raton An

Library of Cong

Generics and bioe
p. cm.
Includes bibl
ISBN 0-8493
1. Drugs —
3. Generic drug
RM301.45.G46
615′.1 — dc20

FOREWORD

Societal decisions reflected in patent law and the Food, Drug, and Cosmetic (FD&C) Act have created in the United States, over a period of about 50 years, three important time periods in the life of a new drug product. The first of these periods is the time prior to approval, when pre-clinical and clinical studies are performed to document safety and efficacy during the IND/NDA process. This period was generally created by the 1938 and 1962 amendments to the FD&C Act. The second period centers on the period of marketing exclusivity that generally occurs after approval of a new drug and prior to the time when generic substitution is permitted. This period is maintained by U.S. patent law and by certain exclusivity provisions of the 1984 Drug Price Competition and Patent Term Restoration amendments to the FD&C Act. The third and last period occurs after termination of patent or exclusivity protection, when multiple manufacturers — generic and innovator — are allowed to market the same drug in different formulations. This domain was created in final form in the U.S. by the 1984 amendments to the FD&C Act.

The societal decisions embodied in the 1984 amendments to the FD&C Act rest on the assumption that several pharmaceutical firms can manufacture different formulations of the same active drug substance that exhibit comparable quality and performance characteristics such that interchangeability between any formulation is likely to produce the same safety and efficacy results. This assumption rests on a science and technology base that (a) permits manufacture of pharmaceutical formulations with identifiable and reproducible quality and performance characteristics; and (b) allows testing of these pharmaceutical formulations to support the conclusion that interchangeable safety and efficacy effects are likely to occur, one bioequivalent formulation to another. The first of these science and technology areas is generally considered in the chemistry, manufacturing and controls portion of a new or abbreviated drug application. The second is considered in the determination of bioequivalence, which is the focus of this text.

From the perspective of both the FDA and pharmaceutical firms, documentation of bioequivalence may be required during any of the three periods in the life of a new drug product. In the IND/NDA phase, documentation of bioequivalence between clinical trial, pilot, and production batches of an innovator formulation may be critical to a reasonable interpretation of clinical trial data and the expectation that the marketed dosage form will be equivalent to the material on which the determination of safety and efficacy was made. After approval, bioequivalence between formulations of the single source innovator product may be equally important, particularly during scale-up and when changes occur in the formulation, site, process or equipment of manufacture. After patent or exclusivity expiration, bioequivalence between the reference listed product and its generic equivalents is not only important but mandatory, based on regulatory requirements of the FD&C Act. Also, changes in the manufacture of the generic equivalent, including changes associated with scale-up, may occur, just as for the pioneer product.

This text focuses on the determination of bioequivalence between formulations that are pharmaceutically equivalent and manufactured using acceptable chemistry, manufacturing and controls and in accordance with Good Manufacturing Practices. The determination of bioequivalence may be made using one or more *in vitro* or *in vivo* modalities, including (1) measurement of drug or active metabolite in an accessible biologic fluid (usually serum or plasma); (2) measurement of a pharmacologic effect; (3) results from a comparative clinical trial; (4) *in vitro* dissolution tests; (5) animal studies; and (6) other methods. Measurement of drug or metabolite in biologic fluid generally offers requisite sensitivity and specificity, although even with this modality questions can arise. Several of these questions —analytical validation, the use of metabolite data, single dose versus steady state studies, the measurement of enantiomers of a drug with a chiral center — are considered in the text. The remaining modalities are generally employed when drug/metabolite concentrations in a biologic fluid are not sufficiently high to permit measurement, or for drug products that are not systemically absorbed, and some of these methods (studies in animals, pharmacodynamic tests) are considered in separate chapters of the text.

Consideration of the modalities available to document bioequivalence indicates a continuum, beginning with chemical and physicochemical tests that focus on identification and strength, continuing through *in vitro* methods, to *in vivo* blood or urine levels studies, to pharmacodynamic methods and concluding, finally, with comparative clinical trials. Unfortunately, metrics and their variance in this continuum tends to increase, so that at the extreme of a clinical trial the ability to detect important differences or even define an endpoint of interest becomes difficult. In this setting, validation of more reliable but perhaps less clinically meaningful endpoints, based for example on physicochemical tests or *in vitro* dissolution, becomes difficult. Some of these issues are considered in the chapter on statistical considerations and in the more general chapters provide FDA and industry perspectives.

While the focus of the text is on generic substitution, many of the principles and challenges are readily extended to the documentation of bioequivalence of clinical trial formulations and to pioneer formulations that are manufactured prior to and after the onset of generic substitution. Documentation of stability in formulation quality and performance may be assessed not only between formulations but also within formulations over time, for example, from the point of manufacture to the time of shelf-life expiry. Many of the issues thus discussed in this text are thus broadly applicable to all points at which assessment of formulation equivalence and therapeutic interchangeability is important.

Roger L. Williams
U.S. Food and Drug Administration
Director, Office of Generic Drugs

PREFACE

The word "generic" is derived from the Latin word "genus" meaning a "general class." Generic drug formulations have been developed and marketed with this concept in mind; however, the difficulty of establishing the bioequivalence of a general class of a specific drug product to a single innovator product was quickly realized. The passage of the Drug Price Competition and Patent Term Restoration Act of 1984 focused much additional attention on the evolving science of generic drug bioequivalence, which has been in a state of constant evolution.

Important evolving areas of this science include, but are not limited to: pharmacokinetics; statistics; dosage form design and quality control; and chemistry and drug analysis in biological fluids. Understanding the importance of distinguishing between different computations of areas under the curve, the application of the two one-sided tests procedure, the distinction between major and minor formulation changes, the significance of propellant types for aerosols, and role of stereoisomers in the evaluation of optically active drugs are all critical to the accurate assessment of drug bioequivalence. Many of these areas have been resolved and the knowledge gained is being applied to the design and analysis of bioequivalence studies. There are still, however, many unresolved topics still under investigation such as *in vivo/in vitro* correlation, role of single vs. multiple dose studies, the use of pharmacodynamic data, the bioequivalence of transdermals, methods for estimating rate of absorption, the role of replicate statistical designs, individual vs. average bioequivalence, etc.

The goal in preparing this text was to present timely information on many bioequivalence topics to individuals actively working in the area. It is hoped that this information will also serve as a reference for other interested scientists.

I thank my colleagues for their work in preparing their chapters, the reviewers for valuable input, and our families for their help and understanding.

THE EDITOR

Andre J. Jackson, Ph.D., is a reviewer at the U.S. Food and Drug Administration, Office of Generic Drugs in the Center for Drug Evaluation and Research.

Dr. Jackson graduated in 1967 from Towson State University and obtained his Ph.D. from the University of Cincinnati in Toxicology in 1972. He did two and one-half years of postdoctoral research in the area of pharmacokinetics with Dr. Edward R. Garrett at the "beehive" in Gainesville, Florida from 1972 to 1975. He worked as a senior research scientist at Bristol Labs in Syracuse, New York from 1975 to 1976. In 1976, he joined the faculty of the School of Pharmacy and Pharmacal Sciences at Howard University in Washington, D.C. as an assistant professor of pharmaceutics. From 1979 to 1984, he held the position of assistant professor of pharmaceutics at the University of Maryland School of Pharmacy. In October 1984, he moved to his present position with the U.S. Food and Drug Administration.

Dr. Jackson has published over 35 research articles, received federal research funding, and has served as an advisor to a number of graduate and postdoctoral students. He has been involved as either project officer or on the evaluation committee for several FDA contracts related to bioequivalence. Dr. Jackson's current duties involve the review of generic drug submissions for the Office of Generic Drugs and present research is focused on the evaluation of suitable methods for measuring and comparing rate of absorption for generic formulations and appropriate methods for determining steady-state in bioequivalence studies, and other areas related to generic drug evaluation.

CONTRIBUTORS

Wade J. Adams, Ph.D.
Drug Metabolism Research
The Upjohn Company
Kalamazoo, Michigan

Mei-Ling Chen, Ph.D.
Division of Bioequivalence
Office of Generic Drugs
U.S. Food and Drug Administration
Rockville, Maryland

Nicholas H.G. Holford, MBCHB, FRACP
Department of Pharmacology
University of Auckland
Auckland, New Zealand

Andre J. Jackson, Ph.D.
Division of Bioequivalence
U.S. Food and Drug Administration
Rockville, Maryland

James Leslie, Ph.D.
Department of Pharmaceutics
University of Maryland School of Medicine
Baltimore, Maryland

Iain J. McGilveray, Ph.D.
Canadian Federal Department of Health
Health Protection Branch
Bureau of Drug Research
Ottawa, Ontario, Canada

Prem K. Narang, Ph.D.
Department of Pharmacokinetics/Dynamics
Adria Laboratories
Columbus, Ohio

Eric D. Ormsby, M.Sc.
Health Canada
Drugs Directorate
Ottawa, Ontario, Canada

Joel S. Owen, R.Ph.
Department of Pharmacal Sciences
School of Pharmacy
Auburn University
Auburn, Alabama

William R. Ravis, Ph.D.
Department of Pharmacal Sciences
School of Pharmacy
Auburn University
Auburn, Alabama

Vinod P. Shah, Ph.D.
U.S. Food and Drug Administration
Center for Drug Evaluation and Research
Rockville, Maryland

Roger L. Williams, M.D.
U.S. Food and Drug Administration
Center for Drug Evaluation and Research
Rockville, Maryland

ACKNOWLEDGMENT TO REVIEWERS

Reza Mehvar, Ph.D.
Drake University
Des Moines, Iowa

Thomas Walle, Ph.D.
Medical University of South Carolina
Charleston, South Carolina

Wayne Colburn, Ph.D.
Harris Labs
Scottsdale, Arizona

Robert J. Wills, Ph.D.
Robert Wood Johnson Medical School
Raritan, New Jersey

Thomas Ludden, Ph.D.
U.S. Food and Drug Administration
Rockville, Maryland

Thomas Karnes, Ph.D.
Virginia Commonwealth University
Richmond, Virginia

Gerald Shiu, Ph.D.
Food and Drug Administration
Rockville, Maryland

J. Brian Houston, Ph.D.
University of Manchester
Manchester, England

K. Sandy Pang, Ph.D.
University of Toronto
Toronto, Ontario, Canada

Carl M. Metzler, Ph.D.
The Upjohn Company
Kalamazoo, Michigan

Ming S. Yip, Ph.D.
Ferring Pharmaceuticals Ltd.
Central, Hong Kong

Marvin C. Meyer, Ph.D.
The University of Memphis
Memphis, Tennessee

Peter Welling, Ph.D.
Parke-Davis Pharmaceutical Research Division
Ann Arbor, Michigan

William H. Barr, Ph.D.
Virginia Commonwealth University
Richmond, Virginia

Mehul Mehta, Ph.D.
U.S. Food and Drug Administration
Rockville, Maryland

Tsai-Lin Lein, Ph.D.
Food and Drug Administration
Rockville, Maryland

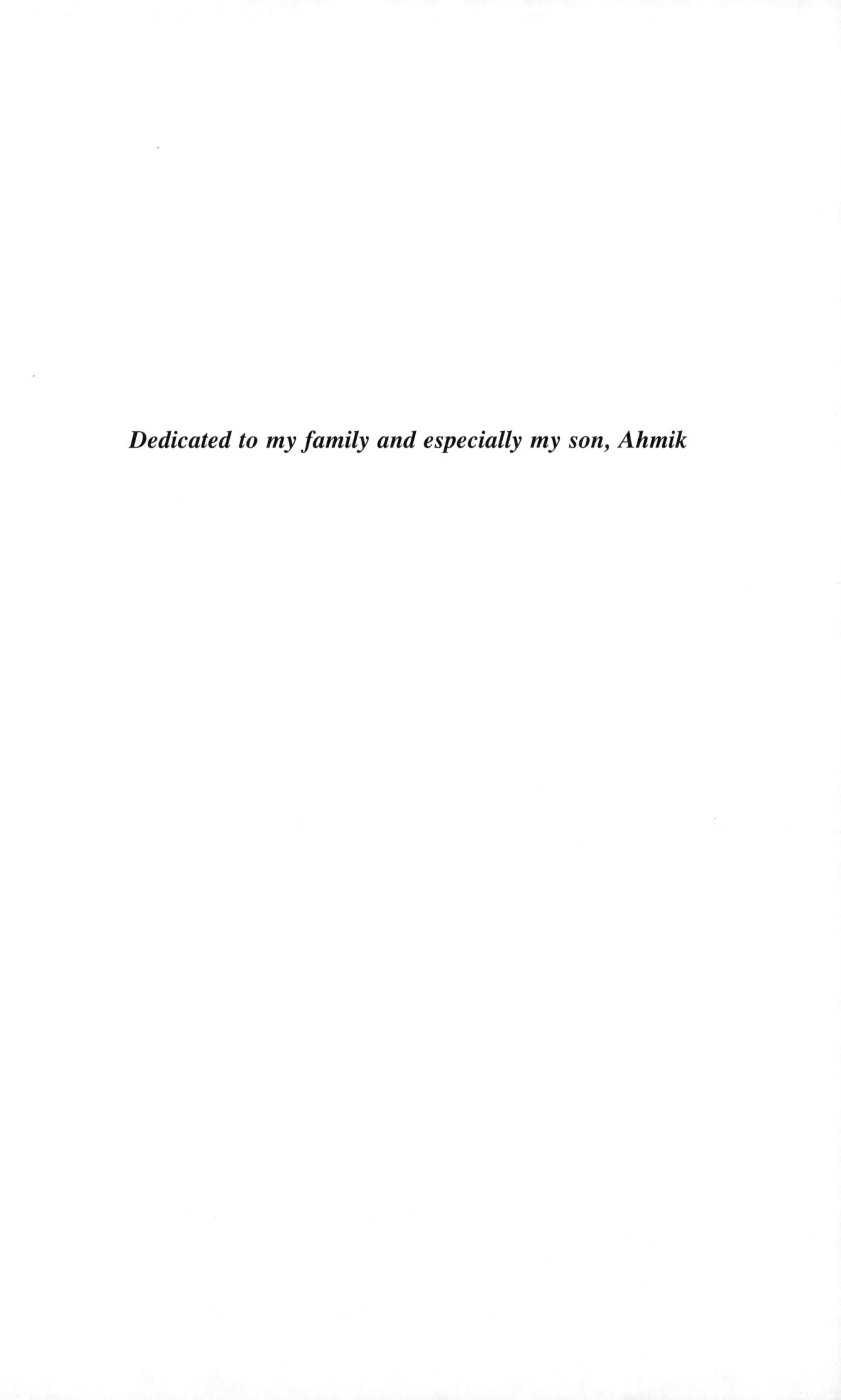

Dedicated to my family and especially my son, Ahmik

CONTENTS

Chapter 1

Statistical Methods in Bioequivalence

Eric Ormsby

CONTENTS

0-8493-6930-4/94/$0.00+$.50

I. INTRODUCTION

The concept of bioequivalence is well established as a surrogate method for determining therapeutic equivalency of drug products among agencies regulating medicines. The two types of drug products to which this concept has been applied are modifications of an existing formulation and generic versions of an innovator's product. There are two main reasons for the popularity of bioequivalence. One is economic, in that the cost of running a bioequivalence study is much less than a full clinical trial. The second reason is the high precision and accuracy in which drugs and metabolites can be measured in blood or plasma so that the complete drug concentration profile can be followed after even a single dose.

It must be recognized that two formulations can never be identical. This can even be extended to two batches of the same formulation or any two tablets within a batch. Therefore, it is the purpose of the bioequivalence study to demonstrate that the profiles produced by the formulations under study do not differ significantly. If the two profiles are indeed superimposable, it is expected that the same therapeutic effect will result. Similarly, even if the profiles do differ, but not significantly, therapeutics will also not be compromised. Thus the basic problem for the regulatory agency is to state what constitutes a significantly different profile for the products being compared. Many conferences[1-4] have been held to foster international harmonization of acceptance standards; yet each agency still has its own set of standards. Further, there is not complete agreement on how to measure superimposition or "closeness" of the profiles.[5-8]

Another confounding factor is that even when the reference formulation is given to the same individual, the identical bioavailability metrics will not be achieved every time. This variation must be accounted for when making inference on the measure of closeness. These two aspects — the actual metrics to determine closeness and the variation in these metrics —highlight the need for sound statistical methodologies to define the standard for closeness and once defined, to optimize the chance of passing the standard.

Over the last two decades, a plethora of papers have been published by workers in statistical methodologies used in the treatment of data from bioequivalence studies. These papers have covered all aspects of statistical methodology from design to inference. The papers span all possible areas of statistical theory — from the Bayesians[9-13] to frequentists, from interval estimation[14-18] to hypothesis testing,[19-22] from nonparametric[23] to parametric analyses, and from robust measures[24] to multivariate theory.[25] It has been confusing but also fascinating that this one concept has allowed statisticians and nonstatisticians alike to compare and contrast different techniques designed to produce one goal — the determination of bioequivalence.

It is not the intention of this chapter to delve too deeply into theoretical statistics, but rather to give practical guidance to the statistical process for investigators intending to conduct bioequivalence studies. This statistical process begins by defining the problem or "what the study must show", developing a method for collecting the necessary information, and deriving an algorithm for the estimation of and inference on the parameters needed to attain the goal. As with any good clinical trial, a summary of the statistical process to be used must be summarized in the study protocol.

Section II describes the purpose of the bioequivalence study. Defining the purpose by setting the acceptance criteria is the major responsibility of the regulatory agency. Section III reviews the important sources of variation in, and distributional assumptions of, the bioavailability metrics most often used. Decision rules and parameter estimation for declaring bioequivalence are presented in Section IV. Section V describes the advantages and disadvantages of the various experimental designs more frequently considered for bioequivalence studies. Section VI discusses other important considerations such as sample size calculations and the implications of outliers. Finally, Section VII discusses some future aspects of bioequivalence.

II. THE PURPOSE OF THE BIOEQUIVALENCE STUDY

The only purpose for a bioequivalence study is to obtain evidence that the test formulation and the reference formulation are indeed "close" enough. Since the results are used to support a claim to a regulatory agency, the agency must state a standard which defines closeness of the profiles for the particular drug product being compared. A regulatory standard is made up of one or more acceptance criteria for each bioavailability metric deemed necessary to characterize the profile. Although the number and type of metrics determining the standard will depend on the particular drug formulation, the underlying statistical concept is the same for each metric making up the standard.

The statistical concept can be expressed as a general probability statement or decision rule for the parameters of the assumed statistical distribution for the bioavailability metric. This statement may be written:

$$\Pr\left\{\Delta_1 \leq f\left(\Theta_t, \Theta_r\right) \leq \Delta_2\right\} \leq 1 - P \qquad \textbf{(1–1)}$$

In words, this equation says that some function comparing the test and reference statistical distribution parameters, $f(\Theta_t,\Theta_r)$, must fall within prescribed limits, Δ_1 and Δ_2, with a certain assurance probability, $1 - P$. The interval spanned by Δ_1 and Δ_2 is called the bioequivalence interval. Therefore, a well-defined standard for a specific drug product will clearly state:

1. Which bioavailability metrics and which of its distribution parameters must meet criteria
2. The width of the bioequivalence interval for each parameter
3. The function of the estimated parameters which is meaningful
4. The assigned assurance probability level

Since the criterion for a parameter is the driving force in designing a study, it will be examined in detail in order to identify where statistics play a role.

A. THE DRUG PRODUCT

A standard must first of all be based on clinical information. For each drug, parameters should be chosen to determine by how much and when the test product can differ from the reference, before therapeutic equivalency would be compromised.

It is reasonable to assume that not all drugs will require the same standards or even the same bioavailability metrics or the same parameters. On the basis of the type of drug, it may be possible to select classes of drugs for which there would be a class standard. These classes may be determined by physiochemical, biopharmaceutical, or pharmacokinetic characteristics; dose-response correlations; or specific indications of the product for which bioequivalence is being claimed. Such classes as drugs with complicated[26] and uncomplicated[27] pharmacokinetics and modified-release[28] formulations have been identified. Different formulations or routes of administration of the same drug would also require different standards such as would be the case for an immediate-release formulation and a modified-release formulation.

It is important to note that the clinical characteristics of the drug and its formulation determine the criteria which make up the standard and therefore determine the type and size of each study to be executed.

B. BIOAVAILABILITY METRICS

The bioavailability metrics of importance in determining a standard are dependent on the drug/formulation and the type of study. Frequently used metrics describing the concentration-time profile are area under the curve (AUC), C_{max}, and T_{max}. The relative importance of these metrics depends on the type of study. There are four common types of studies: single-dose and multiple-dose to steady-state studies each carried out in the fed and fasted state. For single-dose studies a metric of extent through an AUC and a metric of shape through C_{max} is generally considered adequate along with tabulation of T_{max}. C_{max} over an AUC has also been proposed as a better metric for rate comparison,[29-30] especially for drugs with highly variable kinetics. However, a more explicit metric of rate other than C_{max} or T_{max} may be required for some drug products. For multiple-dose studies, additional metrics such as C_{min} and fluctuation $((C_{max} - C_{min})\ \tau/AUC_{\tau})$ may be required. Many studies require reasonable estimation of the terminal elimination rate constant either to be used on its own or, more commonly, to estimate AUC to infinity. Modified-release formulations may need a different metric of shape since C_{max} is highly influenced and variable; perhaps a partial AUC could be used.[31]

Each metric will have its own probability statement such as 1-1 on its statistical parameters; and by considering this, the precision required in measuring that bioavailability metric can be estimated (see Section VI). The metric which will have the most difficulty in passing its criterion is the one to choose to determine sample size.

C. THE FUNCTION OF THE PARAMETERS

Statistics play a major role in determining which parameters of the statistical distribution are best to compare the test and reference profiles. The main emphasis is on estimation of the parameters such that meaningful inferences can be made.

The most common statistical distribution parameter on which to base bioequivalence is a measure of central tendency of the test to reference product bioavailability metric. The usual parameter to measure this location is the mean; and generally the difference in two means is compared, but on a different scale. As will be shown in Section III, the ratio of geometric means or medians is more appropriate for some bioavailability metrics.

The complexity of the actual data summarization from which inference is made can be as simple as the point estimate or as complex as a confidence interval or the appropriate hypothesis tests.

The measure of central tendency is, of course, not the only parameter which can be affected by a formulation. Therefore, an agency may also place a standard on a comparison of the variances which are influenced by formulations (see Section III). Again this comparison may be a ratio, or a difference and its point estimate or confidence interval.

D. THE BIOEQUIVALENCE INTERVAL

The width of the bioequivalence interval (BI) is the main way to capture clinical significance or importance. For the ratio of central tendencies, Δ_1 is generally taken as 80%; or for a difference, 20% of the reference. The origin of this 20% rule is not clear but seems to be consistent with other limits such as United States Pharmacopeia (USP) potency limits.[32] The size of the difference is probably based on summary metrics such as AUC and C_{max} and not on derived rate constants. However, it has been recognized[26] that a narrower interval (e.g., 90 to 111%) might be more appropriate for some drugs such as those with a narrow therapeutic index or those with highly toxic effects. It has also been suggested[33] that drugs which vary greatly day to day within the same individual and do not have a high concentration to effect correlation may have wider limits. This wider BI has also been recommended for metrics which are quite variable.[34] It should be further noted that the bioequivalence interval does not have to be the same for each parameter making up the standard. Some intervals may only have an upper limit when the agency may not be interested that the test product was less than the reference. For instance, less variation in a test product would be better.

Note that the Δ_1 above is expressed as a percentage difference from the reference. This relative difference recognizes the fact that the magnitude of the absolute parameter

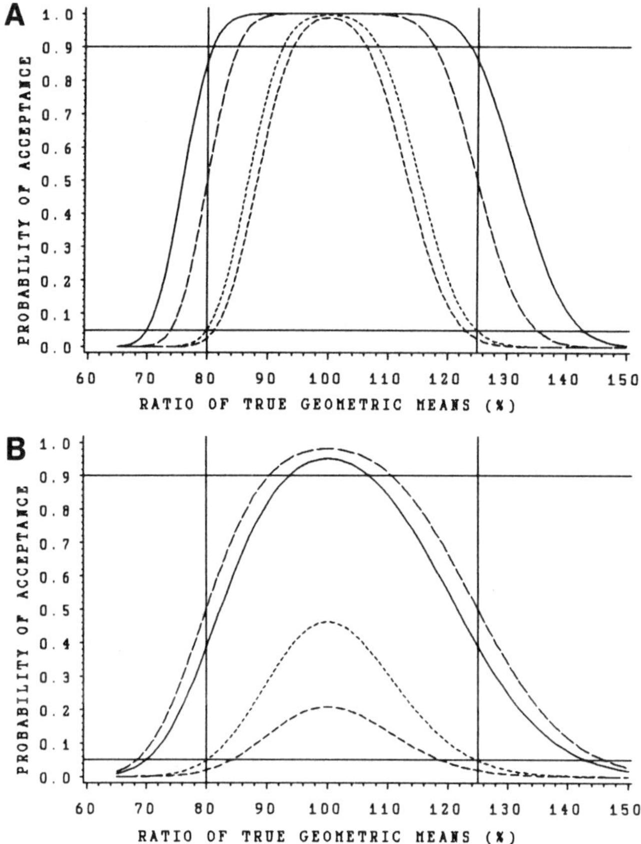

Figure 1–1 Probability of accepting bioequivalence of the ratio of geometric means using different acceptance criteria and residual CVs of **(A)** 15% and **(B)** 30%. —— 90% CI within 70 to 143% BI, ··· 90% CI within 80 to 125% BI, --- 95% CI within 80 to 125% BI, —— mean estimate within 80 to 125% BI.

estimates depends highly on the volunteers in the study and that there could be large differences in the magnitudes of bioavailability metrics across studies. By expressing the results on a relative scale, all studies on a particular drug formulation and all drugs within a class can have the same BI limits. This has important implications on the method of estimation discussed later, which in turn has a direct consequence of defining Δ_2 to be 125% (or 111%) when Δ_1 is 80% (or 90%).

E. THE ASSURANCE PROBABILITY

The amount of assurance the agency requires that the test formulation matches the reference for the parameter tested is measured by $1 - P$. This is the probability that the true difference or ratio of the parameters falls within the safety zone defined by the BI. The smaller the P, the more assurance. The P can be thought of as the consumer risk or the probability of accepting a test formulation parameter as being acceptable, as defined by the criterion, when in fact it is not acceptable. Generally P is set at 0.05 for most parameters which is consistent with an alpha level of 5%. The P may be increased as the importance of the parameter decreases. For instance, if the agency[27] only requires the mean estimate to fall within the BI, then the assurance probability is only 0.50. Similarly, if the 90% confidence interval must fall within the BI, then P is 0.05.

The size of the consumer risk of declaring bioequivalence decreases (i.e., there is less consumer risk) when more criteria are included in any one standard since each criteria is carried out at its own significance level.

F. SUMMARY

The criterion defined in Equation 1–1 has great flexibility in that the limits or the assurance probability, or both, can be changed to suit the clinical importance. The flexibility of the probability statement is illustrated in Figure 1–1. This figure gives the chances of passing various criteria given the true relative differences in geometric means when a standard crossover study is run on 20 volunteers. Note the assurance probabilities are read off the ordinate, where the curve crosses the ratio of geometric means which equals the Δs of the BI. As the true relative difference leaves equality (100%), the chances of passing drops dramatically. The strictest criteria is the 95% confidence interval falling within 80 to 125%. Also note that all criteria are less likely to be passed as the residual variation increases from 15% in Figure 1–1A to 30% in Figure 1–1B.

III. VARIATION AND DISTRIBUTIONAL ASSUMPTIONS

Before executing any study, an investigator must have a sound knowledge of the sources of variation which act on the observed data. This knowledge will direct the investigator to the experimental design which will minimize the influences from specific variability and allow other sources to be estimated. There are sources of variation which the investigator can control, and there are uncontrollable sources which depend greatly on the drug and formulation. Gaffney[35] has discussed estimation of these components of variation as they pertain to bioavailability studies. In order that meaningful statistical parameters can be estimated with maximum precision, knowledge of the theoretical distribution of the bioavailability metrics is also required.

A. SOURCES OF VARIATION

The major source of variation is among subjects (i.e., between subjects). In statistical parlance, this is known as intersubject variance. Subjects have different genes; live in different environments; and are at different stages of their biological, psychological, and social lives. Within a population, the differences in absorption, distribution, metabolism, and elimination of a drug are expressed in a wide range of values for a single bioavailability metric. These estimates can vary 100-fold between subjects for the same drug formulation. The best examples of the wide range of subject differences are observed in persons who are fast and slow metabolizers of a drug because of genetic differences in drug-metabolizing enzymes. Although intersubject variance has great clinical importance, in most bioequivalence studies this plays a minor role. This variation, depicted as σ_B^2, is estimated by the variation in the subjects' means for each of the different bioavailability metrics.

Another source of variation is due to biological differences within each subject. No person's biological functions are identical from day to day or even within a day; for example, metabolism varies throughout a day and seasonally. It follows that even for identical formulations the concentration-time profiles will be different on repeated administrations. Variable first-pass effect, variable absorption, stomach-emptying time, etc. contribute in a major way to this variation.

There is also variation within formulations, within and between batches, although this variation should be minimized through the adherence to *in vitro* testing (e.g., dissolution) during quality control. One problem is that the formulation variation is confounded with biological variation. No matter how we run an experiment we can never distinguish biological variation from formulation variation since the same tablet cannot be given twice and the subject is never identical on different occasions. The total of the formulation and biological variance is called the within-subject or intrasubject variation and will be depicted as σ_w^2. This variation can be estimated for each formulation but only when the formulation is given more than once to the same subject. If there is a large difference between the intrasubject variances for two formulations, it is generally regarded as a formulation problem.

The last major source of differences within subjects between formulations is known as the subject-by-formulation interaction. These differences occur when subjects on one formulation give consistently different values than for the other formulation. An interaction may be significant when a difference in the magnitude of response is seen for different strata in the population (i.e., smokers respond differently than nonsmokers to one of the formulations), or absorption rates may be changed within some subjects because of an interaction with an excipient present in one formulation but not present in the other. Very little is known about this source of variation, but it has received much attention recently with regards to interchangeability and individual equivalence.[36,37]

The sources of variation over which there is direct control are those associated with the analytical assay; sampling time placement; and, to some extent, biological variation. For the analytical assay, it is generally acceptable to use a method which is accurate with precision better than 15% and a lower limit of quantitation with precision better than 20%.[38] If method validation indicates the expected precision to be worse, replicate samples can be employed and averaged to increase precision. If all the samples for one subject compose a single run of the assay, the between run assay variation will be removed from the within-subject comparisons. Single point metrics such as C_{max} and C_{min} usually have more relative variation — as measured by the coefficient of variation (CV) than AUCs. This is because AUCs are linear combinations of the single concentrations over time and the mean of the combination increases at a faster rate than the variance. More samples taken along the profile will reduce the relative error in the AUC.

Sampling time placement depends greatly on the pharmacokinetics of the drug and the formulation. Drugs with a fast absorption rate must have more sampling at the beginning of the profile. It is unacceptable to have the first sampling point as the estimated C_{max}. Further, if an explicit form of absorption rate must be determined, then at least four nonzero concentrations before C_{max} should be obtained. Similarly, the elimination phase of the drug must be characterized in order that AUC to infinity can be obtained. Very little work has been done on optimizing sampling time placement given the pharmacokinetics of the drug and the variation within and between subjects. It is reasonable to require that absorption, distribution, and elimination of the drug be represented by at least four points each. If there is large intersubject variation (>50%), one should add two more times in each of the three phases.

A small amount of biological variation can be controlled through consistent treatment of the subjects within each study day. Break-in phases of 2 days may be necessary to "climatize" subjects to the clinical environment, especially if variable absorption (maybe even variable first pass) is a major source of variation. It must be realized, however, that much of the biological variation cannot be reduced; and this is probably the major source of uncontrollable intrasubject variation.

B. DISTRIBUTION OF PHARMACOKINETIC METRICS

Many large sample studies[39-41] on the pharmacokinetics of drugs indicate that the distribution of bioavailability metrics are skewed to the right (i.e., the right-hand tail is longer than a normal). Other studies indicate that the population may be multimodal which probably depends on genetic polymorphism, and each of these distributions may be skewed to the right. Because distributions are skewed to the right (positive skew), it is reasonable to assume that the distribution is lognormal. This would be expected when a series of biological steps act on an outcome in such a way that each step changes in

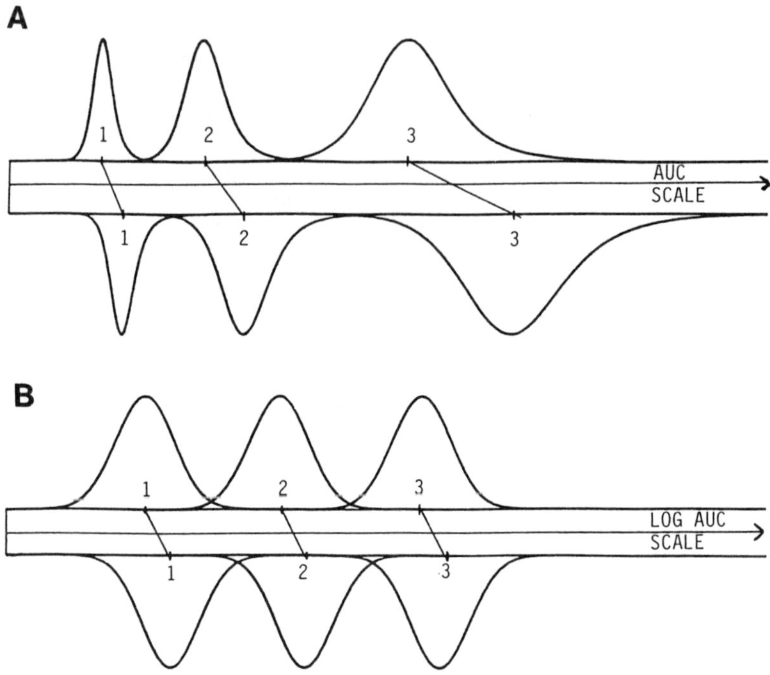

Figure 1–2 Effect of the log transformation on intrasubject comparisons for two formulations having a 20% difference in mean response.

proportion to the amount. A process for generating lognormal deviates is known as "the law of proportionate effect".[42] For this reason the most popular (and well-fitting) pharmacokinetic models are functions of exponentials.

Since even within an individual the drug is acted on by a series of biological steps, the lognormal distribution seems appropriate for intrasubject distributions of bioavailability measures. An example to illustrate how this proportional effect impacts on bioequivalence studies may be helpful.

If clinicians were to be asked what would be the expected drop in AUC if an unknown patient were given a formulation with 20% less drug, their intuitive and generally correct answer would be 20%. Now if a clinician knows the AUC of that particular patient to be 100 units, he would expect the AUC drop of 20% to be 20 units. If a second patient is considered who has an AUC of 1000 units, the expected drop will also be 20%; however, this translates into 200 units. Although the relative difference in AUCs is the same for these two patients, the absolute difference is an order of ten. Thus the magnitude of the patient's drop in AUC depends on that patient's average AUC.

The logarithmic (log) transformation can be used to make the absolute intrasubject differences independent of the patient's AUC since log(80) – log(100) is equal to log(800) – log(1000). It should be noted that it is assumed differences from any cause, not just the formulations, will have a multiplicative effect on the raw scale but become additive on the log scale. The use of the log transformation for concentration-dependent measures of bioavailability is now accepted by all the major regulatory agencies which have documented standards.[26-28,34,43] Some researchers even believe T_{max} is also lognormal; however, due to the discrete time sampling the proportional effect is not apparent. Measures such as fluctuation which are internally corrected for subject effect may or may not be lognormal.

The basis of using the log transformation for statistical purposes is illustrated in Figure 1–2. The first pair of graphs (A) outline the hypothetical lognormal distribution of raw bioavailability metrics, for example, AUC, for three subjects (1, 2, 3). The upper set of distributions are for the reference formulation and the lower set for the test formulation. The distributions have been drawn with the experimental formulation having 20% more extent, and the three subjects have a sequentially twofold increase in means for both formulations. Note that as mean AUC increases across the subjects so does the intrasubject variance (i.e., the distribution spreads out). It should be observed that the CV, the ratio of the standard deviation to the mean, is constant for the six distributions in A. Also the three lines joining the subjects's means for the two formulations are not parallel as AUC increases. The second pair of three distributions (B) represent log transformation of the upper pair of lognormal distributions. All the subject distributions now have the same shape and that the three lines joining the means are parallel, representing equal log differences within all subjects. In addition, the three transformed curves are equidistant within a formulation because the transformation has also removed the twofold effect. When a bioequivalence study is run, random sampling will occur from within each subject's distribution.

C. ESTIMATION OF THE PARAMETERS FROM THE LOGNORMAL DISTRIBUTION

The goal of any bioequivalence study is to compare, using estimates from the data, the closeness of the distribution parameters of the experimental and reference formulations. The most often chosen technique of analysis and estimation is analysis of variance (ANOVA). If the lognormal distribution is assumed, then to meet the assumptions of ANOVA (mainly additivity of the errors) the raw data are log transformed. Logarithms to base e are generally used. Comparisons of the means and variances of the transformed data, which are assumed to follow normal theory, could therefore be made and a conclusion of bioequivalence could be stated by log transforming the BI limits. However, it is somewhat more convenient to express results in the original relative scale because this scale is more familiar.

There are two competing estimates of central tendency of a distribution, the mean and the median. The mean is the expected value of the distribution, while the median is the point at which 50% of the distribution lies above and 50% lies below. If the distribution is symmetric, these two parameters are equal. This is the case with the normal distribution. However, if the assumed distribution is lognormal, the median is always smaller than the mean.

The estimate of the mean of a lognormal distribution based on transformed data is

$$\hat{\mu} = e^{\left(\overline{x} + \frac{1}{2}s^2\right)} \tag{1–2}$$

where $\overline{x}$ and s^2 are the sample mean and variance, respectively, of the transformed data. Land[44] gives an algorithm to form the confidence interval for the difference of two means.

The median of the lognormal distribution from transformed data is estimated:

$$\hat{\tau} = e^{\overline{x}} \tag{1–3}$$

This estimate is also called the geometric mean of the lognormal distribution. An estimator of relative bioavailability is then the ratio of medians or ratio of geometric means which can be obtained:

$$\hat{\Theta} = e^{\left(\overline{x}_E - \overline{x}_R\right)} \tag{1–4}$$

The confidence interval of the difference in $\bar{x}$'s can be inversely transformed to give the confidence interval for the ratio of medians. Liu and Weng[45] use this estimate with a correction factor to estimate the ratio of means.

As noted in Figure 1–2, it is usually better to describe variation in terms of CVs when comparing two lognormal distributions. Standard deviations less than 0.30 derived from the transformed data are good approximations to the CVs of the original scale when multiplied by 100%. The exact formula is

$$CV = \sqrt{e^{\sigma^2} - 1}\ 100\% \qquad \textbf{(1–5)}$$

IV. METHODS FOR DECLARING BIOEQUIVALENCE

There are three basic qualities that a statistical method must possess before it can be used to declare bioequivalence using the decision rule 2-1. It must:

1. Give an unbiased estimate of the comparison of statistical parameters of interest
2. Account for the experimental design
3. Give the overall nominal assigned assurance probability

There are over 20 different methods proposed to declare bioequivalence, but only a few meet the three requirements above. Many cannot take into account the experimental design while others are only for a narrow subset of experimental designs. Some proposed methods produce biased estimates of the parameters. A brief history of bioequivalence determination will illustrate the desired qualities of a bioequivalence method.

A. METHODS FOR BIOEQUIVALENCE

It was quickly recognized[46] that the usual method of formulating the problem through the null hypothesis test of no formulation difference vs. the alternative hypothesis of a formulation difference had two shortcomings when applied to bioequivalence decisions. First, this framework of hypothesis testing can show formulations to have statistically significant differences in parameters which may not be of clinical significance. Second, a study which yields imprecise parameter estimates (inadequate power) would declare the formulations to be bioequivalent but the undetected difference could be truly clinically different.

The second method used by some agencies, to avoid the above problem of the null hypothesis, was to supplement the hypothesis test for formulation differences with a power criterion. The study had to be able to detect a 20% difference with 80% power. However, this procedure also has very poor operating characteristics[22] in that studies with good precision may be rejected more often than studies with the same estimates but worse precision. This is opposite to what a rational procedure should do.

The 75/75 rule, where 75% of the subjects must have test-to-reference percent ratios between 75 and 125%, was another procedure used mainly by the U.S. Food and Drug Administration (FDA). It was criticized for poor characteristics when the intrasubject variances were unequal, and for not possessing a statistical basis.[47-49] However, this method had intuitive appeal and was really the first attempt at declaring individual equivalence.[50]

Westlake[14] proposed using confidence intervals to circumvent the problems with the previous methods. He proposed that reasonable assurance of bioequivalence would be obtained if the confidence interval of the appropriate function of the data should fall entirely within the therapeutically determined BI. He also suggested that the 1–2α% confidence interval would be more in line with the acceptance criteria of new drugs. At the same time Westlake[15] derived a 1–2α% confidence interval which was symmetric about 100%. This symmetrical interval was not well received among the statistical community[51-53] and gives a higher chance of passing than the shortest 1–2α% confidence interval.

The basic problem with the usual hypothesis test outlined above is that it is backward. Instead the alternate hypothesis, not the null, should be bioequivalence defined by the BI. Hauck and Anderson[21] derived a test statistic recognizing this reversal, but their test statistic had poor properties when variances were large. Schuirmann[22] proposed the two one-sided tests procedure which also has the alternative hypothesis of bioequivalence as declared by the BI. The first test tests for subbioavailability while the second one tests for superbioavailability. Since each test is made at the α% level (but for any one study, only one test can make a type I error), the test is said to have an overall error of α%. Also in his paper Schuirmann proved that the same conclusions would be reached using his procedure at an α error for each test and the 1–2α% confidence interval. Thus, if the consumer risk is 5% for each hypothesis test, exact conclusions would be reached if a 90% confidence interval were used.

There have been many other methods in the literature to declare bioequivalence, but for one reason or another they are not widely accepted by all agencies. European guidelines seem to be the most liberal in accepting alternate methods while Canada and the FDA appear to be stricter. Bayesian methods[9-13] have been introduced, but few agencies accept the premise of Bayesian analysis with its prior distribution assumption. A multivariate confidence region[25] was proposed, but as with most multivariate methods is not as powerful as other methods and is rarely submitted for evaluation. Nonparametric[23] and robust[24] methods have been published, but agencies are concerned that important observations are hidden by underweighting and will not come to the attention of reviewers. There are other methods which will be discussed later with regard to population and individual bioequivalence.

B. TYPES OF BIOEQUIVALENCE

From Section III it was shown that the experimental formulation's distribution may differ from that of the reference's:

1. In central tendencies
2. In amount of variation within a person
3. By having interactions with different subjects

If the only interest lies in comparing central tendency, then only average bioequivalence (AB) is being declared. This type of bioequivalence is what has been required presently from most agencies. If in addition to central tendency the confounded form of inter- and intrasubject variances are to be compared, then population bioequivalence (PB) is being declared. This form of bioequivalence is an attempt to control any increased variance in the population caused by the experimental formulation. This type of bioequivalence declaration is important in that if the means and variances are similar, then when a clinician prescribes either formulation the expected response will be within the known limits of variation of the reference. Finally, if the intrasubject variances and the central tendencies for each formulation are compared and if the interaction of the formulation with subjects is to be accounted for, then individual bioequivalence (IB) is being sought. IB declaration is important for interchangeability in that if IB is accepted, similar responses will be obtained if a patient is switched from one formulation to the other.

Example scenarios of the results from a bioequivalence study are illustrated in Figure 1–3. The two vertical broken lines represent the spread of the between-subject means or intersubject variation for two formulations, reference and experimental. The smaller vertical solid lines represent the spread within three subjects or the intrasubject variation, each subject given both formulations. The lines joining the two formulations connect the

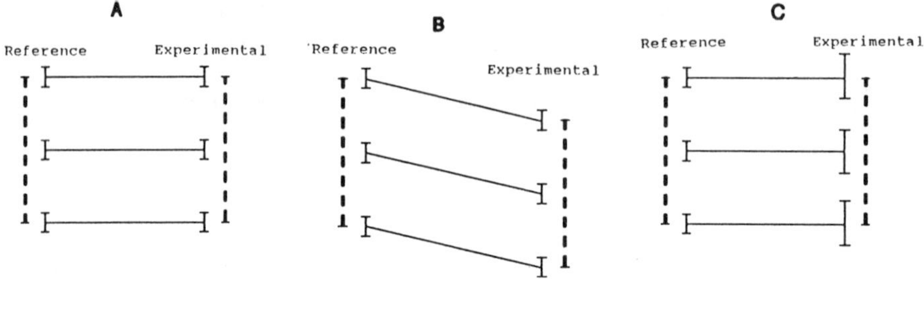

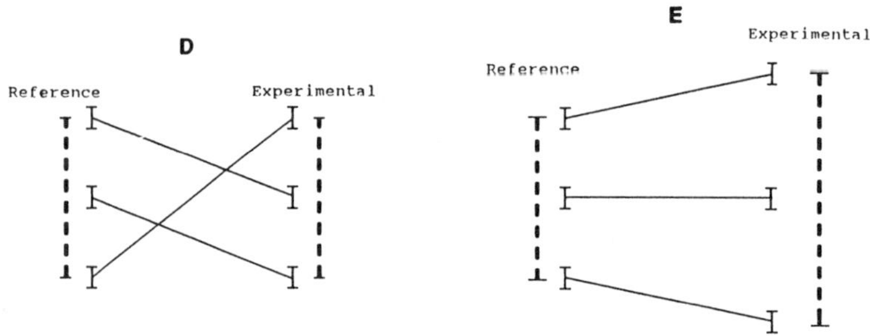

Figure 1–3 Five scenarios depicting how the three types of bioequivalence—average, population, and individual—will declare their respective conclusions (see text for details).

subject's true means. Recall that observations for each subject would be produced by sampling from within the subject's distribution.

In scenario A, the three types of bioequivalence would be accepted since the intersubject spread is the same, the intrasubject variance is the same, and the lines joining the subject's means are parallel, indicating neither subject-by-formulation interaction nor shift in the mean response of the two formulations. However, in scenario B there is a shift in the mean response while the variances stay constant and the interaction is zero. If this shift is large enough, none of the types of bioequivalence should be accepted.

In scenario C the intrasubject variation is increased with the experimental formulation. This increase in variance would imply that a given subject's response would be expected to be more variable on the experimental formulation. The magnitude of this increased intrasubject variation that would be clinically significant has yet to be determined by regulating agencies. If a two-period crossover were run, AB would possibly be accepted since the increase in intrasubject variation is diluted in the error term and can be hidden if sample sizes are large enough. PB and IB, on the other hand, may not conclude bioequivalence since the actual variance parameters are compared.

Scenarios D and E illustrate significant interactions of formulation with subjects. In D, one subject shifts the opposite way of the other two; however, all the other parameters, except this subject-by-formulation interaction, stay the same. In this scenario AB and PB may be accepted but IB would not. In scenario E the interaction has caused an increased intersubject variance for the experimental formulation. This interaction may be detected by both PB and IB methods but not AB methods.

1. Average Bioequivalence

Since the confidence interval and Schuirmann's tests are accepted universally, these methods will be used to illustrate tests for the medians in AB.

The 1–2α% confidence interval for the difference of two arithmetic means on the log scale is

$$\overline{X}_E - \overline{X}_R \pm t_{df,\alpha} SE_{diff} \quad \textbf{(1–6)}$$

where the $\overline{x}$'s are the estimates of the mean for the experimental and reference formulation, SE_{diff} is the appropriate standard error for the difference in means given the experimental design (see equation 1–12), and t is the appropriate *t*-variate for α and the degrees of freedom of the error. If the interval spanned by these limits falls entirely within the BI formed by $Ln(\Delta_1)$ and $Ln(\Delta_2)$, equivalency would be declared for this parameter. Similarly, the confidence limits and the point estimate can be transformed back into the original relative scale by exponentiating each. In this latter case we are making inference on the ratio of medians or geometric means for the two formulation distributions. If all the parameters (e.g., medians for AUC and C_{max}) which make up the standard pass, AB is declared.

The two one-sided tests procedure tests:

$$1. \quad \Pr\left\{t_1 = \frac{\left(\overline{X}_E - \overline{X}_R\right) - Ln\left(\Delta_1\right)}{SE_{diff}}\right\}$$

and

$$2. \quad \Pr\left\{t_u = \frac{Ln\left(\Delta_2\right) - \left(\overline{X}_E - \overline{X}_R\right)}{SE_{diff}}\right\} \quad \textbf{(1 – 7)}$$

If either test yields a probability greater than α, bioequivalence for the parameter tested is rejected. Again, if all the parameters which make up the standard pass this test, AB is declared.

Note that the confidence interval and two one-sided tests procedure use the same quantities in their calculation but the two one-sided test's procedure yields a pair of *p* values.

2. Population Bioequivalence

In addition to AB declaration, PB requires that a comparison of the intrasubject variances pass some standard. The first attempt to compare variances came from Haynes[47] who introduced the Pittman-Morgan test on the pooled variances obtained from a nonreplicated design where pure estimates of intrasubject variance cannot be obtained. The Pittman-Morgan test, tests the null hypothesis of equal variance vs. not equal, and therefore suffers from the same problem which plagued bioequivalence in its infancy — the test is backwards. Furthermore, the test does not take into account the experimental design. Recently Liu[54] and Lui and Chow[55] have derived such a test for either a difference in variances, or a ratio of variances which accounts for period effects and has the proper arrangement of the null and alternative hypotheses. Under their parameterization of the crossover linear model, the comparison of marginal formulation variances is a comparison of intrasubject variances. What has yet to be declared by regulating agencies is the acceptable difference for variances (i.e., to declare the BI for variance comparisons). It would also be reasonable to assume that a one-sided inference could be used for variance comparisons.[56] Sheiner[57] and Schall and Luus[58] propose a combined test for both the mean and the variance comparison; however, they each use a different estimation method and slightly different designs.

The concept of PB leads one to wonder whether a larger difference in average response could be given to the experimental formulation if less variation for the experimental product were shown. This is another concept regulatory agencies must address.

3. Individual Equivalence

As early as 1978[59] concerns were raised that if the purpose of bioequivalence is to determine interchangeability of products, average and even population bioequivalence is not enough. It was not until Ekbohn and Melander[36] published a test for the subject-by-formulation interaction term that interchangeability was addressed. This concept was reiterated by Anderson and Hauck[37,60] and was termed individual equivalence. They also published a nonparametric test (TEIR) for IB based on the usual two-period, two-formulation crossover design; however, their method cannot account for period effects, and will never declare IB for formulations containing drugs with large intrasubject variation which may be independent of formulation unless the BI is widened. The basic principle behind TEIR is that if there are more observed within-subject differences falling outside the BI than would be expected by chance, individual bioequivalence should not be declared. Chinchilli and Esinhart[18] derived a tolerance interval which allows a statement of the kind that $1–\alpha\%$ (95%) of the individuals will have measures within the BI, $100\pi\%$ (99%) of the time. Schall and Luus[58] derived a test based on bootstrapped confidence interval, considering a design where only the reference need be replicated. Sheiner[57] derived a maximum likelihood estimation procedure which is used in a relative risk estimate for IB from a completely replicated crossover design. Endrenyi[61] compared the estimate of within-subject variation between formulations with the within-subject variation within formulations, also for a replicated design. If this ratio is too large, IB cannot be declared.

The problem with many of these proposed methods of declaring PB and IB is that the power of what they can detect has not been adequately determined (i.e., can the method adequately distinguish a twofold increase in intrasubject variance and keep the sample size reasonably small?). Furthermore, the clinical significance or magnitude of these statistical concepts — such as increased intrasubject variation or the presence of a subject-by-formulation interaction — is not well documented, since the regulatory agencies have not required replicated designs. To date there is only a handful of truly replicated bioequivalence studies. Replication is required in order to assess these concepts. Much discussion is expected on individual bioequivalence in the near future once these replicated designs become more common.

C. SUMMARY OF BIOEQUIVALENCE METHODS

Declaration of AB will work reasonably well when the error mean square from the regular two-period, two-formulation crossover is less than 0.04 (CV of 20%). Recalling that this error is made up of all sources of error there does not seem to be much room for a significantly poorer formulation to pass. However, when this error term exceeds 20%, there may be a greater potential to hide (by increasing sample size) a poor formulation either through increased intrasubject variance or through a subject-by-formulation interaction. Thus a replicated design would seem to be warranted for such formulations. This raises another question: How does one know *a priori* how large the error will be in order to run the appropriate design?

The newer approaches to bioequivalence, PB and IB, have raised many questions for the regulatory agencies, mainly: What is the main purpose for running the bioequivalence trial? Only with the replicated designs can the performance of the experimental formulation be completely compared to the performance of the reference.

V. EXPERIMENTAL DESIGN AND ANALYSIS OF VARIANCE

An experimental design describes an unbiased procedure for assigning formulations to subjects. The particular experimental chosen for a bioequivalence study depends on what variances described in Section III are to be estimated and the precision of the comparisons to be made. Further, a good experimental design also minimizes the effect of other sources of variation secondary to the purpose of the study. ANOVA, through a linear model, is the usual method of estimating variances and formulation comparing.

There are two general types of designs which could be used in a bioequivalence study. These are the parallel and the crossover design. Each will be discussed in detail.

A. PARALLEL DESIGN

This type of design is not the one of choice but may be the only alternative in certain situations when the crossover design cannot be used. For instance, if a drug with a long half-life is to be studied, the washout period needed may be too long for the crossover to be effective. For this design a subject is randomized to one and only one of the formulations. Individual bioequivalence cannot be determined using a parallel design since subject-by-formulation interaction cannot be estimated.

A linear model for the parallel design is

$$Y_{ij} = \mu + F_i + \varepsilon_{ij} \qquad \textbf{(1–8)}$$

where Y_{ij} = observation for subject j given formulation i, μ = the overall mean, F_i = the mean effect for formulation i, and ε_{ij} = the residual assumed to be $N(0, \sigma_P^2)$.

The main problem with the design is that the σ_P^2 (the subscripted P indicating a parallel design) is a composite of all sources of variations mentioned in Section III, none of which can be estimated separately. The σ_P^2 is used as the variance term for the standard error of the formulation comparison. It is expected that σ_P^2 will be quite large (greater than 40%), which implies a large number of subjects would have to be recruited.

The log transformation may still be implemented to stabilize the between-group variance. For parallel studies using drugs which may have multimodal distributions the subjects should be screened for rate of metabolism, which may be used as a covariate, or homogeneous subgroups may be formed.

AB can be determined by using the estimated F_i into Equation 1–6 or 1–7, and PB can be determined from the marginal variances for the two formulation groups.

A portion of the intrasubject variance can be estimated if subjects are taken to steady state and concentration profiles are measured on r days. This repeated measures sampling would allow estimation of the subsampling error, but it is not the true intrasubject variance σ_W^2. A pure estimate of σ_W^2 could be obtained only if subjects are taken to steady state on r separate occasions. The appropriate linear model for a repeated measures design is

$$Y_{ijk} = \mu + F_i + V_{j(i)} + \varepsilon_{ijk} \qquad \textbf{(1–9)}$$

where Y_{ijk}, μ, and F_i are defined in Section V.A but $V_{j(i)}$ is subject within formulation term and is distributed $N(0, \sigma_R^2)$ and the ε_{ijk}s contain the subsampling variance. The σ_R^2 is the

Table 1–1 **Four F = P, S crossover designs**

	F = 2		F = 3			F = 4				F = 5				
	Period (P)													
Sequence (S)	**1**	**2**	**1**	**2**	**3**	**1**	**2**	**3**	**4**	**1**	**2**	**3**	**4**	**5**
1	A	B	A	B	C	A	B	C	D	A	B	C	D	E
2	B	A	C	A	B	C	A	D	B	C	A	E	B	D
3			B	C	A	D	C	B	A	E	C	D	A	B
4			C	B	A	B	D	A	C	D	E	B	C	A
5			B	A	C					B	D	A	E	C
6			A	C	B					E	D	C	B	A
7										D	B	E	A	C
8										B	A	D	C	E
9										A	C	B	E	D
10										C	E	A	D	B

Note: The letters in the sequence rows are assigned at random to the formulations. These designs (except the 2, 2, 2 design) are variance and carryover balanced for the given number of formulations.

variance used as the mean square error for the formulation comparisons. This variance is not the true inter-subject variance (σ_B^2) because the subject-by-formulation interaction and some intrasubject variance still remain.

B. CROSSOVER DESIGN

The basic principle behind a crossover design is that subjects generally differ less within themselves when a particular trait is measured repeatedly than they do with other subjects. The immediate consequence is that comparison of formulations are made within subjects. Recall that the intrasubject variance is usually only a small component of the variance from the parallel design. A crossover design is made up of a set of S sequences which describe the order in which all or some of the F formulations are to be given to the subjects in the P periods. Specific crossover designs will be described as F, P, S designs. Subjects are randomized to one of the sequences, and formulations are randomized to the letters defining the group of sequences. The P periods are separated by an adequate washout time, which is determined by the half-life of the drug or the operations of the clinic.

There are many types of crossover designs, but basically they can be divided into two main types: replicated and nonreplicated. By replicated it is meant that at least one formulation is replicated within a sequence and thus within a subject.

1. Nonreplicated Crossover Designs

The simplest nonreplicated crossover designs are constructed when the number of formulations to be tested equals the number of periods, the F = P, S designs. As the number of formulations increases, the number of sequences increases as the factorial of F (i.e., when F = 4, S = 4! = 24). It is generally better to select and replicate a subset of sequences where the subset chosen defines a variance balanced design. A variance balanced design is one where each formulation appears the same number of times in each period such that the variance of the all the formulation comparisons is equal. Such designs for F = 3 to 5 are given in Table 1–1 along with the usual 2, 2, 2 design. The former designs are due to Williams.[62] Note that these designs are balanced for carryover effects (see below) in that each formulation is followed by a different formulation the same number of times. For example, in the 3, 3, 6 design, formulation A is followed by B twice and C twice. Therefore, if A has carryover, B and C are affected by the same magnitude.

When there are more formulations to be compared than periods available, one can consider a class of designs known as the balanced incomplete block designs.[63] These

Table 1–2 **Balanced incomplete block designs for F = 3, 4, and 5**

	F = 3		F = 4				
			Period (P)				
Sequence (S)	1	2	1	2	1	2	3
1	A	B	A	B	A	B	C
2	B	C	B	C	B	C	D
3	C	A	C	D	C	D	A
4			D	A	D	A	B
5			A	C			
6			B	D			
7			D	B			
8			C	A			
9			A	D			
10			D	C			
11			C	B			
12			B	A			

	F = 5								
	Period (P)								
Sequence (S)	1	2	1	2	3	1	2	3	4
1	A	B	A	B	C	A	B	C	D
2	B	C	B	C	D	B	C	D	E
3	C	D	C	D	E	C	D	E	A
4	D	E	D	E	A	D	E	A	B
5	E	A	E	A	B	E	A	B	C
6	A	C	E	B	C				
7	C	E	B	D	E				
8	E	B	D	A	B				
9	B	D	A	C	D				
10	D	A	C	E	A				

designs are given in Table 1–2 for various number of periods and F = 3, 4, and 5. The designs listed are only a subset of the possible sequences for each F and P, but are variance balanced. If the experimental formulations are not to be compared among themselves then each subject should receive the reference formulation. These designs are given in Pigeon.[28]

The linear model for the nonreplicated F, P, S crossover design is

$$Y_{ijkl} = \mu + S_i + V_{j(i)} + F_k + P_l + C_k + \varepsilon_{ijkl} \qquad \textbf{(1–10)}$$

where Y_{ijkl} = observation for subject j in sequence i given formulation k in period l; μ = the overall mean; S_i = effect of sequence i; $V_{j(1)}$ = random effect of subjects within sequence, assumed $N(0, \sigma_B^2)$; F_k = effect of formulation k; P_l = effect of period l; C_k = first-order carryover of formulation k; and ε_{ijkl} = the residual assumed to be $N(0, \sigma_X^2)$.

Assumptions on this model are that observations made on different subjects are independent, and that the variance of an observed Y is $\sigma_B^2 + \sigma_X^2$ and any two observations have a covariance σ_B^2. The subscript X of the residual indicates the residual from a nonreplicated crossover design.

Since these designs are so fundamental to bioequivalence studies, each effect as it appears in the model will be discussed in detail. Special attention will be given to the 2, 2, 2 crossover which is discussed in Grizzle[64] because it is the most often used design.

a. Sequence Effect

The sequence effect measures the differences between the groups of subjects defined by their sequence. In itself it is a nuisance parameter and has little importance in interpreting data. For this reason the sequence effect is often absorbed into the Subject (SEQ) source of error. However, the 2, 2, 2 design is a special case worth noting because a significant sequence effect can be caused by three confounded sources. One, there may be a genuine difference between subjects assigned at random to the two sequences. Two, there may be unequal carryover effect of the two formulations into the next period; or, three, there may be a formulation-by-period interaction. If the cause is the true difference between groups of subjects, formulation comparisons are not biased. If the significant sequence effect is caused from the latter two sources, formulation comparisons are biased. Since these effects are confounded, we never know which are acting. However, it is expected that unequal carryover or formulation-by-period interaction should not exist in a properly designed and executed study. Thus a significant sequence effect in the 2, 2, 2 crossover is generally ignored if no suspicious causes can be found such as nonzero concentrations beginning the second period. The sequence effect in the crossover ANOVA is tested against Subject (SEQ) effect.

b. Subject (SEQ) Effect

Since each subject is assigned only one sequence, subjects are said to be nested within sequence. This Subject (SEQ) effect is tested by the RESIDUAL and should be highly significant. This significance is an indication that the purpose of using the crossover design has been realized in that the between-subject variance is significantly larger than the residual. An estimate of σ_B^2 can be obtained by subtracting the mean squares for Subject (SEQ) from the residual and dividing by the number of periods.

c. Formulation Effect

The comparison of the formulation effect is what is being examined more thoroughly in the bioequivalence criteria. These estimates must be pure formulation estimates in that they do not include any other effect in the model, especially period effects. If the design is balanced in that the same number of subjects are observed for each sequence, the raw formulation means can be used for the formulation comparison. A study should always be designed for this balance. However, should a subject drop out leaving the design unbalanced, the least-squares means are used.

d. Period Effect

A period effect measures the differences between study periods. A well-run study with consistent treatment of subjects should produce no significant period effects. However, a significant period effect does not invalidate the study, but the cause should be investigated.

e. Carryover Effect

The carryover effect measures whether there is a difference between formulations in their effect on subsequent measurements. Carryover effects are termed first-, second-, or up to $P - 1$ order depending on how many periods following administration they are expected to influence. Usually estimating first-order effects is sufficient. As mentioned above, these effects are confounded with the sequence effect in the 2, 2, 2 crossover; and if the carryover effects are unequal for the two formulations, an unbiased estimate does not exist for formulation comparison. For most studies the carryover effect should not be an important factor when an adequate washout period is allowed between doses. One should always use a design which is balanced for carryover (Table 1–1.). If a pure formulation comparison can be derived removing the carryover effect, this estimate should be used.

Table 1–3 **Replicated crossover designs for two formulations**

a. Optimal for carryover estimation

	Period (P)								
Sequence (S)	**1**	**2**	**1**	**2**	**3**	**1**	**2**	**3**	**4**
1	A	A	A	B	B	A	A	B	B
2	B	B	B	A	A	B	B	A	A
3	A	B				A	B	B	A
4	B	A				B	A	A	B

b. Switchback designs

	Period (P)						
Sequence (S)	**1**	**2**	**3**	**1**	**2**	**3**	**4**
1	A	B	A	A	B	A	B
2	B	A	B	B	A	B	A

f. The Residual

This error term is the variation which cannot be explained by the fitting of the effects described above; thus it is sometimes called the residual. It is the summation of all sources of random error described in Section III excluding between-subject variance. Frequently it is called the intrasubject variance estimate for all formulations, but this is a misnomer since the subject-by-formulation interaction is also included. The mean square residual is the estimate of the variance for the formulation comparison. The estimate of the residual CV is directly obtained by using Equation 1–5.

2. Replicated Crossover Designs

Inferred in the above discussion of the nonreplicated designs are problems in estimating pure formulation effects, true intrasubject variances, and subject-by-formulation interaction. These problems can be overcome if replication of formulations is done within a subject. These designs have more periods or sequences than formulations. Such designs are given in Table 1–3 for two formulation comparisons. The first set of three designs, Table 1–3a, are optimal for their respective number of periods, estimation of carryover, and formulation effects; and have minimum variances for both comparisons. If carryover is a real concern, then these designs should be used. Estimation of effects for these designs can be found in Chow and Liu.[65]

The second set of designs in Table 1–3b are called switchback designs. They can also be used and may estimate the subject-by-formulation term better than those designs in Table 3a since formulations are not given in adjacent periods. For estimation of effects in the switchback designs, the reader is referred to Brandt[66] and Carmer.[67]

A very simplified linear model for a replicated design is

$$Y_{ijkl} = \mu + S_i + V_{j(i)} + F_k + P_l + C_k + FV_{j(i)k} + \varepsilon_{ijkl} \tag{1–11}$$

where the first seven terms are defined in Section V.B.1, $FV_{j(i)k}$ is the subject-by-formulation interaction, and the ε_{ijkl} are $N(0, \sigma_W^2)$. The subject-by-formulation term is used as the estimated S^2 in the standard error of the formulation comparison. Equation 1–11 is simplified because it does not include any of the interaction terms of sequence with the other effects or period by formulation.

C. DESIGN CONSIDERATIONS

There are many types of crossover designs depending on the number of sequences, periods, and formulations. Before choosing a design to use, the following should be considered.

1. Does the intrasubject variance for each formulation and the subject-by-formulation interaction need to be estimated explicitly? If they do, then some sort of replicated design is required which usually means only two formulations can be studied at one time. The choice of the replicated design will depend on the precision required in estimating these variances.
2. The more periods used the greater is the chance of dropouts. A regulatory agency will frown on any more than 15% missing values in any one period. Therefore, it is not recommended to use more than four periods. A monetary incentive may be considered if the subject completes all legs of the study. There is also an ethical amount of blood which may be removed over a 6-month period, and with a minimum of 14 samples per period the maximum is reached usually by four periods.
3. How many formulations, strengths, or conditions of dosing need to be studied? The larger the basic design, the more precise is the estimate for residual. If the log transformation is used, there is no reason why different strengths cannot be used in the same study. If food studies are to be run at the same time, a check for homogeneity of the variance should be done. If there are more than four formulations, a balanced incomplete block design may be considered.
4. For what should the design be optimal? Many of the designs discussed are optimal for estimating formulation effects in the presence of unequal carryover effects. However, the chances of carryover, let alone unequal carryover, in a single-dose bioequivalence study are small. Since many of the optimal designs place the same formulations in adjacent periods, the chance of inflating the subject-by-formulation interaction due to autocorrelation is maximized. Also what happens to the optimality of these designs in the presence of missing values or unequal allotment of subjects to sequences?
5. How many subjects can the clinical facility handle in a day before quality will be compromised? If more subjects are required, a study may be broken into consecutive days and have each day as a blocking factor. Also remember the number of subjects must be a multiple of the number of sequences.

VI. OTHER CONSIDERATIONS

A. SAMPLE SIZE

The number of volunteers needed to be recruited into a study depends on which standard the formulation must satisfy. If average equivalence is required, then from Equation 1-6 or 1–7, it can easily be seen how to maximize the chance that the 1–2α% confidence interval will fall entirely within the BI. First is the center point of the interval or the estimated average difference for the parameter in question. The closer the test formulation is formulated to the reference, the smaller this expected difference will be. The farther away from zero the expected difference is, the smaller must be the precision or the standard error of the estimate. The standard error of the difference is

$$SE_{(\bar{x}_E-\bar{x}_R)} = \sqrt{\left(\frac{1}{n_E}+\frac{1}{n_R}\right)S^2} \tag{1–12}$$

Table 1–4 **Sample sizes required to pass average bioequivalence as defined by a BI of 90 to 111% with powers of 0.8 and 0.9**

	Expected Relative Difference in Medians									
	0.92		0.94		0.96		0.98		1.0	
Power	**0.8**	**0.9**	**0.8**	**0.9**	**0.8**	**0.9**	**0.8**	**0.9**	**0.8**	**0.9**
CV (%) 10	258	356	68	92	32	44	20	26	18	22
15	572	792	148	204	68	94	42	56	36	46
20	1006	1392	258	358	118	164	72	96	62	78
25	1554	2152	398	552	182	252	112	148	96	120
30	2208	3058	566	782	258	356	156	208	136	170
35	2960	4100	758	1050	346	478	210	280	180	228
40	3802	5264	972	1346	444	612	268	358	232	292

Table 1–5 **Sample sizes required to pass average bioequivalence as defined by a BI of 80 to 125% with powers of 0.8 and 0.9**

	Expected Relative Difference in Medians							
	0.85		0.90		0.95		1.0	
Power	**0.8**	**0.9**	**0.8**	**0.9**	**0.8**	**0.9**	**0.8**	**0.9**
CV (%) 10	36	48	12	14	8	8	6	8
15	78	106	22	30	12	16	10	12
20	134	186	38	50	26	20	16	20
25	206	284	56	78	28	38	24	28
30	292	404	80	108	40	52	32	40
35	392	540	106	146	52	70	42	52
40	502	694	134	186	66	88	54	66

Table 1–6 **Sample sizes required to pass average bioequivalence as defined by a BI of 70 to 143% with powers of 0.8 and 0.9**

	Expected Relative Difference in Medians											
	0.75		0.80		0.85		0.90		0.95		1.0	
Power	**0.8**	**0.9**	**0.8**	**0.9**	**0.8**	**0.9**	**0.8**	**0.9**	**0.8**	**0.9**	**0.8**	**0.9**
CV (%) 10	28	38	10	12	6	8	6	6	4	6	4	6
15	60	82	18	24	10	12	8	8	6	8	6	6
20	204	144	30	40	16	20	10	14	8	10	8	10
25	160	220	44	60	22	30	14	18	12	14	10	12
30	226	312	62	86	30	42	20	26	16	18	14	18
35	302	418	82	114	40	54	26	34	20	24	18	22
40	388	536	106	144	52	70	32	42	24	30	22	28

where the n_i's are the number of subjects receiving the two formulations and S^2 is the appropriate error term from the ANOVA. Therefore, there are two ways to get more precision: increase n or use the experimental design which minimizes the error term.

Tables 1–4, 1–5, and 1–6 give the number of subjects needed in a 2, 2, 2 crossover to pass AB as declared by Equation 1–6 or 1–7 for BIs of 90 to 111, 80 to 125, and 70 to 143%, respectively. These tables were generated using an exact formula of Diletti et al.[68,69] for the 90% confidence interval approach for determining AB. Similar tables for the two one-sided tests procedure, each at 5%, are given in Phillips.[70] Approximate formulas for the two methods are given in Hauschke et al.[71] for BIs of 80 to 125% and Liu and Chow[72] for BIs ±20%, respectively. The subjects are to be randomly assigned evenly to both sequences.

To find the appropriate cell in the table choose the appropriate BI for the bioavailability metric under test; then choose the expected variation, in terms of a CV, of this metric and the expected relative difference of the test formulation to the reference. Finally, choose a power or probability of passing of either 0.8 or 0.9. If there is a high degree of confidence in the expected variation, the difference, and the study execution, choose 0.8. If little is known about the variation, choose the 0.9 power.

Extra subjects should be added to each sequence to account for dropouts. Two strategies can be used. The first is to add a fixed number of subjects to each sequence, usually adding to each sequence 10% of the calculated n determined from the sample size chart. All subjects are used in this strategy. A second strategy, especially if assaying of samples is expensive, is to only assay the blood if a sequence mate drops out. This strategy assures the study will end with the calculated n. The strategy chosen must be declared in the protocol.

If a standard is made up of more than one parameter, the parameter which is expected to be hardest to pass should determine the sample size. It should be noted that some countries may have a minimum number of subjects (Canada has 12) which must be used. It is also recommended that if it is estimated to use more than 50 subjects, the regulating agency should be contacted. These tables can be used to give very close sample sizes for parallel and other crossover studies.

B. OUTLIERS

As with any other type of studies, there are always values that do not compare well with other results in the bioequivalence study. These curious values which cannot be attributed to missing concentrations in the profile or any extreme concentration in the profile are called outliers. There are many tests to identify outliers,[73] but routine removal from the study is not valid because such outliers can indicate two important and real possible outcomes. One, the profile is a result of a product failure; or, two, this could be the realization of a subject-by-formulation interaction. The main point is that the observation could be very meaningful and should not be discarded unthinkingly.

The only legitimate way of removing a subject's results is to bring the subject back to the study center and repeat both formulations. It is far cheaper to have one subject return than to redo the whole study. If the results are different again we probably have a real subject-by-formulation interaction. Further study of this would be required by the agency. If the two repeated results are similar for the two formulations, then one of the formulations of the initial pair failed and can be identified by comparison with its respective repeat. If it was the reference product that failed, then the test formulation should not be penalized and the subject's results are removed. Usually no more than 5% of the subjects should be considered outliers before the quality of the study would be questioned. If the test formulation failed, then another study may be warranted although it may be wise to do more *in vitro* formulation development before any *in vivo* repeat. Results with and without these outliers should be submitted for review. It should be noted that an *a priori* test for outlier screening should be part of the study protocol and followed even if the study indicates bioequivalence.

C. ADD-ON DESIGNS

All pivotal studies should be designed with the appropriate number of subjects recruited based on the available information on the drug and formulations. Even the results of a study using the expected size can fail the standard; and the sponsor is left with a decision: to reformulate because results were not as expected or to do a larger study. To ignore the first study seems a waste of data; however, some agencies may require this. Canadian guidelines state that if a properly designed study based on reasonable estimates of variability was executed and this study failed, the sponsor has the option of adding to this study the expected number of additional subjects (minimum of 12) required to pass the standard. The combination of studies must meet consistency tests of no significant study-by-formulation interaction and homogeneity of variance from the two studies. Karpinski[74] described the tests required and showed that there is a decreased chance of passing the criteria if two studies with a combined n are run when compared to one study of size n. This decrease is due to the chance of failing the consistency checks. Pilot studies are not to be included in final results.

Bayesian two-stage procedures have been proposed[75-77] in the literature where you start with a small number, peek at the data, and use the estimates from the first stage to determine the sample of the next stage. There is a slight penalty for peeking so more subjects may be required than a one-stage study. These types of studies may be valuable when very little is known about the variation of the bioavailability metric.

Since there is no agreement between agencies on the use of add-ons, there can be no substitute for a well-designed study where estimates of the variation are taken from the literature and the expected mean difference between the formulations is obtained from the laboratory.

VII. SUMMARY AND THE FUTURE

The purpose of this chapter has been to present the major statistical aspects of design, analysis of data, and presentation of results for a bioequivalence study. The investigator must first know *a priori* exactly what regulatory standard the formulation must meet. Without this knowledge no study should ever be executed. The second most important aspect is to understand the drug, the reference formulation, and the test formulation. Understanding the drug is paramount because it generally determines the regulatory standard which must be passed and the size of the study. A careful review of the available literature on the drug to estimate the intrasubject variance, not intersubject variance, will save much money and time.

The newer concept of individual equivalence is appealing but will require many more years of data collection in order to establish statistical concepts such as subject-by-formulation interactions and bioequivalence studies that are sensitive enough to detect different variation in the test formulation that *in vitro* testing cannot.

The challenge of statistics in the future will be to sell new methodologies to regulators, with international harmonization depending on it. Such methods as those based on Bayesian inference, robust statistics, and nonparametric analysis will have to be seriously considered as viable alternatives to the ANOVA methods discussed in this chapter.

ACKNOWLEDGMENTS

I am very grateful to Drs. W. Walope, I. J. McGilveray, and K. Karpinski for their critical reading of the manuscript. I could not have completed it without their gentle nudges and encouragement. I am also grateful to Drs. V. Steinijans and E. Diletti for supplying the three tables on sample sizes.

REFERENCES

1. **Midha, K. K., Ed.,** Bio International '89, *Int. Pharm. J.,* 4(3), 1, 1990.
2. DIA, Workshop on Bioavailability/Bioequivalence: Pharmacokinetic and Statistical Considerations, Bethesda, MD, August 5–7, 1991.
3. **Cartwright, A. C.,** International Harmonization and Consensus of DIA Meeting on Bioavailability and Bioequivalence Testing Requirements and Standards, *Drug Inform. J.,* 25, 471, 1991.
4. **Midha, K. K. and Blume, H. H., Eds.,** *Bio-International, Bioavailability, Bioequivalence, and Pharmacokinetics,* Medpharm, Stuttgart, 1993.
5. **Pabst, G. and Jaegar, H.,** Review of methods and criteria for the evaluation of bioequivalence studies, *Eur. J. Clin. Pharmacol.,* 38, 5, 1990.
6. **McGilveray, I. J. and Ormsby, E. D.,** Harmonization of bioavailability and bioequivalence requirements, *Eur. J. Drug Metab. Pharmacokinet.,* Special Issue No. III, 533, 1991.
7. **Schulz, H.-U. and Steinijans, V. W.,** Striving for standards in bioequivalence assessment: a review, *Int. J. Clin. Pharmacol. Ther. Toxicol.,* 29, 293, 1991.
8. **Steinijans, V. W., Hauschke, D., and Jonkman, J. H. G.,** Controversies in bioequivalence studies, *Clin. Pharmacokinet.,* 22(4) 247, 1992.
9. **Rodda, B. E. and Davis, R. L.,** Determining the probability of an important difference in bioavailability, *Clin. Pharmacol. Ther.,* 28, 247, 1980.
10. **Selwyn, M. R., Dempster, A. R., and Hall, N. R.,** A Bayesian approach to bioequivalence for the 2×2 changeover design, *Biometrics,* 37, 11, 1981.
11. **Flühler, H., Hirtz, J., and Moser, H. A.,** An aid to decision-making in bioequivalence assessment, *J. Pharmacokinet. Biopharm.,* 9, 235, 1981.
12. **Flühler, H., Grieve, A. P., Mandallaz, D., Mau, J., and Moser, H. A.,** Bayesian approach to bioequivalence assessment: an example, *J. Pharm. Sci.,* 72, 1178, 1983.
13. **Selwyn, M. R. and Hall, N. R.,** On Bayesian methods for bioequivalence, *Biometrics,* 40, 1103, 1984.
14. **Westlake, W. J.,** Use of confidence intervals in analysis of comparative bioavailability trials, *J. Pharm. Sci.,* 61, 1340, 1972.
15. **Westlake, W. J.,** Symmetrical confidence intervals for bioequivalence trials, *Biometrics,* 32, 741, 1976.
16. **Mandallaz, D. and Mau, J.,** Comparison of different methods for decision-making in bioavailability assessment, *Biometrics,* 37, 213, 1981.
17. **Locke, C. S.,** An exact confidence interval from untransformed data for the ratio of two formulation means, *J. Pharmacokinet. Biopharm.,* 12, 649, 1984.
18. **Chinchilli, V. M. and Esinhart, J. D.,** Tolerance intervals for assessment of individual bioequivalence, presented to FDA, Division of Biopharmaceutics, Washington, D.C., June 9, 1992.
19. **Patel, H. I. and Gupta, G. D.,** A problem of equivalence in clinical trials, *Biom J.,* 26, 471, 1984.
20. **Rocke, D. M.,** On testing bioequivalence, *Biometrics,* 40, 225, 1984.
21. **Hauck, W. W. and Anderson, S.,** A new statistical procedure for testing equivalence in two-group comparative bioavailability trials, *J. Pharmacokinet. Biopharm.,* 12, 83, 1984. (Erratum *J. Pharmacokinet. Biopharm.,* 12, 657, 1984.)
22. **Schuirmann, D. J.,** A comparison of the two-one sided tests procedure and the power approach for assessing the equivalence of average bioavailability, *J. Pharmacokinet. Biopharm.,* 15, 657, 1987.
23. **Hauschke, D., Steinijans, V. W., and Diletti, E.,** A distribution-free procedure for the statistical analysis of bioequivalence studies, *Int. J. Clin. Pharmacol. Ther. Toxicol.,* 28, 72, 1990.

24. **Yuh L.,** Robust estimation, in *Proc. Bio International '89,* McGilveray, I. J., Dighe, S. V., French, I. W., Midha, K. K., and Skelly, J. P., Eds., McGraw-Hill, Toronto, Canada, 1990, 162.
25. **Chow, S. and Shao, J.,** An alternative approach for the assessment of bioequivalence between two formulations of a drug, *Biom. J.,* 8, 969, 1990.
26. Report C: report on bioavailability of oral dosage formulations, not in modified release form, of drugs used for systemic effects, having complicated or variable pharmacokinetics, Expert Advisory Committee on Bioavailability, Health Protection Branch, Ottawa, Canada, December 1992.
27. Drugs Directorate Guidelines: conduct and analysis of bioavailability and bioequivalence studies. Part A. Oral dosage formulations used for systemic effect, Health Protection Branch, Health and Welfare Canada, 1992.
28. Drugs Directorate Guidelines: conduct and analysis of bioavailability and bioequivalence studies. Part B. Modified release dosage formulations, (Draft) Health Protection Branch, Health and Welfare Canada, 1993.
29. **Endrenyi, L., Fritsch, S., and Wei, Y.,** C_{max}/AUC is a clearer measure than C_{max} for absorption rates in investigations of bioequivalence, *Int. J. Clin. Pharmacol. Ther. Toxicol.,* 29, 394, 1991.
30. **Schall, R. and Luus, H. G.,** Comparison of absorption rates in bioequivalence studies of immediate release drug formulations, *Int. J. Clin. Pharmacol. Ther. Toxicol.,* 30, 153, 1992.
31. **Chen, M.,** An alternative approach for assessment of rate of absorption in bioequivalence studies, *Pharm. Res.,* 9, 1380, 1992.
32. **McGilveray, I. J.,** Bioequivalence: a Canadian regulatory perspective, Chapter 13, in *Pharmaceutical Bioequivalence,* Welling, P. G., Tse, F. L. S., and Dighe, S. V., Eds., Marcel Dekker, New York, 1991, 383.
33. **Benet, L. Z.,** Highly variable drugs, presentation at Bio '92, Bad Homburg, Germany, 1992.
34. Commission of the European Communities, Committee on Proprietary Medicinal Products (CPMP) Working Party on Efficacy, Note for Guidance Investigation of Bioavailability and Bioequivalence, December 1991.
35. **Gaffney, M.,** Variance components in comparative bioavailability studies, *J. Pharm. Sci.,* 81, 315, 1992.
36. **Ekbohn, G. and Melander, H.,** The subject-by-formulation interaction as a criterion of interchangeability of drugs, *Biometrics,* 45, 1249, 1989.
37. **Anderson, S. and Hauck, W. W.,** Consideration of individual bioequivalence, *J. Pharmacokinet. Biopharm.,* 18, 259, 1990.
38. Conference report of analytical validation: bioavailability, bioequivalence and pharmacokinetic studies, *Pharm. Res.,* 9, 588, 1992.
39. **Steinijans, V. W., Eicke, R., and Ahrens, J.,** Pharmacokinetics of theophylline in patients following short-term intravenous infusion, *Eur. J. Clin. Pharmacol.,* 22, 417, 1982.
40. **Friedman, D. J., Greenblatt, E. S., Burstein, J. S., Harmatz, J. S., and Shader, R. I.,** Population study of triazolam pharmacokinetics, *Br. J. Clin. Pharm.,* 22, 639, 1986.
41. **Ormsby, E. D.,** Log transformation, in *Proc. Bio International '89,* McGilveray, I. J., Dighe, S. V., French, I. W., Midha, K. K., and Skelly, J. P., Eds., McGraw-Hill, Toronto, Canada, 1990, 157.
42. **Shimizu, K. and Crow, E. L.,** History, genesis, and properties, in *Lognormal Distributions: Theory and Applications,* Vol. 88, Crow, E. L. and Shimizu, K., Eds., Marcel Dekker, New York, 1988, chap. 1.
43. Meeting of Generic Drug Advisory Committee to the FDA, Washington, D.C., September 1991.

44. **Land, C. E.,** An evaluation of approximate confidence interval estimation methods for lognormal means, *Technometrics,* 14, 145, 1972.
45. **Liu, J. and Weng, C.,** Estimation of direct formulation effect under log-normal distribution in bioavailability/bioequivalence studies, *Stat. Med.,* 11, 881, 1992.
46. **Metzler, C. M.,** Bioavailability — A problem in equivalence, *Biometrics,* 30, 309, 1974.
47. **Haynes, J. D.,** Statistical simulation study of new proposed uniformity requirement for bioequivalence studies, *J. Pharm. Sci.,* 70, 673, 1981.
48. **Cabana, B. E.,** Assessment of 75/75 rule: FDA viewpoint, *J. Pharm. Sci.,* 72, 98, 1983.
49. **Haynes, J. D.,** FDA 75/75 rule: a response, *J. Pharm. Sci.* 72, 99, 1983.
50. **Dobbins, T. W. and Thiyagarajan, B.,** A retrospective assessment of the 75/75 rule in bioequivalence, *Stat. Med.,* 11, 1333, 1992.
51. **Kirkwood, T. B. L.,** Bioequivalence testing — A need to rethink, *Biometrics,* 37, 589, 1981.
52. **Mantel, N.,** Do we want confidence intervals symmetric about the null value?, *Biometrics,* 33, 759, 1977.
53. **Westlake, W. J.,** Response to Kirkwood, *Biometrics,* 37, 591, 1981.
54. **Liu, J.,** Bioequivalence and intrasubject variability, *J. Biopharm. Stat.,* 1, 205, 1991.
55. **Lui, J. and Chow, S.,** On the assessment of variability in bioavailability/bioequivalence studies, *Commun. Stat., Part A,* 21, 2591, 1992.
56. **Bofinger, E.,** Expanded confidence intervals, one-sided tests, and equivalence testing, *J. Biopharm. Stat.,* 2(2), 181, 1992.
57. **Sheiner, L. B.,** Bioequivalence revisited, *Stat. Med.,* 11, 1777, 1992.
58. **Schall, R. and Luus, H. G.,** On population and individual bioequivalence, *Stat. Med.,* 12, 1109, 1993.
59. **Hwang, S., Huber, P. B., Hesney, M., and Kwan, K. C.,** Bioequivalence and interchangeability, *J. Pharm. Sci.,* 67, IV "Open Forum", 1978.
60. **Hauck, W. W. and Anderson, S.,** Types of bioequivalence and related statistical considerations, *Int. J. Clin. Pharmacol. Ther. Toxicol.,* 30, 181, 1992.
61. **Endrenyi, L.,** A procedure for the assessment of individual bioequivalence, unpublished manuscript, 1993.
62. **Williams, E. J.,** Experimental designs balanced for the estimation of residual effects of treatments, *Aust. J. Sci. Res. Ser. A,* 2, 149, 1949.
63. **Westlake, W. J.,** The use of balanced incomplete block designs in comparative bioavailability trials, *Biometrics,* 30, 319, 1974.
64. **Grizzle, J. E.,** The two-period change-over design and its use in clinical trials, *Biometrics,* 21, 467, 1965. (Correction: *Biometrics,* 30, 327, 1974.)
65. **Chow, S. C. and Liu, J. P.,** On assessment of bioequivalence under a higher-order crossover design, *J. Biopharm. Stat.,* 2(2), 239, 1992.
66. **Brandt, A. E.,** Tests of significance in reversal or switchback trials, *Iowa State Coll. Agric. Exp. Stn. Res. Bull.,* 234, 60, 1938.
67. **Carmer, S. G.,** Analysis of crossover designs for bioequivalency testing, in Proc. of the Biopharmaceutical Section of the American Statistical Association, Chicago, 1986, 171.
68. **Diletti, D., Hauschke, D., and Steinijans, V. W.,** Sample size determination for bioequivalence assessment by means of confidence intervals, *Int. J. Clin. Pharmacol. Ther. Toxicol.,* 29, 1, 1991.
69. **Diletti, D., Hauschke, D., and Steinijans, V. W.,** Sample size determination: extended tables for the multiplicative model and bioequivalence ranges of 0.9 to 1.11 and 0.7 to 1.43, *Int. J. Clin. Pharmacol. Ther. Toxicol.,* 30, 287, 1992.

70. **Phillips, K. F.,** Power of the two one-sided tests procedure in bioequivalence, *J. Pharmacokinet. Biopharm.,* 18, 137, 1990.
71. **Hauschke, D., Steinijans, V. W., Diletti, D., and Burke, M.,** Sample size determination for bioequivalence using a multiplicative model, *J. Pharmacokinet. Biopharm.,* 20, 557, 1992.
72. **Liu, J. and Chow, S.,** Sample size determination for the two one-sided tests procedure in bioequivalence, *J. Pharmacokinet. Biopharm.,* 20, 101, 1992.
73. **Chow, S. C. and Tse, S. K.,** Outlier detection in bioavailability/bioequivalence studies, *Stat. Med.,* 9, 549, 1990.
74. **Karpinski, K. F.,** Add-on subject design, in *Proc. Bio International '89,* McGilveray, I. J., Dighe, S. V., French, I. W., Midha, K. K., and Skelly, J. P., Eds., McGraw-Hill, Toronto, Canada, 1990, 138.
75. **Racine-Poon, A., Grieve, A. P., Flühler, H., and Smith, A. F. M.,** A two-stage procedure for bioequivalence studies, *Biometrics,* 43, 847, 1987.
76. **Freeman, P. R.,** The performance of the two-stage analysis of two-treatment, two-period crossover trials, *Stat. Med.,* 8, 1421, 1989.
77. **Durrleman, S. and Simon, R.,** Planning and monitoring of equivalence studies, *Biometrics,* 46, 329, 1990.
78. **Pigeon, J. G. and Raghavaras, D.,** Crossover designs for comparing treatments with a control, *Biometrika,* 74, 321, 1987.

Chapter 2

Role of Single- and Multiple-Dose Studies in the Estimation of Bioequivalency

Andre J. Jackson

CONTENTS

I. BACKGROUND AND INTRODUCTION

The role of single- (sd) and multiple-dose (md) studies in pharmacokinetics has been well established. By varying the route and method of administration, single-dose studies have been used to determine the pharmacokinetic parameters required to describe drug absorption, distribution, metabolism, and elimination.[1] Published reports have described numerous methods of estimating model-dependent (e.g., intercompartmental rate constants)[2-4] and model-independent parameters such as clearance, mean residence time, and sojourn time using single-dose data.[5-7] Although not always conclusive, single-dose studies do provide some clues as to whether a drug exhibits nonlinear kinetics within the proposed therapeutic range, confirmation of which would be obtained from multiple-dose studies. The administration of two or more single doses separated in size by a factor of two or more can be used to assess the nonlinearity of such parameters as: (1) normalized area under the curve, (2) consistency of clearance, and (3) fraction of drug excreted.[8] Single-dose studies have also proved useful in investigating the formation and excretion of drug metabolites.[9] A few drugs such as isoproteronol (when used to relieve an acute asthma attack) and nitroglycerin (to relieve angina) are known to be effective following a single dose.[10]

However, since most drugs are therapeutically effective only after multiple-dose administration, it is essential that one understand how the body handles drugs at steady state. Multiple-dose and steady-state experiments are essential whenever the therapeutically effective use of the drug requires dosing the patient to steady-state concentrations.[11] Comparing the results from single- and multiple-dose studies also provides information on chronic or time-dependent drug effects such as enzyme induction, unusual accumulation, or drug-induced alterations in disposition.[11] The duration of multiple dosing in relation to the drug terminal half-life is the critical factor for ascertaining attainment of steady-state conditions. A drug dosed at its half-life will achieve 87.5% of its steady-state concentration after three doses.[10] Attainment of steady state is normally confirmed by the comparison of several consecutive C_{min} values (trough drug levels recorded at each dosing interval just prior to the next dose) or $AUC_{(0-\tau)}$ values (area for a dosing interval at steady state), following multiple dosing to confirm that successive C_{min}s or AUCs are not significantly changing. Information obtained from the single- and multiple-dose studies is used to establish a multiple-dosing regimen consistent with the drug's therapeutic index so that the compound can be effective with minimal toxicity.

A complicating factor even for a drug with linear kinetics is the presence of an active metabolite that is eliminated more slowly than its precursor.[12] It has been shown that drugs with slowly eliminated (i.e., excretion-rate limited) metabolites may produce a higher than predicted accumulation ratio since the final ratio results from the combined parent and metabolite concentrations.[12]

Several additional pharmacokinetic relationships have proved useful in predicting multiple-dose kinetics from single-dose data. Most notably, the area under the curve from time zero to infinity following a single dose is equal to the area under the curve from time zero to the conclusion of the dosing interval at steady state.[1] It has also been shown that at steady state the concentration maximum (C_{max}) becomes larger and the time for that maximum (T_{max}) becomes earlier, compared to single dosing.[1]

Although single-dose data may be used to predict steady-state behavior for many therapeutic agents, there are some drugs for which prediction is not possible, such as those drugs which exhibit time- or concentration-dependent kinetics. The nonlinear kinetics may be a consequence of absorption, first-pass metabolism, binding, excretion, or biotransformation.[13] Many of these drugs such as phenytoin[14] and the salicylates[15] have had their nonlinear kinetics thoroughly investigated. Some major consequences of concentration dependent kinetics are (1) nonproportional increase in AUC with increasing dose (i.e., a disproportionally large increase in the steady-state blood concentration is observed following an increase in the dose), (2) decreasing drug clearance with increasing dose and dose rate, (3) decreasing percentage of drug metabolized via a Michaelis-Menten pathway with increasing dose and dose rate, and (4) increasing time required to reach steady state with increasing dose rate.[16]

Besides drugs with nonlinear kinetics, there are other drugs such as metoprolol and bepridil with linear kinetics (i.e., they maintain a linear dose/plasma concentration relation), but whose multiple-dose kinetics still are not readily predicted from single-dose data.[17] For metoprolol, the fraction absorbed following oral dosing appears to increase by about 25% with repeated administration, while for bepridil the clearance-to-availability ratio is reported to be halved upon multiple dosing. Consequently, a reliable prediction of steady-state levels for these drugs cannot be made based on single-dose data.

To establish bioequivalency, one must first determine that the drug products are *pharmaceutical equivalents;* that is, they contain the same active ingredient(s), are of the same dosage form, and are identical in strength and route of administration. To be considered bioequivalent, the test and reference drug products should not exhibit any significant differences in either the rate or the extent of absorption when the therapeutic moiety is administered at the same molar dose under similar experimental conditions, in either a single dose or multiple doses.[18] Therefore according to the Code of Federal Regulations (CFR), either type of study design (sd or md) may be used to establish equivalency, although steady-state studies are more costly and difficult to conduct. Unfortunately, drug pharmacokinetics/pharmacodynamics may make steady-state studies unfeasible (as in the case of haloperidol, which should only be given once daily to healthy normal subjects).[19] The fact that bioequivalence studies are usually done in healthy normal volunteers rather than in patients also limits the feasibility of multiple-dose administration for many drugs. Any study used to establish bioequivalency should be predictive of steady-state performance, since (as stated above) few drugs are administered therapeutically as only a single dose.[10] Thus, the reasons for using single- and multiple-dose studies in bioequivalency testing are somewhat different than they are for drug development. During drug development, multiple-dose studies are used mainly to confirm or refute evidence of dose proportionality obtained from single-dose studies and to establish an appropriate therapeutic dosing regimen.

Recently, in 1988 a Food and Drug Administration (FDA) task force on bioequivalence considered the adequacy of single-dose studies in defining bioequivalence.[20] The following conclusion was published by the task force: "The task force believes that as a general rule a single-dose study is adequate. Multiple-dose studies should be performed only when a single-dose study is not a reliable indicator of bioavailability, e.g., because of the kinetics of the drug." These findings have been expanded in a recent presentation to the Generic Drug Advisory Committee.[21] The information presented to the committee dealt with additional concerns about the pharmacokinetics of linear and nonlinear drugs. A summary conclusion on single vs. multiple dosing issued by the committee stated: "For drugs that are poorly soluble or exhibit saturable transport, a single dose study is adequate. Single dose studies provide sufficient information to assess bioequivalency for drugs with saturable first-pass and no indication of interaction between metabolite(s) and drug being absorbed. Single dose studies are generally adequate in predicting steady-state behavior for drugs that either exhibit saturable distribution and/or elimination." The committee's major concern regarding the use of multiple-dose studies was that they do not provide as sensitive a measure of differences in rate of absorption between formulations compared to single-dose studies.

In the Code of Federal Regulations,[22] conditions are listed for which a multiple-dose study may be required to determine bioavailability. These conditions include: (1) when there is a difference in the rate of absorption but not in the extent of absorption, (2) when there is excessive variability in bioavailability from subject to subject, (3) when the concentration of the active drug ingredient or its metabolite(s) in the blood resulting from a single dose is too low for analysis, or (4) when the drug is a controlled-release dosage form. It has been recently brought to this author's attention that this section of the CFR is being revised under a new heading that will make these regulations applicable only to new chemical entities. Nevertheless, the current regulations raise several important scientific issues regarding drug bioequivalency. This chapter will assess the utility of single-dose studies in estimating the bioequivalency of both linear and nonlinear drugs, using the current confidence interval method.[23]

Bioequivalency is determined by using the confidence interval approach (two one-sided tests procedure) to statistically evaluate observed differences in rate and extent of absorption between the test and reference treatment means for C_{max} and $AUC_{(0-\infty)}$. Factors critical to determining the confidence intervals about the means are (1) the numerical difference between the test and reference means or their ratios, (2) the number of subjects used in the study, and (3) the intrasubject variance of the data.[23] The choice of a single- or multiple-dose study design will have a different effect on each bioequivalency parameter of interest (i.e., $AUC_{(0-\infty)}$, C_{max}, and T_{max}), depending on whether the drug exhibits linear or nonlinear kinetics.

II. BIOEQUIVALENCY CONSIDERATIONS: LINEAR KINETICS

Most currently marketed drugs exhibit linear kinetics. Fewer than 40 are known to have a degree of nonlinearity sufficient to produce clinical consequences.[13] Although the kinetics of linear drugs at steady state are predictable from single-dose data, the values obtained for at least two of the bioequivalence parameters of interest (C_{max}, T_{max}) will change in going from single to multiple dosing, as previously discussed. Single-dose $AUC_{(0-\infty)}$, on the other hand, has been shown to be predictive of multiple-dose $AUC_{(0-\tau)}$.[1] The theoretical basis for this predictive capability is contained in the following relationships:

$$AUC(0-\infty) = FD_o/VK \qquad \textbf{(2-1)}$$

$$AUC(0-\tau) = FD_o/VK \qquad \textbf{(2-2)}$$

where F is the fraction absorbed, D_0 is dose, and VK is clearance.

Equation 2–1 describes area under the curve in a one-compartment model following a single dose and is equivalent to Equation 2–2 which describes area under the curve at steady state from time 0 to time τ (conclusion of the dosing interval).

Table 2–1 presents single- and multiple-dose estimates for C_{max} and T_{max} based on published simulated data. These data show that even with sizable error included, the theoretical relationships discussed above remain valid. At steady state, drug accumulation combined with an earlier T_{max} results in a higher C_{max} value than that observed following single-dose administration.[1] Each of these kinetic outcomes affects the confidence interval values used in determining bioequivalency as shown in Table 2–2. For C_{max}, the width of the interval either decreased or showed no change while the range for $AUC_{0-\infty}$ always decreased in going from single to multiple dosing. The range width and upper and lower limits for the confidence intervals for T_{max} increased in going from single to multiple dosing and in general were highly variable, which argues against using T_{max} for the determination of bioequivalency. Therefore, this parameter will be excluded from any further discussion of single vs. multiple dosing.

Experimental data for several drug products evaluated by the FDA Division of Bioequivalence support the results obtained using the simulated data. Acceptability of volunteers for these studies was based on their medical histories, physical examinations, and clinical laboratory tests. There was a 1 to 2 week washout period between study phases. A synopsis of the study details is presented in Tables 2–3 and 2–4. The data in Table 5 for C_{max} clearly show a decrease in the range of the 90% confidence intervals obtained from multiple-dose studies compared with those obtained from single-dose studies. This observed decrease may be accounted for as follows:

1. Drug accumulation during multiple dosing yields a steady-state C_{max} value which provides data mainly on previously absorbed drug rather than on drug absorbed from the most recent dose.[24]

Table 2–1 **Summary of bioavailability parameters following the simulation of single- (50 mg) and multiple-dose (50 mg/6 h) drug administration in the linear one-compartment body model with either 0.2 or 0.6 fractional standard deviation added to each concentration**

	Reference[a]		Test[b]	
Parameters	**0.2 FSD**	**0.6 FSD**	**0.2 FSD**	**0.6 FSD**
Single dose				
T_{max} (h)	3.97 (1.59)	4.62 (2.32)	2.32 (0.90)	2.13 (1.05)
C_{max} (μg/ml)	19.04 (1.40)	25.48 (5.28)	24.66 (1.92)	34.77 (5.26)
$AUC_{0-\infty}$ (μg/ml × h)	259.69 (16.65)	248.94 (50.77)	256.68 (29.23)	238.50 (43.15)
Multiple dose				
T_{max} (h)	1.67 (0.83)	2.87 (1.76)	1.70 (1.03)	2.02 (1.33)
C_{max} (μg/ml)	48.06 (4.42)	68.08 (5.57)	54.25 (5.26)	83.00 (8.69)
$AUC_{0-\infty}$ (μg/ml × h)	222.75 (15.15)	232.23 (39.29)	243.62 (16.43)	261.16 (40.41)

Note: FSD = SD/predicted concentration. All values are mean (± SD). All tabular values are mean (± SD).

[a] $k_a = 0.35/h$; $k_{10} = 0.2/h$; V = 1L; $k_{21} = 0.6/h$; $k_{12} = 0.5/h$.

[b] $k_a = 0.75/h$; $k_{10} = 0.2/h$; V = 1L; $k_{21} = 0.6/h$; $k_{12} = 0.5/h$.

From Jackson, A. J., *Biopharm. Drug Dispos.*, 8, 483, 1987. With permission of John Wiley & Sons.

Table 2–2 **The 90% confidence intervals for the parameters T_{max}, C_{max}, and $AUC_{0-\infty}$ for the simulated one-compartment linear Model**

	T_{max}		C_{max}		$AUC_{0-\infty}$	
FSD = 0.6						
md	(41.5	99.2)	(116.2	127.6)	(103.2	121.7)
sd	(24.6	67.6)	(125.2	147.7)	(85.6	106.0)
FSD = 0.2						
md	(72.0	131.1)	(107.4	118.3)	(105.5	113.2)
sd	(41.3	75.6)	(124.8	134.2)	(93.9	103.8)

The results are given for single- (sd) 50 mg and multiple-dose (md) 50 mg/6 h simulations with either 0.2 or 0.6 fractional standard deviation added to each concentration. From Jackson, A. J., *Biopharm. Drug Dispos.*, 8, 483, 1987. With permission of John Wiley & Sons.

2. The intrasubject variability decreases for most of the drugs as reflected by the lower standard error.
3. The difference between test and reference C_{max} values decreases for most drugs at steady state.

The $AUC_{0-\infty}$ values for erythromycin and procainamide in Table 2–6 exhibited a decrease in the standard error and in the 90% confidence interval ranges for multiple vs. single dosing. The other drugs displayed similar confidence interval ranges for single vs. multiple dosing with the upper and lower limits also comparable. This supports earlier findings using simulated data[25] which indicated a minimal change in $AUC_{0-\infty}$ confidence intervals for linear drugs when going from single to multiple dosing.

Based on both the data in Table 5 and the conclusions of the Generic Drug Advisory Committee, single-dose studies are predictive of the extent of absorption, since both single- and multiple-dose studies yielded comparable confidence intervals (CIs) for AUC. On the other hand, "the rate of absorption" as measured by the 90% CI for C_{max} is only properly determined from single-dose data, since accumulation of drug to steady state results in inappropriate measurement of this parameter.[26] The greater the accumulation ratio, the smaller the CI limits and ranges for a defined level of intrasubject variation in k_a during absorption. Thus, most multiple-dose studies meet the confidence interval criterion of 80 to 120% on the normal scale or 80 to 125% following log transformation for C_{max} even when the single-dose studies do not.[25,27] One author has suggested that the bioequivalence range of C_{max} be widened to 70 to 130% for some immediate-release products.[27] However, it was not clear whether this proposed change was to apply only to single-dose studies, as scientific rigor would require.

As shown above, only single-dose studies provide an accurate measurement of rate of absorption (i.e., using C_{max}) for immediate-release generic drug products; and it is recommended that the current bioequivalency regulations in the CFR be changed accordingly.

III. BIOEQUIVALENCY CONSIDERATIONS: DRUGS WITH NONLINEAR KINETICS

A recent review discussed the clinical implications of nonlinear kinetics.[13] Many of the drugs studied in the review article have been previously discussed in this chapter. The relationship between nonlinear kinetics and bioequivalency is primarily affected by rate of absorption, fraction absorbed, and intrinsic clearance. Figure 2–1 gives the results for some simulations using the models described therein. These data clearly point out that the

Table 2–3 **Summary of single-dose study characteristics for Erythromycin, Nifedipine, Procainamide, Metoclopromide, and Quinidine**[a]

	Erythromycin	Nifedipine	Procainamide	Metoclopramide	Quinidine I
Subjects	24	24	24	27	26
Dose	250-mg[b] Delayed release capsule	20-mg Capsule	500-mg[b] Sustained release (SR) tablet	10-mg Tablet	324-mg[b] SR tablet
Reference Drug	Eryc Parke-Davis	Procardia Pfizer	Procan Parke-Davis	Reglan A. H. Robins	Quinaglute Berlex
Assay-CV	11.6% at 0.6μg/ml	3.3% at 5.0 ng/ml	3.8% at 0.1 μg/ml	2.5% at 5.0 ng/ml	4.6% at 0.1 μg/ml
Linearity	0.15–1.09 μg/ml 0.78–3.0 μg/ml	5.0–400 ng/ml	0.1–5.0 μg/ml	2.0–100 ng/ml	0.1–4.0 μg/ml

[a] Analysis of unpublished bioequivalence data submitted to the Division of Bioequivalence, Food and Drug Administration.
[b] Single- and multiple-dose studies done with same lot of test drug.

Table 2–4 **Summary of Multiple-dose Study Characteristics for Erythromycin, Nifedipine, Procainamide, Metoclopromide, and Quinidine**[a]

	Erythromycin	Nifedipine	Procainamide	Metoclopramide	Quinidine I
Subjects[b]	24	22	20	26	19
Dose	250-mg[c] Enteric capsule q.i.d.	10-mg Capsule t.i.d.	500-mg[c] SR tablet q.i.d.	10-mg Tablet q.i.d.	324-mg[c] SR tablet t.i.d.
Reference	Eryc	Procardia	Procan	Reglan	Quinaglute
Drug	Parke-Davis	Pfizer	Parke-Davis	A. H. Robins	Berlex
Assay-CV	11.6% at 0.6μg/ml	7.7% at 5.0 ng/ml	6.2% at 0.05 μg/ml	17.6% at 2.0 ng/ml	6.6% at 0.2 μg/ml
Linearity	0.15–1.09 μg/ml 0.78–3.0 μg/ml	2.0–300 ng/ml	0.05–5.0 μg/ml	2.0–30 ng/ml 30–150 ng/ml	0.1–4.0 μg/ml

[a] Analysis of unpublished bioequivalence data submitted to the Division of Bioequivalence, Food and Drug Administration.
[b] Single- and multiple-dose studies were done in different subjects.
[c] Single- and multiple-dose studies done with same lot of test drug.

Table 2–5 **Single-dose (sd) and multiple-dose (md) Test (T) and reference (R) C_{max} values (±CV), standard error (SE), 90% confidence interval (CI), and range for the drugs in Table 2–4**

	C_{maxT}	C_{maxR}	Diff C_{max}	SE	90% CI	Range
Erythromycin						
sd	1.16 μg/ml (66.3)	1.08 μg/ml (62.0)	0.08	3.0	(88–126)	38
md	2.10 μg/ml (31.9)	1.98 μg/ml (37.8)	0.12	0.13	(94–117)	23
Metoclopramide						
sd	51.09 μg/ml (30.4)	50.47 μg/ml (28.3)	0.62	2.42	(93–109)	16
md	55.28 μg/ml (26.3)	53.12 μg/ml (26.6)	2.16	1.50	(99–108)	9
Nifedipine						
sd	139.00 μg/ml (69.0)	165.00 μg/ml (51.0)	26.00		(59–110)	51
md	87.77 μg/ml (39.6)	94.03 μg/ml (48.7)	7.33	9.33	(86–114)	28
Quinidine (SR)						
sd	1.48 μg/ml (38.3)	1.14 μg/ml (34.5)	0.35	0.09	(117–144)	27
md	2.44 μg/ml (29.3)	1.97 μg/ml (24.5)	0.47	0.12	(113–134)	21
Procainamide						
sd	1.20 μg/ml (19.2)	0.95 μg/ml (16.6)	0.25	0.05	(117–134)	17
md	2.07 μg/ml (17.9)	2.07 μg/ml (11.6)	0.00	0.05	(98–109)	11

Table 2–6 **Single-dose (sd) and multiple-dose (md) test (T) and reference (R) AUC values (±CV), standard error (SE), 90% confidence interval (CI), and range for the drugs in Table 2–4**

	AUC μg/ml × h T	AUC μg/ml × h R	Difference AUC	SE	90% CI	Range
Erythromycin						
sd	3.35 (47.7)	3.26 (51.9)	0.09	0.22	(91–114)	23
md	7.98 (36.7)	8.67 (43.6)	0.69	0.44	(83–100)	17
Metoclopramide						
sd	381.7 (34.8)	364.1 (34.5)	18.48	13.8	(98–111)	13
md	1,639.7 (33.1)	1,550.8 (31.2)	104.83	55.64	(100–112)	12
Nifedipine						
sd	327.0 (20.2)	359.0 (18.9)	30.56	18.26	(83–100)	17
md	192.9 (42.0)	194.1 (48.2)	0.32	6.78	(94–106)	12
Quinidine						
sd	17.3 (18.6)	14.5 (28.4)	2.82	0.96	(108–130)	22
md	18.6 (32.0)	17.0 (26.3)	1.61	0.94	(100–119)	19
Procainamide						
sd	9.1 (16.6)	9.0 (20.8)	0.1	0.26	(95–105)	10
md	10.23 (15.6)	10.24 (12.1)	0.01	0.21	(96–103)	7

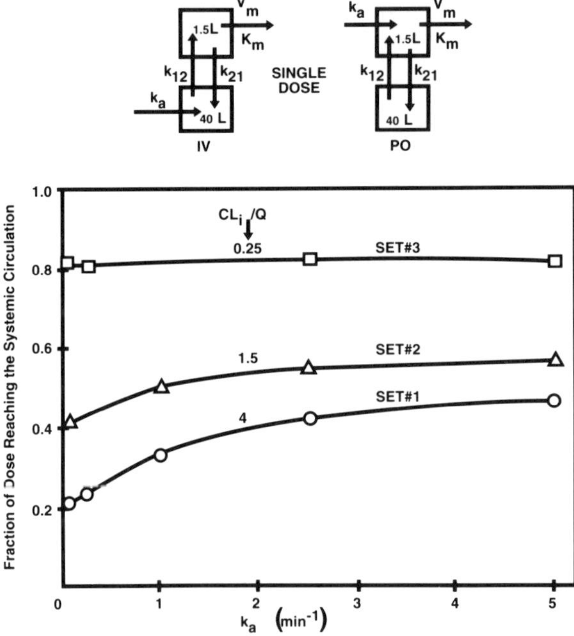

Figure 2–1 Plots of bioavailability vs. first-order input rate constant, k_a. Data were simulated by numerical integration using the models shown above the figure. (Redrawn from Wagner, J. G., Effect of first-pass Michaelis-Menten metabolism on performance of controlled release dosage forms, in *Oral Sustained Release Formulations: Design and Evaluation,* Pergamon Press, New York, 1988, 114. With permission of copyright holder McGraw-Hill.)

larger the ratio CL_i/Q (intrinsic clearance/blood flow), the larger the increase in AUC with increasing k_a.[28] However, the effect of k_a on the simulations in Figure 2–1 was minimal when CL_i/Q = 1.5 or less. The intercept on the graph origin indicates the minimum bioavailability for first-order conditions.

Phenytoin and propranolol, drugs with low and high CL_i/Q values, respectively, have been investigated using both simulated and experimental data to determine how their bioequivalency (CIs) are affected by changes in rate and extent of absorption of a formulation. For phenytoin C_{max}, multiple-dose studies produced narrower 90% CIs with higher upper and lower limits compared to single dose using either experimental or simulated data for multiple-dose studies (Tables 2–7 and 2–8).[29] For $AUC_{0\text{-}\infty}$, the confidence interval obtained from the simulated multiple-dose data was wider and its upper limit was higher compared to single dosing; while for the experimental data, only product "B" completely followed this pattern. This contrasts with the phenytoin C_{max}, where the experimental and simulated data were in total agreement. The phenytoin results, especially for C_{max}, with higher upper and lower limits, are different from those seen for linear drugs. Thus, these data demonstrate that only multiple-dose studies should be used to assess bioequivalency parameters for drugs such as phenytoin which exhibit saturable elimination within the therapeutic dosage range.

The observation that an increase in bioavailability occurs with an increase in k_a most often for drugs with larger CL_i/Q ratios poses an interesting question for immediate-release formulations at or above the level of saturation: Is the observed treatment mean difference in C_{max} following single-dose administration equal to that observed at steady state?[28] This was investigated by simulating data for a drug with a CL_i (Vm/Km) = 25 l/h, which clearly

Table 2–7 **The 90% confidence interval for the test vs. reference bioavailability parameters obtained from the simulation of a nonlinear model for phenytoin**

	T_{max}		C_{max}		$AUC_{0-\infty}$	
CV = 54%						
Nonlinear II						
sd	(105.8	139.1)	(81.8	98.6)	(99.4	100.0)
md	(103.1	155.4)	(88.7	101.1)	(93.1	102.8)

Note: The simulation was done with 54% coefficient of variation added to the respective k_a values for the test and reference.

From Jackson, A. J., *Biopharm. Drug Dispos.*, 10, 489, 1989. With permission of John Wiley & Sons.

Table 2–8 **Estimated 90% confidence intervals for T_{max}, C_{max}, and $AUC_{0-\infty}$ following the administration of phenytoin sodium capsules as either single or multiple dose in two different groups of subjects**

Dose	T_{max}		C_{max}		$AUC_{0-\infty}$	
Product A						
100 mg	(102.5	168.9)	(80.1	107.8)	(92.8	112.1)
300 mg/d	(84.0	149.9)	(97.8	112.8)	(100.0	113.1)
Product B						
100 mg	(68.0	179.5)	(72.4	98.8)	(90.4	104.1)
300 mg/d	(78.2	139.8)	(87.1	106.8)	(83.4	105.4)

Note: Data is presented for two formulations A and B and the intervals are expressed as the per cent difference between the test and reference means.

From Jackson, A. J., *Biopharm. Drug Dispos.*, 10, 489, 1989. With permission John Wiley & Sons.

showed nonlinear kinetics over the therapeutic range. Data were simulated using a modified first-pass model (first-order elimination from the central compartment and transfer to liver was faster than return to plasma) for oral (p.o.) input given in Figure 2–1. Parameters for the simulations were k_{12} = 0.4/h, k_{21} = 0.1/h, and k_{10} = 0.2/h. Following the calculation of the plasma curves corresponding to the respective k_a, V_{max}, and K_m values, 15% random assay error was added to each concentration value prior to the estimation of C_{max} and AUC. Parameter values for the model with their statistical variance are given in Table 2–9. Simulations 1, 2, and 3 were categorized according to the differences between their test and reference k_a values (20, 53, and 102%, respectively) as:

	Simulation 1	Simulation 2	Simulation 3
k_a test	0.42/h	0.537/h	0.707/h
k_a reference	0.35/h	0.35/h	0.35/h

The k_a values comprising the populations were generated from a bivariate normal distribution (correlation 0.60) with the reported mean k_a value and coefficient of variation of 50%. V_{max} and K_m values were also generated from a bivariate normal distribution with correla-

Table 2–9 **Mean C_{max}, % difference, standard error (SE), 90% confidence interval (CI) based on Log transformed data, and interval range**

Dose (μg)	Test (μg/ml)	Reference (μg/ml)	Difference %	SE	CI	Range
1,000 sd	122	115	6.0	0.036	(98–112)	13
1,000/8 h md	701	679	3.7	0.055	(93–112)	19
2,000 sd	254	247	2.8	0.038	(95–109)	13
2,000/8 h md	1,419	1,383	2.6	0.054	(93–111)	18
10,000 sd	1,299	1,252	3.7	0.036	(97–110)	13
10,000/8 h md	7,269	7,018	3.5	0.055	(93–112)	19

Note: Data simulated (simulation 1) with mean kat = 0.42/h, kar = 0.35/h (CV = 0.50 and correlation = 0.60), V_{max} = 5,000 μg/h (CV = 0.25), K_m = 0.2 μg/ml (CV = 0.25 with K_m and V_{max} correlation = 0.9).

tion 0.90 between the final estimates, and was assumed constant between treatment periods. The fraction absorbed was assumed to be 1.0 with simulated doses of 1,000, 2,000, and 10,000 μg. The multiple-dosing regimen specified dosing every 8 h. For each comparison 36 subjects were simulated. Results from the simulations are presented in Tables 2–9 to 2-14. Simulation 1 indicates linearity for C_{max} and $AUC_{0-\infty}$ between the 1000 and 2000 μg doses, and there was a good prediction of the multiple-dose confidence interval for C_{max} from the single dose at these doses. However, there was little agreement between single- and multiple-dose CIs for $AUC_{0-\infty}$ at any dosing level. This was apparently related to the increase in the standard error since the mean AUC values were smaller at steady state for the 10,000 μg/8 h dose. The decrease in the mean AUC values at steady state was related to the presence of the linear pathway in the model. Figure 2–2 is a plot of the fraction of the dose excreted (by linear and nonlinear pathways) vs. dose administered following single and multiple dosing. The data show that as the dose is increased, sd and/or md, a smaller fraction is eliminated via the nonlinear pathway compared to the linear pathway. Following multiple dosing, greater than 95% of elimination occurs via the linear pathway, indicating a linear relationship between the mean AUC values and dose (i.e., steady-state AUC values are equal to $AUC_{0-\infty}$). However, the presence of the nonlinear elimination pathway results in the standard error of the mean being larger following multiple dosing compared to single dosing, thus rendering the single-dose AUC confidence interval a poor predictor of the confidence interval at steady state (Table 2–10).

In simulation 2, mean C_{max} values were linear for doses between 1000 and 2000 μg for single and multiple dosing. Mean $AUC_{0-\infty}$ values were nonlinear for the single dose but linear for the multiple dose, reflecting the diminished contribution of nonlinear elimination at steady state. For both C_{max} and $AUC_{0-\infty}$, single-dose confidence intervals were poor predictors of the steady-state confidence intervals. This appeared to again result from an increase in the standard error in going from single to multiple dosing.

Simulation 3, with differences in mean k_a values of over 100%, again showed linearity at the two lower doses and nonlinearity at 10,000 μg. In contrast to simulations 1 and 2, the multiple-dose CI for C_{max} was not predicted by the single-dose data at any dose level. In fact, in all cases, the range for the C_{max} multiple-dose CI increased compared to that computed for the single dose as a result of increases in the standard errors and the higher reference mean values. A similar lack of predictability was observed for $AUC_{0-\infty}$ due to the greater differences observed between treatment means and increase in standard error in going from single to multiple dosing. Therefore, it appeared that single-dose data were able to accurately predict the steady-state CI for C_{max} only at the lowest dose administered in each case.

Table 2–10 **Mean AUC, % difference, standard error (SE), 90% confidence interval (CI) for log-transformed data, and confidence interval range for drug with same parameters given in Table 2–9**

Dose (μg)	Test (μg/ml × h)	Reference (μg/ml × h)	Difference %	SE	90% CI	Range
1,000 sd	3,360	3,328	0.96	0.013	(99–103)	4
1,000/8 h md	4,391	4,233	3.70	0.057	(93–113)	20
2,000 sd	7,950	7,914	0.45	0.011	(98–102)	4
2,000/8 h md	8,996	8,672	3.70	0.054	(94–112)	18
10,000 sd	46,989	47,045	0.12	0.013	(97–102)	5
10,000/8 h md	45,906	44,149	3.50	0.051	(112–131)	19

Table 2–11 **Mean C_{max}, % difference, standard error (SE), 90% confidence interval (CI), and interval range for drug with mean kat = 0.53/h (CV = 50% and correlation = 0.6) and with remaining parameters the same as in Table 2–9**

Dose (μg)	Test (μg/ml)	Reference (μg/ml)	Difference %	SE	CI	Range
1,000 sd	117	121	3.30	0.026	(93–101)	8
1,000/8 h md	693	685	1.10	0.074	(86–110)	24
2,000 sd	257	247	4.00	0.044	(96–111)	15
2,000/8 h md	1378	1396	1.30	0.068	(86–108)	22
8,000 sd	1255	1254	0.079	0.040	(92–105)	13
8,000/8 h md	7226	6959	3.800	0.066	(90–113)	23

Table 2–12 **Mean AUC, % difference, standard error (SE), 90% confidence interval (CI), and confidence interval range for the simulations from Table 2–11**

Dose (μg)	Test (μg/ml × h)	Reference (μg/ml × h)	Difference %	SE	90% CI	Range
1,000 sd	3,415	3,433	0.5	0.013	(97–101)	4
1,000/8 h md	4,277	4,240	0.9	0.066	(87–109)	22
2,000 sd	7,917	8,023	1.30	0.013	(94–100)	6
2,000/8 h md	8,712	8,705	0.08	0.065	(87–109)	21
10,000 sd	46,349	46,510	0.30	0.019	(96–103)	7
10,000/8 h md	44,571	41,128	5.20	0.098	(91–127)	36

The single-dose CI, however, did a poor job of predicting the steady-state $AUC_{0-\infty}$ CI. Even though the lower doses appeared to be linear, the results at the higher doses were unpredictable. The reasons for this lack of agreement appear to be related to the changes observed both in the standard errors and in the proximity of means following single vs. multiple dosing. In addition, the presence of the linear pathway did not significantly improve the capability of predicting steady-state behavior of the bioequivalence parameters from single-dose data. These problems merit further investigation using both experimental and simulated data.

Data obtained from the administration of single and multiple doses of immediate- and controlled-release propranolol to normal individuals also raise concerns as to the usefulness of single-dose (sd) data in predicting steady-state multiple-dose (md) relationships.

Table 2–13 **Mean C_{max}, % difference, standard error (SE), 90% confidence interval (CI), and interval range for drug with mean kat = 0.70/h (CV = 50% and correlation = 0.6) and with remaining parameters the same as in Table 2–9**

Dose (mg)	Test (μg/ml)	Reference (μg/ml)	Difference %	SE	CI	Range
1,000 sd	119	107	11.2	0.076	(97–125)	28
1,000/8 h md	668	640	4.3	0.114	(87–129)	42
2,000 sd	247	230	7.4	0.070	(95–120)	25
2,000/8 h md	1375	1282	7.2	0.099	(93–130)	37
8,000 sd	1252	1172	6.8	0.056	(98–119)	21
8,000/8 h md	7414	6974	6.3	0.097	(99–117)	35

Table 2–14 **Mean AUC, % difference, standard error (SE), 90% confidence interval (CI), and confidence interval range for the simulations from Table 2–13**

Dose (mg)	Test (μg/ml × h)	Reference (μg/ml × h)	Difference %	SE	90% CI	Range
1,000 sd	3,295	3,124	5.4	0.051	(97–115)	18
1,000/8 h md	4,214	3,950	6.6	0.114	(90–131)	41
2,000 sd	7,616	7,610	0.08	0.039	(93–106)	13
2,000/8 h md	8,469	7,962	6.30	0.099	(92–129)	37
8,000 sd	46,349	46,510	0.30	0.019	(96–103)	7
8,000/8 h md	43,294	41,128	5.20	0.098	(91–127)	36

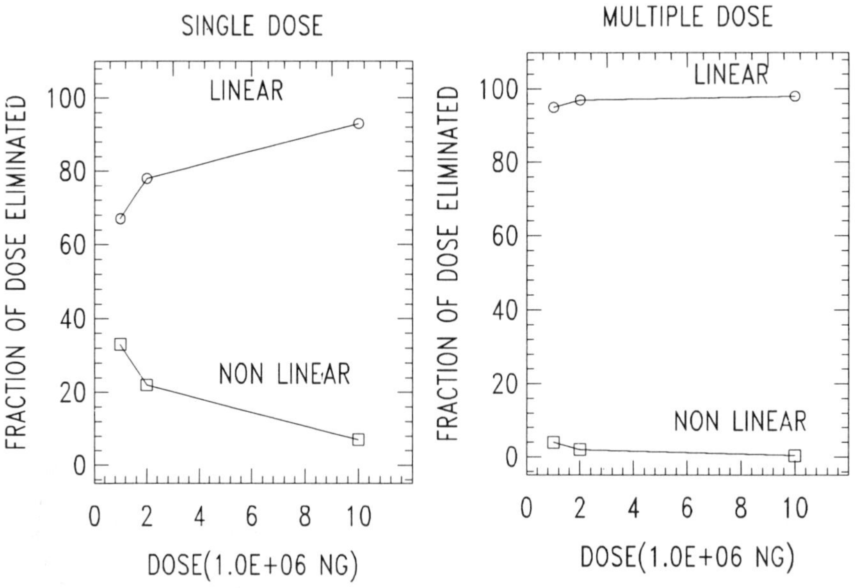

Figure 2–2 Plot of the fraction of the dose excreted via the linear and nonlinear pathways as a function of dose following single- and multiple-dose administration based on the modified (i.e., linear elimination from the central compartment) first-pass model in Figure 1.

The studies below were done on several different propranolol products with the immediate-release formulation administered as a single 80-mg tablet. The multiple doses were either 2 × 40-mg tablets or 4 × 20-mg tablets given every 8 h. Study details were as follows:

	Controlled release		**Immediate release**		
	sd	**md**	**sd**	**md-1**	**md-2**
Subjects	24	28	18	24	36
Assay % CV	9.6% (interday)		11% (interday)		
Linear range	0.5–200 ng/ml		1.0–200 ng/ml		

Results from the studies presented in Tables 2–15 and 2–16 for C_{max} and $AUC_{0\text{-}\infty}$, respectively, show a decrease in the range of the CI limits for C_{max} and AUC in going from single to multiple dosing. This observed decrease was apparently due to the smaller difference between the observed means at steady state since the standard error actually increased in the multiple-dose studies. Therefore, at the dosage levels for propranolol (which has a reported CL_i = 444 l/h[16]) used in these studies the multiple-dose CIs were also not well predicted by the single-dose data. In contrast to the simulated study data, the experimental data which had a higher CL_i appeared to behave in an almost linear fashion within the therapeutic range investigated. Had the study been performed on the 90-mg propranolol strength, perhaps more of the potential for nonlinearity would have been evident.

Differences between the single- and multiple-dose study results used to estimate the bioequivalence of phenytoin, a nonlinear drug that does not exhibit a first-pass effect, were also observed (Table 2–7). Details of the phenytoin study were as follows:

	sd	**md**
Dose	100 mg	300 mg/d (28 d)
Subjects	16	12
Assay CV	5.8% (interday)	5.8% (interday)
Linear range	0.2–2.5 μg/ml	0.2–2.5 μg/ml

Larger differences were observed between the test and reference mean values and standard errors for the single-dose data than for the multiple-dose data, a pattern previously observed with the simulated data for phenytoin.[29]

IV. CONTROLLED-RELEASE FORMULATIONS

Single- and multiple-dose studies play a major role not only in the determination of bioequivalency for controlled-release products, but also in the evaluation of their pharmacokinetic characteristics. Single-dose studies performed on controlled-release products have been used mainly to evaluate dose dumping rather than to predict steady-state performance, since the degree to which multiple-dose performance can be predicted from single-dose data (even for a drug with linear kinetics) depends on the level of drug accumulation which occurs.[26] Treatment differences observed following a single dose may be at variance with those observed at steady state. For example, Phyllocontin® and Theo-Dur® — sustained-release theophylline products — differed 40% in mean plasma C_{max} following a single dose, but exhibited only a 10% difference at steady state.[31]

Table 2–15 **Mean C_{max}; difference in C_{max}; standard error (SE); 90% confidence interval (CI); and range for Propranolol (sustained release), Propranolol (immediate release), and Dilantin**

Dose (mg)	Test (μg/ml)	Reference (μg/ml)	Difference	SE	90% CI	Range
Propranolol						
SR 160 sd	23.7	23.7	0	0.036	(87–117)	30
SR 160/d md	44.7	41.6	2.49	2.60	(96–117)	21
IR 80 sd	68.6	60.1	8.50	6.58	(96–132)	37
IR 4 × 20/8 h md	153	169	16.0	9.8	(81–100)	19
IR 2 × 40/8 h md	150	145	5.0	12.51	(89–118)	29
Phenytoin						
IR 100 sd	1.25	1.29	0.04	0.08	(85–107)	22
IR 100/8 h md	10.2	9.49	3.9	0.4	(98–114)	16

Table 2–16 **Mean AUC; difference in AUC; standard error (SE); 90% confidence interval (CI); and range for Propranolol (sustained release), Propranolol (immediate release), and Dilantin**

Dose (mg)	Test (μg/ml × h)	Reference (μg/ml × h)	Difference	SE	90% CI	Range
Propranolol						
SR 160 sd	522.8	596.9	74.04	0.043	(85–121)	36
SR 160/d md	662.7	642.0	18.50	37.07	(96–112)	16
IR 80 sd	391	383	8.00	28.45	(87–114)	27
IR 4 × 20/8 h md	733	783	50.0	41.18	(85–102)	17
IR 2 × 40/8 h md	682.2	682.6	0.43	48.3	(88–112)	24
Phenytoin						
IR 100 sd	37.0	36.1	0.9	2.1	(92–112)	20
IR 100/8 h md	191.7	193.4	1.62	8.66	(91–107)	16

Several studies on controlled-release indomethacin, 75-mg capsule, further illustrate the difficulties in predicting multiple-dose performance from single-dose data for controlled-release products.[32] A summary of the confidence interval data for two such studies follows:

	sd		md	
	AUC	C_{max}	AUC	C_{max}
Study 1	88–98	69–93	91–100	80–98
Study 2	93–106	79–96	95–104	75–97

In both studies the AUC sd confidence intervals closely matched those obtained at steady state; whereas for C_{max}, this was less true, especially in study 1 where the single dose indicated that the test was absorbed much slower than the reference. However, following multiple dosing the test rate of absorption (C_{max}) is much closer to that for the reference.[25] In study 2, the range increased somewhat from single to multiple dosing. These data clearly show that only multiple-dose studies can adequately evaluate the bioequivalence of controlled-release drug products, since prediction of steady-state performance from single-dose data is not always reliable. Another complicating factor which precludes the exclusive use of single-dose data is that most generic controlled-release products do not have the same formulation, and they may not always provide an absolutely constant release rate. Furthermore, these products contain more drug per dose than the comparable immediate-release formulation does, which raises concerns related to subject safety such as dose-dumping.

Also of concern are the CFR guidelines for the evaluation of controlled-release products *in vivo*.[30] According to 21 CFR 320.25, "The purpose of an *in vivo* bioavailability study involving a drug product for which a controlled-release claim is made is to determine if all of the following conditions are met:

1. The drug product meets the controlled-release claims made for it.
2. The bioavailability profile established for the drug product rules out the occurrence of any dose-dumping.
3. The drug product's steady-state performance is equivalent to that of a currently marketed non-controlled-release or controlled-release drug product that contains the same active drug ingredient and that is subject to a full new drug application."

Conditions 1 and 3 are normally evaluated by doing head-to-head single- and multiple-dose bioequivalence studies comparing the candidate dosage form with the marketed standard. Current methods for accomplishing the second objective are not as well defined. The head-to-head studies used to determine bioequivalence are inadequate for making quantitative comparisons of dose-dumping. It has been proposed that dose-dumping be investigated by comparing the AUC values of the generic controlled-release formulation to a marketed immediate-release dosage form following single-dose administration.[33] Though at best this comparison is only qualitative, in practice this approach appears to work, with the steady-state study being pivitol by verifying that the proper blood levels are maintained by the test controlled-release dosage form.

Using the multiple-dose study to estimate equivalence instead of product performance (i.e., dose-dumping) presents some of the same difficulties encountered above in the use of md C_{max} values to estimate the rate of absorption of immediate-release products (i.e., loss of sensitivity of the parameter due to the effects of drug accumulation). Even though C_{max} does not provide a sensitive measure of absorption rate for CR products, it does indicate whether the product has attained a desirable maximum concentration.

A rigorous use of single-dose studies would allow a more quantitative examination of both the drug absorption rate and of dose-dumping in controlled-release products, especially those that exhibit a significant level of drug accumulation (e.g., accumulation ratio of 1.2 or greater).[26] Perhaps controlled-release generic formulations need to be compared to the approved immediate-release reference product only if there is evidence of dose-dumping (area above C_{max} which is outside the desirable effective range) from a previous head-to-head biostudy conducted between the test and reference controlled-release dosage forms. From the previous arguments it must be concluded that more emphasis should be placed on the single-dose study in evaluating absorption rate, since multiple-dose C_{max} values can be influenced by the degree of drug accumulation. Multiple-dose studies should be used primarily to measure product performance in attaining and maintaining therapeutic plasma levels.

ACKNOWLEDGMENT

The author would like to acknowledge the help of Dr. Shriniwas V. Nerurkar in the analysis of the simulation data, and the many helpful suggestions of Larry A. Ouderkirk in the preparation of this chapter.

REFERENCES

1. **Gibaldi, M. and Perrier, D.,** One-compartment model, in *Pharmacokinetics,* Swarbrick, J., Ed., Marcel Dekker, New York, 1975, 1.
2. **Zhi, J.,** Initial slope technique to estimate first- and zero-order drug absorption rate constants, *J. Pharm. Sci.,* 77, 816, 1988.
3. **Rowland, M., Benet, L. Z., and Reigelman, S.,** Two-compartment model for a drug and its metabolite: application to acetylsalicylic acid pharmacokinetics, *J. Pharm. Sci.,* 59, 364, 1970.
4. **Wagner, J.,** Linear pharmacokinetic equations allowing direct calculation of many needed pharmacokinetic parameters from the coefficients and exponents of polyexponential equations that have been fitted to the data, *J. Pharmacokinet. Biopharm.,* 4, 443, 1976.
5. **Segre, G.,** The sojurn time and its prospective use in pharmacology, *J. Pharmacokinet. Biopharm.,* 16, 657, 1988.
6. **Wagner, J.,** Types of mean residence times, *Biopharm. Drug Dispos.,* 9, 41, 1988.
7. **Cheng, H. and Jusko, W. J.,** Mean residence time concepts for pharmacokinetic systems with nonlinear drug elimination described by the Michaelis-Menten equation, *Pharm. Res.,* 5, 156, 1988.
8. **Wagner, J. G.,** Dosage regimen calculations, in *Fundamentals of Clinical Pharmacokinetics,* Wagner, J. G., Ed., Drug Intelligence Publications, Hamilton, IL, 1975, 129.
9. **Cheng, H. and Jusko, W. J.,** An area function method for calculating the apparent elimination rate constant of a metabolite, *J. Pharmacokinet. Biopharm.,* 17, 125, 1989.
10. **Rowland, M. and Tozer, T. N.,** Therapeutic response and toxicity, in *Clinical Pharmacokinetics Concepts and Applications,* Rowland, M. and Tozer, T. N., Eds., Lea & Febiger, Philadelphia, 1980, 155.
11. **Jusko, W. J.,** Guidelines for collection and analysis of pharmacokinetic data, in *Applied Pharmacokinetics,* 2nd ed., Evans, W. E., Schentag, J. J., and Jusko, W. J., Eds., Applied Therapeutics, Spokane, WA, 1986, 9.
12. **Devane, C. L. and Jusko, W. J.,** Drug and metabolite concentrations combined in predicting steady-state concentrations from test doses, *Biopharm. Drug Dispos.,* 4, 19, 1983.
13. **Ludden, T. M.,** Nonlinear pharmacokinetics: clinical implications, *Clin. Pharmacokinet.,* 20, 429, 1991.
14. **Sawchuk, R. J. and Rector, T. S.,** Steady-state plasma concentrations as a function of the absorption rate and dosing interval for drugs exhibiting concentration-dependent clearance: consequences for phenytoin therapy, *J. Pharmacokinet. Biopharm.,* 7, 543, 1979.
15. **Levy, G. and Tsuchiya, T.,** Salicylate accumulation kinetics in man, *N. Engl. J. Med.,* 287, 430, 1972.
16. **Wagner, J. G.,** Modeling first-pass metabolism, in *Pharmacokinetics: Mathematical and Statistical Approaches to Metabolism and Distribution of Chemicals and Drugs,* Vol. 145, Pecile, A. and Rescigno, A., Eds., Plenum Press, New York, 1987, 129.
17. **Graves, D. A.,** Failure of single-dose kinetics to predict steady state, *Drug Intell. Clin. Pharm.,* 22, 917, 1988.
18. Bioavailability and Bioequivalence Requirements, 21 Code of Federal Regulations, 320.1(e), 139, 1991.
19. Guidance for Conducting an *in vivo* Bioequivalence Study on Haloperidol, Division of Bioequivalence, Food and Drug Administration, 1987.
20. Report by the Bioequivalence Task Force, Bioequivalence Hearing Conducted By Food and Drug Administration (1986), 18, Washington, D.C., 1988.

21. Division of Bioequivalence, Generic Drug Advisory Committee Meeting, Washington, D. C., September 26–27, 1992.
22. Guidelines on the Design of a Multiple-Dose *in vivo* Bioavailability Study, 21 Code of Federal Regulations, 320.27(a)3, 148, 1991.
23. **Schuirmann, D. J.,** A comparison of the two one-sided tests procedure and the power approach for assessing the equivalence of average bioavailability, *J. Pharmacokinet. Biopharm.,* 15, 657, 1987.
24. **Tozer, T. N.,** Personal communication, Generic Drug Advisory Committee Meeting, Washington, D.C., September 26–27, 1992.
25. **Jackson, A. J.,** Prediction of steady-state bioequivalence relationships using single dose data I-linear kinetics, *Biopharm. Drug Dispos.,* 8, 483, 1987.
26. **Tahtawy, A., Jackson, A. J., and Ludden T.,** American Association of Clinical Pharmacology and Therapeutics, (Abstr.), Hawaii, March 1993.
27. **Steinijans, V. W., Sauter, R., Jonkman, H. G., Schulz, H. U., Stricker, H., and Blume, H.,** Bioequivalence studies: single vs. multiple dose, *Clin. Pharmacol. Ther. Toxicol.,* 27, 261, 1989.
28. **Wagner, J. G.,** Effect of first-pass Michaelis-Menten metabolism on performance of controlled release dosage forms, in *Oral Sustained Release Formulations: Design and Evaluation,* Yacobi, A., Ed., Pergamon Press, New York, 1988, 95.
29. **Jackson, A. J.,** Prediction of steady-state bioequivalence relationships using single dose data II-nonlinear kinetics, *Biopharm. Drug Dispos.,* 10, 489, 1989.
30. Guidelines for the Conduct of an *in vivo* Bioavailability Study, 21 Code of Federal Regulations, 320.25, f, (i, ii, iii), 146, 1991.
31. **Mucklow, J. C. and Kuhn, S.,** The rise and fall of serum theophylline concentration: a comparison of sustained-release formulations in volunteers with rapid theophylline clearance, *Br. J. Clin. Pharmacol.,* 20, 589, 1985.
32. Indomethacin Controlled-Release Products, Bioequivalence studies submitted to Division of Bioequivalence, Summary of study details available through Freedom of Information, Division of Bioequivalence, Rockville, MD, 1989–1992.
33. **Vallner, J. J., Honigberg, I. L., Kotzan, J. A., and Stewart, J. T.,** A proposed general protocol for testing bioequivalence of controlled-release drug products, *Int. J. Pharm.,* 16, 47, 1983.

Chapter 3

Role of Metabolites in Bioequivalency Assessment

Mei-Ling Chen and Andre J. Jackson

CONTENTS

I. INTRODUCTION

Metabolism of xenobiotics is essential for detoxification and removal of foreign substances from the body. In general, the defensive mechanisms are to convert the xenobiotic into one or more polar compounds so that the metabolites can readily be eliminated from the body. Similarly, drug metabolism is traditionally viewed as the metabolic processes which inactivate the therapeutic moiety and results in the degradation product(s) that possess little pharmacological activity relative to the parent drug. This concept of drug metabolites as inert substances derived from the parent compounds may be true in some cases. In other cases, however, many drugs have been found to give rise to their metabolite(s) exhibiting various degrees of therapeutic activity or different types of adverse reactions.[1-4]

The importance of metabolites in new drug development cannot be overemphasized. In order to maximize the desired effects of a drug while minimizing its untoward effects in the patient population, a thorough understanding of pharmacokinetics/dynamics of the drug and its metabolites is required for rational drug development and proper dosing. Despite this, questions have been raised as to the role of metabolites in bioequivalence determinations.[5-8] The contention lies in the fact that evaluation of bioequivalence between formulations addresses different issues than the development of new drugs. While the goal of drug development necessitates the documentation of safety and efficacy data, bioequivalence determinations assess the equivalency of formulations with the same chemical entity that has previously been demonstrated to be both safe and effective. This review is aimed at examining the genuine role of metabolites in bioequivalence evaluations.

II. CONCEPTS OF BIOEQUIVALENCE

A. REGULATORY REQUIREMENTS OF BIOEQUIVALENCE

The Federal Food, Drug, and Cosmetic Act of 1984 establishes that evaluation of bioequivalence between formulations be made on the basis of the rate and extent of drug absorption.[9] In this context, bioequivalence refers to the comparison of bioavailabilities of different products which stems from the assumption that the level of drug circulating in the blood predicts the clinical efficacy of the drug product.

To demonstrate bioequivalence of formulations, sponsors are usually required to conduct an *in vivo* randomized, crossover study in which the test and reference formulations are administered to a small population (typically 20 to 30 normal human subjects).[10,11] The concentration-time profiles of the drug and/or metabolite(s) in biological fluid, such as blood or urine, are constructed following drug administration. The rate and extent of drug absorption are then estimated by the pharmacokinetic parameters derived from the profiles of the subjects. The extent of absorption is usually represented by the area under the serum/plasma concentration-time curve from time zero to infinity ($AUC_{0-\infty}$). While the metric(s) used for the rate of absorption in bioequivalence determination has long been subject to criticism, it is currently expressed by peak concentration (C_{max}) and time to reach the peak (T_{max}) obtained from the serum/plasma profiles.[6,12-16]

B. BIOEQUIVALENCE CRITERIA

The current statistical methodology used by the Food and Drug Administration (FDA) for assessment of bioequivalence involves the use of a two one-sided tests procedure to determine the comparability of the average values of pharmacokinetic parameters measured after the administration of the test and reference products.[17] This procedure entails the calculation of a confidence interval for the ratio (or difference) between the test and reference average. The confidence intervals are constructed at the $\alpha = 0.05$ level of significance.

For years, the FDA has adopted a range of ±20% as the standard equivalence criterion for the relative difference between the averages of the test and reference product.[18] However, it is noted that the Office of Generic Drugs (OGD) in the FDA has recently recommended logarithmic transformation for AUC and C_{max}. The rationale for using log-transformed data in the evaluation of bioequivalence has been discussed in the FDA guidance.[19] Meanwhile, in line with this change, an equivalence criterion of 80 to 125% has been adopted for approval of generic drugs.[19]

III. USE OF METABOLITES IN BIOEQUIVALENCE ASSESSMENT

Conceivably, there are two possible purposes for which metabolite data may be employed for evaluation of bioequivalence. One reason for the need of metabolite level data is when the parent drug has a relatively short half-life and/or the parent drug levels are too low to be measured. In this case, analysis of the parent drug is limited or precluded, and thus bioequivalence evaluation would have to rely on the metabolite data. The other reason for using metabolite data rests on the basis that the metabolite is the additional or sole source for therapeutic or pharmacological activity. For the former case, irrespective of whether the metabolite under consideration has pharmacological activity or not, it will serve as the surrogate marker for the parent drug to assess pharmaceutical quality of the formulation.

Allopurinol, a hypouricemic agent prescribed in gout, provides a good example for the combined purposes as mentioned above. Serum half-lives of allopurinol and its metabolite, oxipurinol, were reported as 39 ± 11 min and 13.6 ± 2.8 h after the i.v. administration of 300 mg of allopurinol.[20] The serum concentrations of allopurinol fell so rapidly that within 6 h of dosing, allopurinol levels were generally below the sensitivity of the assay. In contrast, oxipurinol (the metabolite of allopurinol), also effective in diminishing production of uric acid, has a relatively long half-life compared to the parent drug.[21,22] In this case, the measurement of the active metabolite which exists in high concentrations certainly facilitates understanding of the therapeutic effects of the drug.

The question of whether metabolite data can be used to predict bioequivalence of formulations needs to be addressed from both pharmacokinetic and pharmacodynamic standpoints.

A. PHARMACOKINETIC CONSIDERATIONS[23-25]

Literally, establishment of bioequivalence relies on the comparison of the rate and extent of drug absorption between the test and reference formulations. Since the parent drug is the species absorbed into the body, it is contended that the parent drug should be of particular concern in bioequivalence assessment.[5] While metabolite information can aid in the evaluation of bioequivalence, the formation of metabolite(s) is, in many cases, a sequence secondary to the absorption of the parent drug.[7] Hence, it is speculated that the appearance of metabolite(s) in the blood, in most cases, would be so remote from the absorption process of the parent drug that metabolite data would not be useful for distinguishing small differences existing, if any, between formulations in the bioequivalence arena.

On the other hand, the use of metabolite data has been advocated in bioequivalence determinations for the following reasons. The appearance of metabolites in the blood generally reflects the absorption pattern exhibited by the parent drug, inasmuch as the metabolites are the derivatives of the parent compound. For instance, if the parent drug of formulation A is absorbed faster relative to formulation B, the appearance of the metabolite from formulation A would be earlier than formulation B within the same individual, and vice versa. Hence, metabolite data would provide similar information as with its parent drug regarding bioequivalence of the formulations.

Theoretical considerations are given below to examine the predictability of metabolite(s) for parent drug in the assessment of bioequivalence.

1. Rate of Absorption

Chen and Jackson[7,26] have studied the effect of pharmacokinetic models of metabolites on the equivalence determination of rate of drug absorption for conventional or immediate-release dosage forms. Using the current estimates (i.e., C_{max} and T_{max}) for rate of absorption, the authors conducted a series of simulations for drugs with linear pharmacokinetics. The simulations apply to primary metabolites arising from metabolizing organs or first-pass metabolism. It is assumed that the metabolites formed by first-pass metabolism will not be subject to sequential elimination within the first-pass tissue. Moreover, luminal metabolism is considered as a first-pass effect; and thus metabolites formed in the gut lumen are available for absorption. The following sections summarize the authors' findings according to the characteristics of drugs.

a. Linear Kinetics Without First-Pass Effect

The metabolite models (Figure 3–1) used in the simulations described the formation of a single metabolite with the elimination of metabolite being rate-limited by its formation in the body (FRL) or by its excretion from the systemic circulation (ERL).[23] Interestingly, results of the simulation indicated that bioequivalence determination using C_{max} of the parent drug and metabolite was independent of metabolite models, as evaluated by the confidence interval approach. In other words, metabolite kinetics have no bearing on the equivalence determination with respect to the rate of absorption between formulations.

Chen and Jackson[7] further explored the influence of formulation, subject, and assay variability on the performance of the parent drug and metabolite.[7] Simulation results

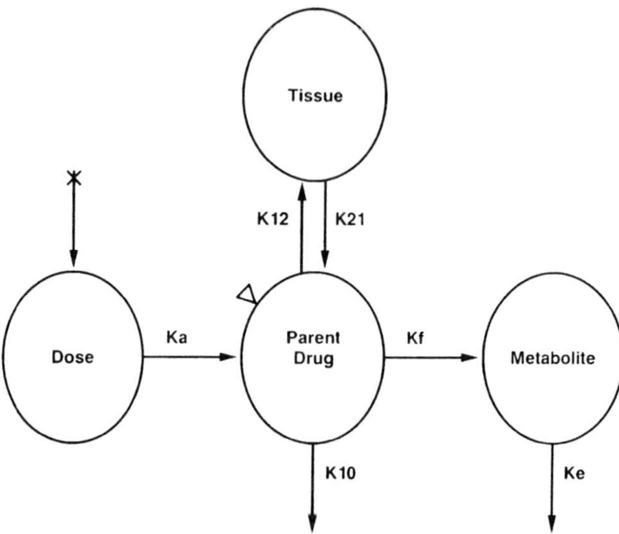

Figure 3–1 Compartmental metabolite model used for simulation of drugs exhibiting linear kinetics without first-pass effect, where k_a = first-order absorption rate constant, k_{12} and k_{21} = intercompartment transfer constants, k_{10} = first-order elimination rate constant for parent drug from central compartment, k_f = formation rate constant of metabolite, and k_e = first-order elimination rate constant for metabolite. (From Chen, M. L. and Jackson, A. J., *Pharm. Res.,* 8, 25, 1991. With permission of Plenum Publishing.)

revealed a consistently wider confidence interval for C_{max} of the parent drug relative to metabolite, irrespective of the metabolite models or error structure specified in the simulations. Accompanied with this decrease in the confidence limits of C_{max} from the parent drug to metabolite was a reduction of residual error (or the so-called "intrasubject variability") estimated from the analysis of variance. Perusal of the real data from bioequivalence studies on these drugs has been found to substantiate the simulated results (Table 3–1).[7]

The authors attributed the above findings to the differences in the origin of variability for C_{max} of the parent drug and metabolite. From the pharmacokinetic point of view, regardless of metabolite kinetics, assuming a one-compartment model the peak concentration of a drug and its metabolite can be described simply by the following two equations:

$$C_{max}(p) = \frac{k_a FD}{V(k_a - k)}\left(e^{-k.t\max(p)} - e^{-ka.t\max(p)}\right) \qquad \textbf{(3–1)}$$

$$C_{max}(m) = A.e^{-k.t\max(m)} + B.e^{-ke.t\max(m)} - C.e^{-ka.t\max(m)} \qquad \textbf{(3–2)}$$

where $C_{max}(p)$ and $C_{max}(m)$ are the peak concentration of the parent drug and metabolite, respectively; $t_{max(p)}$ and $t_{max(m)}$ are the corresponding peak time for parent drug and metabolite; F is the fraction of the administered dose D that is absorbed following oral administration; V is the volume of distribution of parent drug; k is the elimination rate constant of parent drug; k_e is the elimination rate constant of metabolite; and A, B, and C are coefficients representing functions of the various rate constants and fractions formed from the parent drug that are systemically available.

Table 3–1 **Summary data of bioequivalence studies on C_{max} parameter for drugs following linear kinetics and without first-pass effect**

Parent drug/ metabolite	Dose	Subject no.	Mean C_{max}(μg/ml) Reference	Test	Intrasubject variability[a]	90% CI[b]	CI width
Acetohexamide	500 mg	24	36.66	34.19	0.237	(81, 105)	24
Hydroxyhexamide		24	24.41	24.93	0.131	(95, 108)	13
Allopurinol	300 mg	20	1.57	1.70	0.319	(91, 126)	35
Oxypurinol		20	5.90	5.80	0.068	(95, 102)	7
Procainamide	500 mg	22	2.84	2.97	0.133	(98, 111)	13
N-acetylprocainamide		22	0.93	0.93	0.09	(96, 105)	9

[a] Intrasubject variability is expressed by the root mean square of the error term divided by the reference mean.

[b] Confidence interval (CI) is expressed as the percentage of the reference mean.

From Chen, M. L. and Jackson, A. J., *Pharm. Res.*, 8, 25, 1991. With permission of Plenum Publishing.

According to Equations 3–1 and 3–2, the variance of C_{max} for the parent drug originates from k_a and k; and that for metabolite derives from k, k_e, and k_a. In the case of an immediate-release dosage form, k_a is probably significantly larger than k or k_e. Under such conditions, the last term $C.e^{-ka.tmax(m)}$ in Equation 3–2 is relatively small compared with the preceding two terms, $A.e^{-k.tmax(m)}$ or $B.e^{-ke.tmax(m)}$; and hence the contribution of k_a to the overall variability of metabolite C_{max} becomes negligible.

Similarly, for a drug exhibiting two-compartment model (Figure 3–1), the following equations describe the peak concentration for the parent drug and its metabolite:

$$C_{max}(p) = \frac{k_a FD(k_{21} - k_a)}{V(\alpha - k_a)(\beta - k_a)} e^{-ka.t\,max(p)} + \frac{k_a FD(k_{21} - \alpha)}{V(k_a - \alpha)(\beta - \alpha)} e^{-\alpha.t\,max(p)} + \frac{k_a FD(k_{21} - \beta)}{V(k_a - \beta)(\alpha - \beta)} e^{-\beta.t\,max(p)} \quad \textbf{(3–3)}$$

$$C_{max}(m) = A'e^{-\lambda 1.t\,max(m)} + B'e^{-\lambda 2.t\,max(m)} + C'e^{-\lambda 3.t\,max(m)} + D'e^{-ka.t\,max(m)} \quad \textbf{(3–4)}$$

where $\alpha + \beta = k_{12} + k_{21} + k_{10}$, $\alpha\beta = k_{21}k_{10}$; $\lambda_1 + \lambda_2 + \lambda_3 = k_f + k_{10} + k_{12} + k_{21} + k_e$, $\lambda_1\lambda_2 + \lambda_2\lambda_3 + \lambda_1\lambda_3 = k_{21}(k_f + k_{10} + k_{12}) + k_e(k_f + k_{10} + k_{12}) + k_{21}k_e - k_{21}^2$, $\lambda_1\lambda_2\lambda_3 = k_{21}k_e(k_f + k_{10} + k_{12} - k_{21})$; and A′, B′, C′, and D′ are coefficients representing functions of the various rate constants and fractions formed from parent drug that are systemically available. For immediate release drug products, it can be readily demonstrated that $k_a > \alpha > \beta$ and $k_a > \lambda_1 > \lambda_2 > \lambda_3$. Hence, while the variance of C_{max} for the parent drug resides in k_a, α, and β, the variance of C_{max} for metabolite mainly comes from λ_1, λ_2, and λ_3, rather than k_a.

The above hypothesis is further supported by the data from an *in vivo* bioequivalence study on procainamide HCl capsules (Figures 3–2 and 3–3). An estimation of relative magnitudes of residual error for the three rate constants, k_a, k_e, and k_f (formation rate constant of metabolite), obtained from the fitted data in the study showed a much greater intrasubject variability for k_a relative to k_f and k_e (Table 3–2). It appears that a significantly higher variability results for C_{max} of the parent drug than for the metabolite due to the dominance of k_a in its estimation.

Chen and Jackson[7] concluded that the C_{max} of the metabolite fails to predict the potential variability in k_a and thus cannot be used to differentiate the input rate of drugs that follow linear kinetics and without first-pass effect.[7] In order to reach an informed conclusion with respect to bioequivalence for this class of drugs, therefore, it is imperative that parent drug data be employed for evaluation whenever possible.

b. Linear Kinetics with First-Pass Effect

Simulations conducted for drugs exhibiting linear kinetics with first-pass effect employed triamterene as a model drug (Figure 3–4).[26,27] Since preliminary results had demonstrated the independence of metabolite models (FRL vs. ERL) on the absorption rate of parent drugs, simulations thereafter were mainly focused on the error structure in the model.

Varying magnitudes of random errors were assigned to the relevant parameters in the model — including rate constants k_a, k_s, k_f, k_{10} and k_e — with the only assumption that the intrasubject variability of k_a is always larger than or comparable to the rest of the rate constants. The intersubject coefficients of variation (CVs) for various rate constants

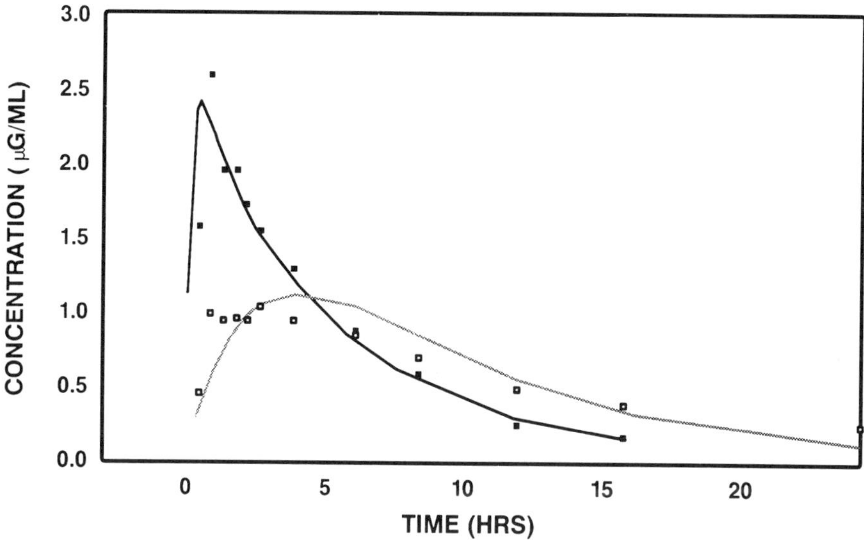

Figure 3–2 Mean plasma concentrations of procainamide (■) and its metabolite, *N*-acetylprocainamide (□), in subject 16 following a single 500-mg Pronestyl capsule. (From Chen, M. L. and Jackson, A. J., *Pharm. Res.*, 8, 25, 1991. With permission of Plenum Publishing.)

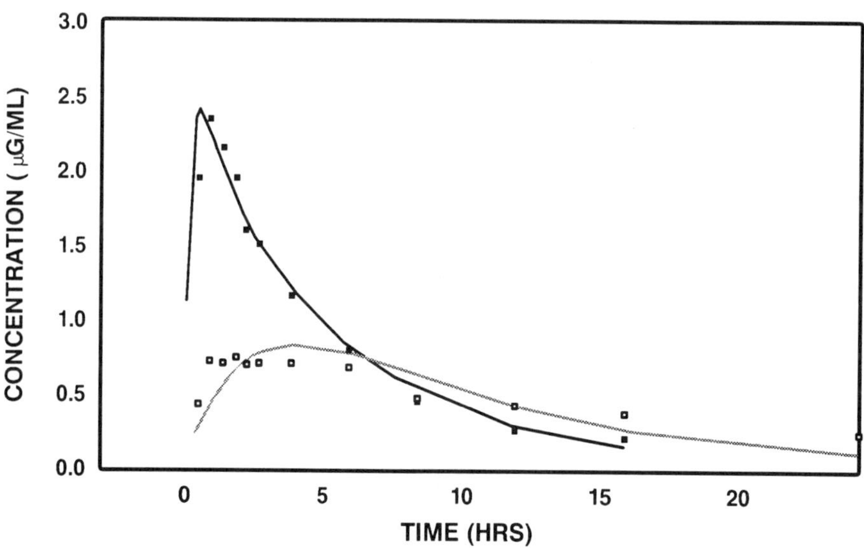

Figure 3–3 Mean plasma concentrations of procainamide (■) and its metabolite, *N*-acetylprocainamide (□), in subject 16 following a single 500-mg generic procainamide HCl capsule. (From Chen, M. L. and Jackson, A. J., *Pharm. Res.*, 8, 25, 1991. With permission of Plenum Publishing.)

ranged from 20 to 60%. The correlation coefficients for each rate constant within an individual varied from 0.25 to 0.95 between the test and reference product. As with the cases for linear kinetics without first-pass effect, the simulation results showed that in most instances the residual error (or intrasubject variability) for C_{max} is greatly diminished

Table 3–2 **Summary of rate constants for fitted data from a bioequivalence study administration of a single 500-mg procainamide**

Rate constant	Mean (% CV) Test	Mean (% CV) Reference	Mean difference (%)	Intrasubject variability[a]
k_a, per h	2.17 (110.3)	1.36 (142.9)	0.81 (59.6)	1.209
k_f, per h	0.71 (57.1)	0.63 (48.0)	0.08 (12.7)	0.307
k_e, per h	0.26 (35.0)	0.31 (35.6)	0.05 (16.1)	0.299

[a] Intrasubject variability is expressed by the root mean square of the error term divided by the reference mean.

From Chen, M. L. and Jackson, A. J., *Pharm. Res.*, 8, 25, 1991. With permission of Plenum Publishing.

from the parent drug to metabolite, which leads to a narrower confidence interval for the metabolite relative to the parent drug. These findings were not dependent on the fraction of total body clearance that furnishes the metabolite via first-pass route to the general circulation.[28]

An exceptional situation occurs when the intrasubject variance of k_a is low and of k_e is high. Under such circumstances, the confidence limits for the metabolite would be wider than those for the parent drug.

In an attempt to explore alternative situations by which a higher residual error may be observed for the metabolite than the parent drug, additional simulations were done assuming a much lower intrasubject CV for k_a relative to k_s. As expected, the simulation

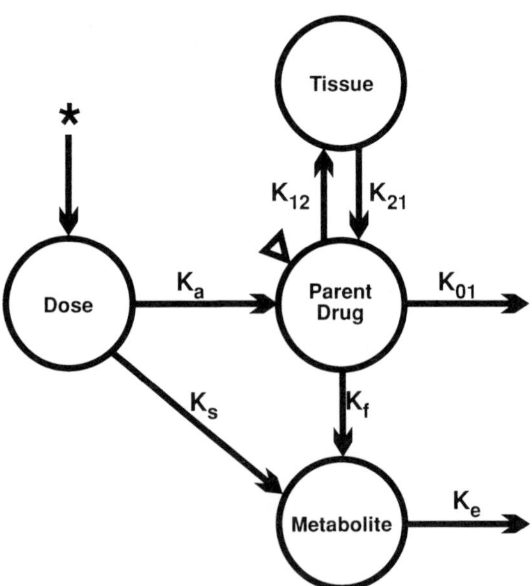

Figure 3–4 Triamterene model used for simulation of drugs exhibiting linear kinetics with first-pass effect, where k_a = first-order absorption rate constant, k_s = first-order rate constant for the fraction metabolized via first-pass effect, k_f = formation rate constant for metabolite from parent drug, k_{12} and k_{21} = intercompartment transfer constants, k_{10} = first-order elimination rate constant for parent drug from central compartment, and k_e = first-order elimination rate constant for metabolite.

showed an increase in residual error for C_{max} of the metabolite in comparison to the parent drug, and a tighter interval is obtained for the parent drug rather than the metabolite.

Table 3–3 lists summary statistics on the C_{max} parameter for *in vivo* bioequivalence studies on drugs following linear kinetics with first-pass effect.[29] The experimental data are in close agreement with the simulation results. Wider intervals were observed for the parent drug than for the metabolite in most cases, with the exception of imipramine and nortriptyline which yielded opposite results. It appears that imipramine and nortriptyline may represent the cases where either the intrasubject variability is small for k_a but large for k_e or the within-individual variability is high for the first-pass route of the drug.

One may suspect that the presence of first-pass metabolism which occurs immediately following absorption of the drug will enhance the sensitivity of metabolite data in the prediction of equivalency of rate of absorption between formulations. In view of the simulation results, however, the above hypothesis is only true for this class of drugs with a high degree of within-subject variability in the first-pass metabolism pathway. The ramification of the simulation results is that the assessment of bioequivalency in the rate of absorption for this type of drug would have to be based on both C_{max} values of the parent drug and metabolite, if metabolite data are pertinent to the determination of clinical efficacy and/or safety of the drug product.

c. Nonlinear Kinetics

Table 3–4 presents summary statistics for C_{max} parameter from single-dose bioequivalence studies on nonlinear drugs.[29] For verapamil, as with linear drugs, the confidence interval of C_{max} for the parent drug was wider than that for the metabolite. However, in the case of propranolol, comparable range of confidence limits were obtained for both parent drug and metabolite. Compared with diltiazem, the desacetyl metabolite exhibited a wider interval and yet the desmethyl metabolite yielded a narrower interval. It is unclear, at present, whether the conclusions drawn from drugs following linear pharmacokinetics could be extended to drugs with nonlinear kinetics. Simulations for this class of drugs are currently under way in the FDA.

d. Controlled-Release Dosage Forms

Table 3–5 shows C_{max} data from single-dose bioequivalence studies for controlled-release dosage forms.[29] Comparison of a conventional/immediate-release (Table 3–4) and a controlled-release (Table 3–5) product with identical drug entity revealed the distinctly different pharmacokinetic behavior between the two dosage forms. This is reflected by the difference in the relative magnitude of the confidence limits for verapamil/propranolol vs. their metabolite counterpart.

Drugs in controlled release dosage forms have distinct release profiles compared with those in conventional/immediate-release dosage forms. It is speculated that for controlled-release drug products, since absorption process is rate limited by the release of drugs from the formulation and metabolite formation is immediate to the existence of parent drug, metabolite data may be useful in the prediction of bioequivalence between formulations.

2. Extent of Absorption

Houston[30] used a first-pass metabolite model (Figure 3–5) to illustrate the distinction between the AUC of the parent drug (AUC[p]) and AUC of metabolite (AUC[m]) for bioavailability/bioequivalence studies. Assuming that liver is the only metabolizing organ, the AUC of the parent drug and metabolite can be derived as:

$$AUC(p) = fa \cdot F_H \cdot D/CL \qquad \textbf{(3–5)}$$

$$AUC(m) = fa \cdot fm \cdot F_H(m) \cdot D/CL(m) \qquad \textbf{(3–6)}$$

Table 3–3 **Summary data of bioequivalence studies on C_{max} parameter for drugs following linear kinetics with first-pass effect**

Parent drug/ metabolite	Dose	Subject no.	Mean C_{max} (ng/ml) Reference	Test	Intrasubject variability[a] (%)	90% CI[b]	CI Width
Triamterene	75 mg	23	143.0	161.6	27.9	(99, 127)	28
Hydroxy-triamterene sulfate		23	1928.0	1902.2	17.1	(90, 107)	17
Doxepin	100 mg	38	55.9	50.4	28.4	(79, 102)	23
Desmethyldoxepin		38	11.9	11.0	16.2	(86, 99)	13
Isosorbide dinitrate	20 mg	20	27.0	30.9	64.8	(79, 150)	71
Isosorbide-2-mononitrate		20	38.4	43.9	21.0	(103, 126)	23
Isosorbide-5-mononitrate		20	181.9	199.1	19.3	(99, 120)	21
Metoprolol	100 mg	34	140.3	150.0	17.4	(100, 114)	14
Hydroxymetoprolol		31	144.7	154.1	9.3	(103, 110)	7
Amitriptyline	50 mg	24	24.8	25.6	18.5	(94, 112)	18
Nortriptyline		24	9.8	9.8	12.0	(94, 106)	12
Imipramine	100 mg	22	57.1	58.7	14.3	(95, 110)	15
Desipramine		21	21.5	21.4	19.2	(89, 110)	21
Nortriptyline	75 mg	26	31.0	29.9	11.7	(91, 102)	11
Hydroxynortriptyline		26	26.7	26.2	19.3	(89, 107)	18

[a] Intrasubject variability is expressed by the root mean square of the error term divided by the reference mean.

[b] Confidence interval (CI) is expressed as the percentage of the reference mean.

Table 3–4 **Summary data of single-dose bioequivalence studies on C_{max} parameter for drugs following nonlinear kinetics**

Parent drug/ metabolite	Dose	Subject no.	Mean C_{max} (ng/ml)		Intrasubject variability[a] (%)	90% CI[b]	CI Width
			Reference	Test			
Diltiazem	120 mg	30	176.9	170.9	15.9	(90, 103)	13
Desacetyldiltiazem		30	10.1	9.8	29.4	(85, 110)	25
Desmethyldiltiazem		30	34.1	33.4	10.8	(94, 103)	9
Propranolol	80 mg	30	47.7	57.3	27.0	(105, 138)	33
4-Hydroxypropranolol		30	12.8	14.7	26.9	(100, 132)	32
Verapamil	120 mg	28	127.5	138.5	35.8	(92, 125)	33
Norverapamil		28	38.4	43.9	21.2	(92, 111)	19

[a] Intrasubject variability is expressed by the root mean square of the error term divided by the reference mean.

[b] Confidence interval (CI) is expressed as the percentage of the reference mean.

Table 3–5 **Summary data of single-dose bioequivalence studies on C_{max} parameter for drugs in controlled-release dosage forms**

Parent drug/ metabolite	Dose	Subject no.	Mean C_{max} (ng/ml) Reference	Test	Intrasubject variability[a] (%)	90% CI[b]	CI Width
Procainamide	500 mg	24	1.3	1.4	15.4	(98, 113)	15
N-Acetylprocainamide		24	0.6	0.6	11.6	(95, 106)	11
Propranolol	160 mg	24	23.8	23.7	12.5	(87, 117)	30
4-Hydroxypropranolol		21	1.7	1.9	33.7	(89, 127)	38
Verapamil	240 mg	12	116.5	110.8	14.4	(86, 104)	18
Norverapamil		12	149.3	151.7	28.0	(85, 118)	33

[a] Intrasubject variability is expressed by the root mean square of the error term divided by the reference mean.

[b] Confidence interval (CI) is expressed as the percentage of the reference mean.

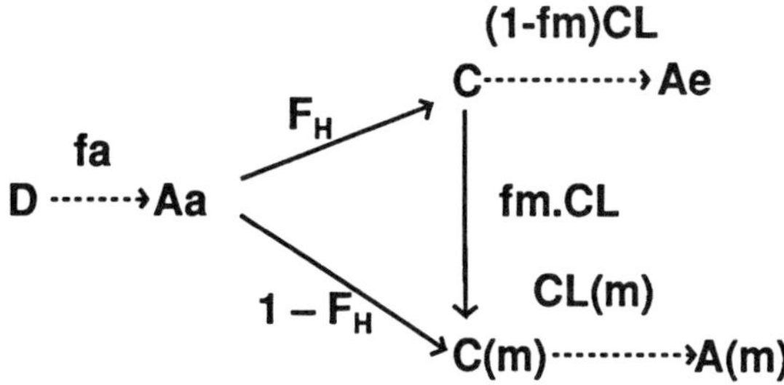

Figure 3–5 Schematic representation for an orally administered drug which undergoes a certain degree of first-pass metabolism in the liver, where D = dose, fa = fraction of drug absorbed, Aa = amount of drug at the absorption site, F_H = fraction of dose absorbed which escapes the liver during the absorption phase, k_a = absorption rate constant of the drug, C = concentration of drug in plasma at any time, C(m) = concentration of metabolite in plasma at any time, fm = fraction of absorbed drug converted to metabolite, CL = clearance of the drug, CL (m) = clearance of the metabolite, Ae = amount of drug excreted in the urine, A(m) = amount of metabolite excreted in the urine.

where fa is the fraction of drug absorbed from the absorption site; F_H is the fraction of drug escaping first-pass metabolism; D is the dose; CL is the systemic clearance of drug; CL(m) is metabolite clearance; fm is the fraction of absorbed drug converted to the metabolite of interest; and $F_H(m)$ is the systemic availability of metabolite, which may be conceived as the ratio of the amount of metabolite leaving the liver to the amount of the metabolite formed.

In a crossover bioequivalence study, since dose is a constant and clearances of each subject are assumed to be unchanged from one treatment to the other, it follows that:

$$\frac{AUC(p)_T}{AUC(p)_R} = \frac{fa_T \cdot F_{H(T)}}{fa_R \cdot F_{H(R)}} = \frac{F_T}{F_R} \tag{3–7}$$

where subscripts T and R denote the test and reference formulations, respectively. It is readily shown by Equation 3–7 that the ratio of AUC(p) represents the relative bioavailability of the two formulations (F_{rel}). In contrast, the use of AUC(m) in bioequivalence studies will yield:

$$\frac{AUC(m)_T}{AUC(m)_R} = \frac{fa_T \cdot fm_T \cdot F_{H,T}(m)}{fa_R \cdot fm_R \cdot F_{H,R}(m)} \tag{3–8}$$

Equation 3–8 can be reduced to:

$$\frac{AUC(m)_T}{AUC(m)_R} = \frac{fa_T}{fa_R} \tag{3–9}$$

provided that $fm_T = fm_R$ and $F_{H,T}(m) = F_{H,R}(m)$. It can be seen that instead of F_{rel}, the ratio of AUC(m) only gives the estimate of relative fraction absorbed (fa,rel) between formulations. Accordingly, Houston[30] concluded that the use of AUC(m) in bioequivalence studies as a substitute for AUC(p) is not justified.

On the contrary, Tucker et al.[31] suggested that equivalency with respect to the extent of drug absorption in a linear system may be assessed by the measurements of AUC from the parent drug or metabolite, regardless of the biological activity of the metabolite. The authors considered F_H to be constant for each individual when switching formulations with the same drug entity. If this is the case, using the first-pass metabolite model proposed by Houston, Equation 3-7 will be reduced to fa,rel, an identical formula as Equation 3–9. Consequently, irrespective of the chemical species measured, both AUC ratios estimate the relative fraction of dose absorbed into the body, if the drug contents (and therefore, the doses) are the same between formulations.

It appears that there is a common assumption inherent in the theories between Houston and Tucker; i.e., clearance in each individual is constant. Tucker's extension that F_H is also constant may be true for low-clearance drugs rather than high-clearance drugs. It is speculated that as clearance increases, the assumption of a constant F_H may not be valid. For high-clearance drugs, small changes in clearance within each individual from one formulation to another will result in large changes in F_H since the two variables are reciprocally related.

B. PHARMACODYNAMIC CONSIDERATIONS

It is indisputable that bioequivalence evaluations should rely on the pharmacokinetic data of active metabolites if the parent drug is a prodrug which rapidly degrades in the body or possesses little pharmacological activity and clinical effect. Drugs such as clofibrate and clorazepate are in this category, and bioequivalency is evaluated based on their respective active metabolites: *p*-chlorophenoxyisobutyric acid for clofibrate and desmethyldiazepam for clorazepate.[32,33]

The need to consider metabolite(s) in bioequivalence decisions cannot be overemphasized based on pharmacodynamic consideration. The contribution of important metabolite(s) to the overall assessment of bioequivalence should rest on the following factors:

1. Significant potency for the metabolite compared with the parent drug
2. Significant steady-state plasma concentration ratio between the metabolite and parent drug, and/or
3. Significant concentration ratio between the metabolite and parent drug at the site of action

From a pharmacodynamic standpoint, there is no doubt that measurement of active metabolite(s) assures the efficacy and safety of the drug product. However, for years the question of whether metabolite(s) data should be used to define or augment bioequivalence determinations from the parent drug remains a controversial issue.[5-8]

1. Areas of Controversy

Concerns arise partly from the absence of an apparent relationship for most drugs between blood levels and pharmacodynamic response.[3,34-38] The presence of several metabolites with varying degrees of potency and possibly different spectra of pharmacological activity from the given drug, as well as the complex nature of disease states, renders it extremely difficult to correlate the blood concentration of the drug or metabolite(s) with the relevant therapeutic effect.[38-40] Furthermore, since demonstration of biological activity is frequently derived from *in vivo* or *in vitro* screening in animals rather than in humans, it is perhaps difficult to understand the relative contributions of the parent drug vs. metabolites in the treatment of the underlying disease(s).

Another reason against the use of metabolite data for bioequivalence testing is that the parent drug is the true determinant of formulation performance as far as the absorption of the chemical entity is concerned. Granted that the activity of the metabolite(s) has been established as important for the assessment of bioequivalence, problems often arise with respect to measurement of the metabolite. Not only is the appearance rate of the metabolite often compounded with metabolism and release from tissue, but also the study design for the parent drug may not be necessarily optimal for the metabolite.[7,41]

Despite all the arguments, the general belief is that relative pharmacological activity of the parent drug vs. metabolite reflects the clinical effect; and thus measurement of active moieties should be an important key to drug development, be it a new drug or a generic drug. Therefore, use of the metabolite in addition to the parent drug should be essential to the determination of bioequivalence if the metabolite has a significant contribution to the clinical effect.

2. Clinical Significance

The presence of active metabolites, though not directly related to formulation, may enhance the overall clinical effect of drugs. The clinical effect, including both efficacy and toxicity, may be estimated by the pharmacodynamic factors listed in the preceding section. This is especially true for those drugs with narrow therapeutic indices (Table 3-6).[42-47] Judging from the steady-state concentration ratio and potency ratio between the major metabolite and parent drug, it is readily seen that in most cases the measurement of metabolites constitutes an integral part in bioequivalency evaluation of these drugs.

IV. CONCLUSIONS

The genuine role of drug metabolites in the assessment of bioequivalence has been addressed from pharmacokinetic and pharmacodynamic viewpoints. Even if the target species for comparison in bioequivalence studies is the parent drug, the knowledge of metabolite pharmacokinetics aids in the evaluation of bioequivalence. While this may be true when the analysis of the parent drug is limited, it is essential when the parent drug only acts as a prodrug and the metabolite is the therapeutically active moiety. Alternatively, if both parent drug and metabolite are active, the value of the metabolite should be weighed by the potency and concentration ratio of the parent drug vs. metabolite. In this regard, particular attention should be given to the drugs with narrow therapeutic indices.

When the metabolite is active, the need of measurement of metabolite levels for determination of bioequivalence is largely dependent on the pharmacokinetics of the drug and the metabolite of interest. Both simulations and experimental data for drugs exhibiting linear kinetics without complication of first-pass effect clearly demonstrate the lack of power for the metabolite to discriminate formulation difference in the rate of absorption. For linear drugs with first-pass effect, in addition to the parent drug, metabolite data are pertinent to the equivalence evaluation of absorption rate provided that the metabolite is the first-pass product and high intrasubject variability exists for the first-pass route of the drug. Similarly, experimental data for nonlinear drugs and controlled-release dosage forms revealed that metabolite data may be required for assessment of bioequivalence.

As for the extent of absorption, from pharmacokinetic consideration, metabolite(s) data can be employed in the equivalency determination of low-clearance drugs. For high-clearance drugs, however, the use of metabolite AUC as a substitute of parent drug AUC is questionable.

ACKNOWLEDGMENT

The authors wish to express their thanks to Drs. K. Sandy Pang and J. Brian Houston for their review of the chapter and their insightful suggestions.

Table 3–6 **Representative drugs with narrow therapeutic indices and their active metabolites(s)**

Drug	Metabolite(s)	Therapeutic level (P)	Steady-state conc ratio (M/P)	Potency Ratio (M/P)
Amiodarone	Desethylamiodarone	0.5–2.5 μg/ml	1.0	
Carbamazepine	Carbamazepine-10,11-epoxide	4–10 μg/ml	0.2–0.25	1.0
Imipramine	2-OH-Imipramine	100–300 ng/ml	0.27 ± 0.19	
	Desipramine		2.0 (Enuretic boys)	
			0.83 (Adults)	
	2-OH-Desipramine		0.38 (OH-DMI/DMI)	
Nortriptyline	10-OH-Nortriptyline	50–140 ng/ml	1.4 ± 0.86	0.5
Primidone	Phenobarbital	5–10 μg/ml	>1	
	Phenylethylmalonamide		0.74 ± 0.38	
Procainamide	*N*-Acetylprocainamide	3–14 μg/ml	1.8 ± 0.59 (Fast acetylator)	0.7–0.9
			0.6 ± 0.09 (Slow acetylator)	
Quinidine	3-OH-Quinidine	2–6 μg/ml	0.29	
Thioridazine	Mesoridazine	1–1.5 μg/ml	2.0	4.0
	Sulphoridazine		0.3–0.5	5.0

Note: P = Parent drug; M = Metabolite.

REFERENCES

1. **Drayer, D. E.,** Pharmacokinetically active drug metabolites: therapeutic and toxic activities, plasma and urine data in man, accumulation in renal failure, *Clin. Pharmacokinet.,* 1, 426, 1976.
2. **Guentert, T. W.,** Pharmacokinetics of benzodiazepines and of their metabolites, in *Progress in Drug Metabolism,* Vol. 8, Bridges, J. W. and Chasseaud, L. F., Eds., Taylor & Francis, London, 1984, chap. 5.
3. **Eadie, M. J.,** Formation of active metabolites of anticonvulsant drugs: a review of their pharmacokinetic and therapeutic significance, *Clin. Pharmacokinet.,* 21, 27, 1991.
4. **Ebihara, A. and Fujimura, A.,** Metabolites of antihypertensive drugs: an updated review of their clinical pharmacokinetic and therapeutic implications, *Clin. Pharmacokinet.,* 21, 331, 1991.
5. Pharmaceutical Manufacturers Association (PMA), Pharmacokinetics of drug metabolites, presented at Drug Metabolism Workshop, Bethesda, MD, April 27–28, 1989.
6. Rate of absorption in bioequivalency determinations, in *Proc. Bio-International '89, Issues in the Evaluation of Bioavailability Data,* McGilveray, I. J., Dighe, S. V., French, I. W., Midha, K. K., and Skelly, J. P., Eds., Toronto, Canada, Oct. 1-4, 1989, 13.
7. **Chen, M. L. and Jackson, A. J.,** The role of metabolites in bioequivalency assessment. I. Linear pharmacokinetics without first-pass effect, *Pharm. Res.,* 8, 25, 1991.
8. International Pharmaceutical Federation (FIP), Importance of metabolites in assessment of bioequivalence, presented at Bio-International '92, Bioavailability, Bioequivalence and Pharmacokinetic Studies Conference, Bad Homburg/Frankfurt, Germany, May 20–22, 1992.
9. U.S. Department of Health and Human Services, Food and Drug Administration, *Federal Food, Drug and Cosmetic Act,* as Amended and Related Laws, 86–1051, Section 505(j)(7)(B); codified as 21 USC (U.S. Code) 355(j)(7)(B), U.S. Government Printing Office, Washington, D.C., 1986, 66.
10. Food and Drug Administration, Bioequivalence requirements and *in vivo* bioavailability procedures, *Fed. Reg.,* 42, 1624, 1977.
11. Food and Drug Administration, Bioavailability and Bioequivalence Requirements, 21 Code of Federal Regulations (CFR), 1992, 320.
12. **Khoo, K., Gibaldi, M., and Brazzell, R. K.,** Comparison of statistical moment parameters to C_{max} and T_{max} for detecting differences in *in vivo* dissolution rate, *J. Pharm. Sci.,* 74, 1340, 1985.
13. **Jackson, A. J. and Chen, M. L.,** Application of moment analysis in assessing rates of absorption for bioequivalency studies, *J. Pharm. Sci.,* 76, 6, 1987.
14. **Aarons, L.,** Assessment of rate of absorption in bioequivalence studies, *J. Pharm. Sci.,* 76, 853, 1987.
15. **Chen, M. L.,** Assessment of rate of absorption in bioequivalence studies, presented at Generic Drugs Advisory Meeting, Food and Drug Administration, Bethesda, MD, September 26–27, 1991.
16. **Chen, M. L.,** An alternative approach for assessment of rate of absorption in bioequivalence studies, *Pharm. Res.,* 9, 1380, 1992.
17. **Schuirmann, D. J.,** A comparison of the two one-sided tests procedure and the power approach for assessing the equivalence of average bioavailability, *J. Pharmacokinet. Biopharm.,* 15, 657, 1987.
18. U.S. Department of Health and Human Services, Food and Drug Administration, *Approved Drug Products with Therapeutic Equivalence Evaluations,* 12th ed. U.S. Government Printing Office, Washington, D.C., 1992, viii.

19. Division of Bioequivalence, Office of Generic Drugs, Food and Drug Administration, Guidance on Statistical Procedures for Bioequivalence Studies Using a Standard Two-Treatment Crossover Design, 1992.
20. **Hande, K., Reed, E., and Chabner, B.,** Allopurinol kinetics, *Clin. Pharmacol. Ther.,* 23, 598, 1978.
21. **Elion, G. B., Callahan, S., Nathan, H., Bieber, S., Rundles, R. W., and Hitchings, G. H.,** Potentiation by inhibition of drug degradation: 6-substituted purines and xanthine oxidase, *Biochem. Pharmacol.,* 12, 85, 1963.
22. **Spector, T. and Johns, D. G.,** Stoichiometric inhibition of reduced xanthine oxidase by hydroxypyrazolo (3,4-D) pyrimidines, *J. Biol. Chem.,* 245, 5079, 1970.
23. **Houston, J. B.,** Drug metabolite kinetics, *Pharmacol. Ther.,* 15, 521, 1981.
24. **Pang, K. S.,** A review of metabolite kinetics, *J. Pharmacokinet. Biopharm.,* 13, 633, 1985.
25. **St-Pierre, M. V., Xu, X., and Pang, K. S.,** Primary, secondary and tertiary metabolite kinetics, *J. Pharmacokinet. Biopharm.,* 16, 493, 1988.
26. **Chen, M. L. and Jackson, A. J.,** The role of metabolites in bioequivalency assessment. II. Linear pharmacokinetics with first-pass effect, unpublished data, 1993.
27. **Hasegawa, J., Lin, E. T., Williams, R. L., Sorgel, F., and Benet, L. Z.,** Pharmacokinetics of triamterene and its metabolites in man, *J. Pharmacokinet. Biopharm.,* 10, 507, 1982.
28. **Pang, K. S. and Kwan, K. C.,** A commentary: methods and assumptions in the kinetic estimation of metabolite formation, *Drug Metab. Dispos.* 11, 79, 1983.
29. Division of Bioequivalence, Office of Generic Drugs, Food and Drug Administration, Bioequivalence Study Data on File.
30. **Houston, J. B.,** Analytical issues in bioequivalency determinations: importance of metabolites in bioequivalence, in *Proc. Bio-International '89, Issues in the Evaluation of Bioavailability Data,* McGilveray, I. J., Dighe, S. V., French, I. W., Midha, K. K., and Skelly, J. P., Eds., 1989, 97.
31. **Tucker, G. T., Rostami, A., and Jackson, P. R.,** Metabolite measurement in bioequivalence studies. I. Theoretical considerations, presented at Bio-International '92, Bioavailability, Bioequivalence and Pharmacokinetic Studies Conference, Bad Homburg/Frankfurt, Germany, May 20–22, 1992.
32. Division of Bioequivalence, Office of Generic Drugs, Food and Drug Administration, Guidance on *in vivo* Bioequivalence Study and *in vitro* Dissolution Testing for Clofibrate, 1986.
33. Division of Bioequivalence, Office of Generic Drugs, Food and Drug Administration, Guidance on *in vivo* Bioequivalence Study and *in vitro* Dissolution Testing for Clorazepate, 1987.
34. **Levy, R. H., Wilensky, A. J., and Friel, P. N.,** Other antiepileptic drugs, in *Applied Pharmacokinetics: Principles of Therapeutic Drug Monitoring,* 2nd ed., Evans, W. E., Schentag, J. J., and Jusko, W. J., Eds., Applied Therapeutics, Spokane, WA, 1986, 540.
35. **Gengo, F. and Green J. A.,** Beta blockers, in *Applied Pharmacokinetics: Principles of Therapeutic Drug Monitoring,* 2nd ed., Evans, W. E., Schentag, J. J., and Jusko, W. J., Eds., Applied Therapeutics, Spokane, WA, 1986, 735.
36. **Schottelius, D. and Fincham, R. W.,** *Clinical Application of Serum Primidone Levels in Antiepileptic Drugs: Quantitative Analysis and Interpretation,* Pippenger, C. E., Penry, J. K., and Kutt, H., Eds., Raven Press, New York, 1978, 273.
37. **Kutt, H.,** Clinical pharmacology of carbamazepine in antiepileptic drugs: quantitative analysis and interpretation, Pippenger, C. E., Penry, J. K., and Kutt, H., Eds., Raven Press, New York, 1978, 297.

38. **DeVane, C. L.,** Cyclic antidepressants, in *Applied Pharmacokinetics: Principles of Therapeutic Drug Monitoring,* 2nd ed., Evans, W. E., Schentag, J. J., and Jusko, W. J., Eds., Applied Therapeutics, Spokane, WA, 1986, 852.
39. **Lapierre, Y. D.,** Are all benzodiazepines clinically bioequivalent, *Prog. Neuro-Psychopharmacol. Biol. Psychiatry,* 7, 641, 1983.
40. **Anderson, P., Bondesson, U., and Sylven, C.,** Clinical pharmacokinetics of verapamil in patients with atrial fibrillation, *Eur. J. Clin. Pharmacol.,* 23, 49, 1982.
41. **McGilveray, I. J., Ormsby, E., and Midha, K. K.,** Metabolites in bioequivalence: examples and problems, presented at Bio-International '92, Bioavailability, Bioequivalence and Pharmacokinetic Studies Conference, Bad Homburg/Frankfurt, Germany, May 20–22, 1992.
42. *Goodman and Gilman's The Pharmacological Basis of Therapeutics,* 8th ed., Gilman, A. G., Rall, T. W., Nies, A. S., and Taylor, P., Pergamon Press, New York, 1990.
43. **Evans, W. E., Schentag, J. J., and Jusko, W. J., Eds.,** *Applied Pharmacokinetics: Principles of Therapeutic Drug Monitoring,* 2nd ed., Applied Therapeutics, Spokane, WA, 1986.
44. **Tomson, T. and Bertilsson, L.,** Potent therapeutic effect of carbamazepine-10,11-epoxide in trigeminal neuralgia, *Arch. Neurol.,* 41, 598, 1984.
45. **Reidenberg, M. M., Drayer, D. E., Levy, M., and Warner, H.,** Polymorphic acetylation of procainamide in man, *Clin. Pharmacol. Ther.,* 17, 722, 1975.
46. **Elson, J., Strong, J. M., Lee, W.-K., and Atkinson, A. J., Jr.,** Antiarrhythmic potency of *N*-acetylprocainamide, *Clin. Pharmacol. Ther.,* 17, 134, 1975.
47. **Rakhit, A., Holford, N. H. G., Guentert, T. W., Maloney, K., and Riegelman, S.,** Pharmacokinetics of quinidine and three of its metabolites in man, *J. Pharmacokinet. Biopharm.,* 12, 1, 1984.

Chapter 4

Analytical Aspects of Bioequivalency Testing

James Leslie

CONTENTS

I. INTRODUCTION

For valid conclusions to be drawn from the results of bioequivalency testing, measured drug concentrations must be accurate, precise, and specific for the intact drug and bioactive metabolites. Modern methods of drug analysis in biological matrices — high-performance liquid chromatography (HPLC); gas-liquid chromatography (GLC); and immunoassays, particularly radioimmunoassay (RIA) — are capable of providing accurate and precise data over the range of concentrations needed to meet the requirements for bioequivalency testing. There are no specific regulatory or compendial requirements for analysis of drugs and related compounds in biological matrices, but a number of recently published articles address the issues of validation and performance of bioanalytical methods.[1-5] One of these articles describes a complete validation and report of a bioanalytical study.[5] The report of a conference sponsored jointly by the American Association of Pharmaceutical Scientists, U.S. Food and Drug Administration, Federation International Pharmaceutique, Health Protection Branch (Canada), and Association of Official Analytical Chemists to reach a consensus on the requirements of assays in bioequivalence, pharmacokinetic, and clinical studies has been published.[6] Bioanalytical methods must be thoroughly validated prior to use and applied in a controlled manner to ensure that they will perform satisfactorily. Performance should be monitored during sample analysis to confirm that predetermined specifications are met.

0-8493-6930-4/94/$0.00+$.50

Most bioequivalency studies require analysis of drugs and metabolites in human plasma or serum, but sometimes in other biological matrices such as whole blood or urine. This chapter focuses on plasma or serum, but the same discussion can be directed with appropriate modification to other biological matrices. Bioanalytical analyses involve the quantification of organic molecules of widely differing chemical and physical properties; and the assay of each compound has to be evaluated on an individual basis, taking into consideration the complexity of the assay and the target concentrations. A presentation of the requirements of an assay for bioequivalency testing including the topics of sensitivity, accuracy, reproducibility, selectivity, and data reduction is given in this chapter.

Some comparisons of the analysis of drugs in biological matrices to the analysis of drugs in dosage forms and bulk powders are mentioned to show that acceptance criteria applied to dosage form analyses are not necessarily applicable to the evaluation of bioanalytical methods. The differences in criteria are due to the complexity of the assays and the fact that the application of bioanalytical data is to biological systems which are highly variable, whereas dosage form analysis is applied to physicochemical systems that have much less variability.

II. ASSAY SELECTION AND DEVELOPMENT

Unlike the analysis of drugs in dosage forms and bulk powders, there are no compendial or official methods for the analyses of drugs in biological matrices. In fact, many methods are developed and applied as part of submissions to regulatory agencies and may not be available in the scientific literature. A critical stage, therefore, in a bioequivalency experiment is to develop and validate a bioanalytical assay. Assay development is the process in which a series of experiments is performed to find the conditions necessary to measure the analyte of interest, and requires a knowledge of the physical and chemical properties of the drug so that the development process can be individualized in a rational manner. Details of the factors involved in assay development have been presented.[7]

Published methods may be used with modification, if necessary. However, the existence of a method in the literature does not mean that it can be considered to have been validated. In fact, as has been pointed out,[2,8] methods published in the literature rarely include consistent validation data. Complete validation of a method obtained from the literature must be conducted in the laboratory performing the analyses for the bioequivalency experiment in a manner similar to the validation of a newly developed method. On the other hand, newly developed methods need not be cross validated or correlated with published methods. Cross validation is sometimes performed if, for example, there are doubts about the specificity, as in radioimmunoassay, when it might be desirable to cross validate the method against a method such as mass spectrometry which can be demonstrated to be specific. The implications for bioequivalency conclusions about any differences noted must be considered on a case-by-case basis. For example, in the difficult assay for thorazine it was noted that although the drug concentrations obtained by radioimmunoassay were 30 to 40% higher than when assayed by gas chromatography-mass spectrometry (GC-MS), the two sets of results yielded the same conclusions with regard to bioequivalency of thorazine formulations.[9] Interlaboratory correlation of a method is rarely needed in bioequivalency studies since each study is a discrete experiment in which the analysis is performed within a single laboratory. This is in contrast to multisite clinical studies in which analysis may be performed in different laboratories, possibly even by different procedures. Under these circumstances a correlation between the results obtained in the different methods must be demonstrated.

A brief overview of the analytical methods suitable for the assay of drugs and related compounds in biological matrices for bioequivalency studies is presented below. Appropriate references should be consulted for detailed methodologies.

A. HIGH-PERFORMANCE LIQUID CHROMATOGRAPHY (HPLC)[10-14]

HPLC is the current method of choice for analysis of drugs in biological fluids in bioequivalency studies. The method is simple in concept, and reliable modern equipment makes it convenient to perform. A liquid, the mobile phase, is pumped through a column of a tightly packed material during which time the components of the analytical mixture are separated. Reversed-phase chromatography in which the column packing is less polar than the mobile phase is most commonly used. The effluent is monitored by a suitable detector, and the height or area of the resulting peaks is quantified electronically. The method is applicable to many compounds because (1) different packing polarities ranging from ionic to 18 carbon nonpolar are available and (2) the mobile phase can be readily modified in the type and concentration of the organic component (acetonitrile, methanol, tetrahydrofuran are commonly used) and the pH of buffers added to it. The use of different methods of detection such as ultraviolet absorption, fluorescence, and electrochemical contribute significantly to the flexibility and sensitivity of the method. Concentrations in the low nanogram per milliliter (ng/ml) range can be quantified.

Biological samples containing the drug must generally be pretreated before injection into the HPLC system. Methods most commonly used in this pretreatment include (1) precipitation of proteins in serum or plasma samples, (2) liquid-liquid extraction, and (3) liquid-solid (solid-phase) extraction. The method of pretreatment can have a significant impact on the accuracy, precision, and selectivity of the assay. An internal standard is usually added to the sample at the beginning of the analysis to compensate for solvent transfer losses and volume changes during sample processing.

Chromatograms of extracts from biological samples usually exhibit a number of peaks in addition to those of the analytes and internal standard. A typical chromatogram of an extract of a drug from a biological matrix is shown in Figure 4–1. The extra peaks are due to the presence of endogenous compounds in the biological matrix and are often even larger than the analyte peaks. The peaks of interest must be sufficiently resolved from other peaks, and be sharp and symmetrical for good sensitivity and accuracy. Baseline separation of drug peaks from those of endogenous compounds is not always necessary as long as peak heights, rather than areas, are measured and there is resolution such that the neighboring peak does not contribute significantly to the drug peak height. A computer-simulated chromatogram, Figure 4–2, illustrates this point. When reviewing bioanalytical data there should be a qualitative review of the chromatography and instrument settings before looking at the quantitative criteria for acceptability.[3]

The data obtained are the heights (or areas) of the peaks of interest, and the ratio of the peak height of the analyte to that of the internal standard is calculated. The concentrations of the analyte in the unknowns are determined by a comparison of the peak height ratios for the unknowns to those of calibrators processed simultaneously with the samples.

B. GAS-LIQUID CHROMATOGRAPHY (GLC)[10,11,15,16]

Although HPLC is the current method of choice, GLC is an acceptable method for analysis of drugs. As in HPLC the analytes must first be extracted from the biological matrix, but in GLC the extract is redissolved in a volatile solvent and a portion injected into the GLC system. The sample mixture is vaporized and swept by a flow of carrier gas through a column containing a packing material. Flexibility of the method for different compounds is provided by the availability of packings of various polarities and the temperature (isothermal or temperature gradient) at which the separations can be achieved. The components of the mixture separate as they pass through the column and are monitored by a suitable detector and quantified electronically. Detection techniques of different degrees of sensitivity and specificity such as flame ionization and nitrogen-phosphorus and electron capture add flexibility to the method, particularly when the drug can be derivatized prior to injection into the GLC system.

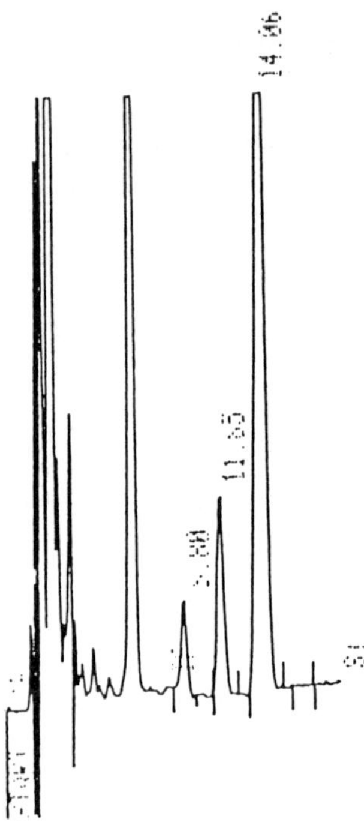

Figure 4–1 HPLC chromatogram obtained for theophylline in serum after precipitation of proteins by perchloric acid. Peak at 11.65 min is theophylline, and that at 14.06 min is the internal standard. (Unpublished data.)

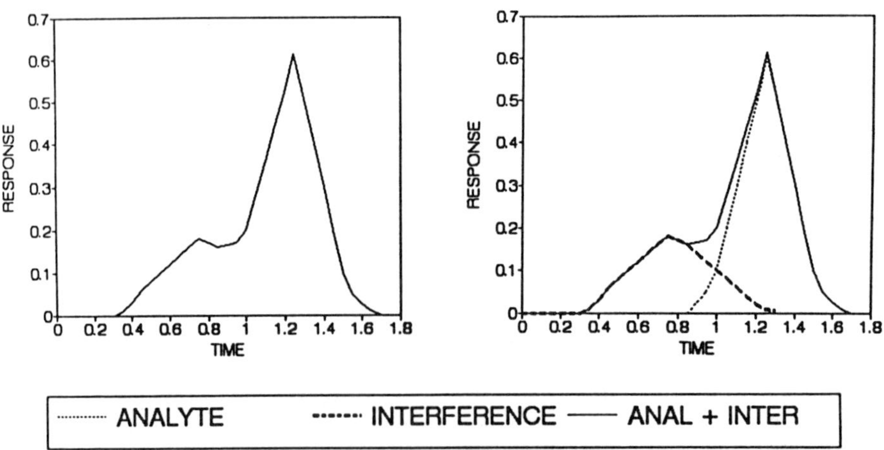

Figure 4–2 Simulated chromatogram showing relative effects on an interfering peak on analyte peak height and area.

An internal standard is added to the samples at the beginning of the analysis, and the data obtained is a peak height (or area) ratio of analytes to internal standard. As in HPLC the chromatograms exhibit a number of peaks in addition to the analytes and internal standard. In fact, the discussion about the chromatograms for HPLC can be equally applied to GLC.

C. RADIOIMMUNOASSAY (RIA)[17-19]

The specificity of antibody-antigen interactions combined with the sensitivity of the measurement of radioactivity provide a method, known as radioimmunoassay, for the determination of drugs in biological fluids. In contrast to HPLC and GLC it is not usually necessary, unless some purification or concentration steps are needed, to isolate the analytes from the plasma or serum.

An antibody that will combine with the drug is required. Since drugs are small molecular weight organic compounds, they themselves do not promote formation of antibodies when injected into an animal; thus they are first conjugated to a high molecular weight compound and then used to elicit an immune response. Antibodies may be obtained by cell hybridization techniques (monoclonal antibodies) or by injecting the drug conjugated to a high molecular weight compound into an animal (polyclonal antibodies). Under favorable circumstances antibodies are obtained that "recognize" the drug and bind to it in a specific manner by noncovalent interactions. Monoclonal antibodies are single molecular forms of an antibody whereas polyclonal antibodies are mixtures of different molecular species. Both monoclonal and polyclonal antibodies have been used in drug analysis, and, as an example, radioimmunoassay methods using both types of antibodies have been used for the quantification of fluphenazine.[20,21]

The assay procedure is to incubate a small volume of the serum containing the analyte with small volumes of the diluted antiserum and tracer quantity of the radioactive (usually ^{125}I or tritium) labeled drug. Calibrators and unknowns are processed simultaneously with a constant amount of antibody and radioactive analyte using a predetermined optimal set of conditions. Because of the nature of the antibody-drug interaction and its sensitivity to a number of physical and chemical factors, incubations are performed at least in duplicate. The unbound analyte and radioactive analyte are separated from those bound to the antibody by a suitable technique, and the radioactive analyte measured is in an appropriate radiation counter. It is desirable to collect at least 10,000 counts for each incubation tube processed to obtain acceptable counting statistics (1% relative standard deviation). Concentrations in the low picogram per milliliter range can be measured.

D. OTHER METHODS

HPLC, GLC, and RIA are by far the most commonly used assay methods in bioequivalence studies. Other methods which are sometimes used include mass spectrometry (MS)[22] and immunoassays[17] other than RIA such as enzyme-multiplied immunoassay technique (EMIT), fluorescent-induced polarization (FIP), and enzyme-linked immunoabsorbent assay (ELISA). Microbiological assays[23,24] are useful for the quantification of antibiotics, particularly for those antibiotics which are a mixture of molecular entities.

III. ANALYTICAL EXPERIMENTAL PROTOCOL

Once an assay has been developed and validated for a specified analyte, a standard operating procedure (SOP) for the analysis of the bioequivalency samples is written and analyses performed according to this procedure. Any changes which could significantly affect the assay results (e.g., substituting a different type of column, making a major change in wavelength in HPLC, making a new batch of antibody in RIA, or changing the extraction procedure) require at least a partial revalidation. The degree of revalidation depends on the factors which influence the results and is best judged by the analyst familiar with the method.[2]

In bioequivalency experiments reference and test product(s) are administered to a group of volunteers according to a random crossover design under a set of conditions specified in a clinical protocol. Samples of blood (or urine) are obtained from the subjects at specified times; and whole blood, plasma, serum, or urine are stored under predetermined conditions to await analysis. The next task therefore is to analyze the set of samples drawn from each volunteer according to the assay SOP. Analytical samples may be processed totally randomly or subject by subject in a series of analytical runs. Since the objective of the experiment is to compare concentrations of the drug from a test product to those from a reference product, it is desirable to analyze one subject's samples in a single run to minimize the effect of interrun assay variability.[4] Samples are generally assayed singly in chromatographic procedures whereas in radioimmunoassays specimens are incubated at least in duplicate because of the less reliable end point compared to chromatographic assays. The effect of assay variability on the results of bioequivalency testing has been discussed[25] when it was concluded that assay variability makes a minor contribution to the overall variability in bioequivalency testing.

The analytical run consists of processing a set of standards and subject samples with quality control samples interspersed among the samples to monitor assay performance. Five to eight standard concentrations (not including zero) in the biological matrix has been recommended[6] although more may be needed for a wide concentration range or for characterization of a nonlinear standard curve. Single point calibrations as used in dosage form analysis[26] are not acceptable in bioequivalence studies because of the range of concentrations of the samples. The concentration intervals should be spaced so as to adequately define the calibration line without undue emphasis on high or low concentrations. In radioimmunoassays it is conventional to vary successive concentrations by a factor of two, presumably because of the logarithmic functions used in the data reduction. In chromatographic assays, gradually increasing concentration intervals are used as the calibration concentrations increase. The concentration range should be chosen such that the measured drug concentrations from the maximum through the washout phase should be in the overall concentration range and not, for example, in the range covered by only a few concentration values.

At least two sets of three concentrations (high, medium, and low on the standard line) of quality control samples should be included.[3,6,8] Acceptance criteria for analytical runs based on results obtained for the standards and controls should be established *a priori*. It has been suggested that four out of six controls should be within 20% of their nominal values with the two unsatisfactory controls being of different concentrations for a run to be considered satisfactory.[2] However, other approaches to acceptability which depend on the accuracy and precision of the individual assay have been proposed.[1,3]

IV. ACCURACY

Obviously, results must be accurate. Accuracy is defined how close a measured value is to the true value. Absolute accuracy is how close the measured value is to a known or independently determined standardized concentration. In the analysis of drugs in biological matrices it is not possible to determine absolute accuracy because no such standards are available. Reference standards are approximated in therapeutic drug monitoring where commercial companies make available control samples which have been analyzed by a number of reference laboratories using a variety of methods.[27] The availability of these controls is limited to a relatively small number of drugs for most of which there is no longer any need for bioequivalency testing and in any case would have inappropriate concentrations. Nevertheless, experience in analyzing these control samples has shown that the results are method dependent, emphasizing the difficulty of defining absolute accuracy in assaying bioanalytical samples.

Accuracy in bioanalytical chemistry is more often expressed on a relative basis,[2] i.e., the measured values of standards are compared to the concentrations in solutions spiked with known amounts of the drug. In effect, therefore, it is difficult to determine absolute accuracy in a bioanalytical procedure; however, with accurate weighings of authenticated reference standards and accurate volumetric or gravimetric dilutions, an acceptable measure of accuracy can be achieved. In this process there could be systematic errors which cancel. For example, a common procedure during assay validation is to perform the analytical run on a set of replicate standards along with the standards. The standard line is used to back calculate the concentrations of the other standards, and the deviation from the spiked values is considered to be a measure of accuracy. This process could lead to a spurious measurement of accuracy because consistent biases in the method would cancel. It also depends on how accurately the standards were prepared. It is advisable in this procedure to use standards prepared independently from the control or validation samples for which accuracy is being assessed.[3]

In bioequivalence testing the accuracy within analytical runs (intrabatch) and between analytical runs (interbatch) is of interest. The terms intraday and interday variability which are often used rather than intrabatch and interbatch imply that the runs are completed in a day or only one run is made each day; thus the terms intrabatch and interbatch are preferred.[1]

Accuracy is determined during the validation process by analysis of replicate sets of the biological matrix spiked with the analyte. There are many ways in which the experiment to assess accuracy can be performed but a typical procedure to determine intrabatch accuracy might be to perform an analytical run according to sequence:

S1, S2, S3, S4, S5, S6, C1, C3, C6, C1, C3, C6, S1, S2, S3, S4, S5, S6, C1, C3, C6, C1, C3, C6, S1, S2, S3, S4, S5, S6, C1, C3, C6, C1, C3 and C6

in which S represents standards with concentrations 1, 2, 3, etc., and C represents control samples (independently prepared from the standards in the same matrix) corresponding to concentrations 1, 3, and 6. S1 to S6 and C1 to C3 are in order of increasing concentration. The first six standards are used to construct a calibration line, the parameters of which are used to calculate the concentrations of all the other standards and samples. The means are computed for the calculated concentrations of the control samples and the standards, and are compared to the nominal values.

The interbatch accuracy could be assessed by repeating the analysis sequence described above in two additional independent analytical runs using freshly prepared standards, but using portions of the same control samples. The mean concentration of each standard is calculated for the three runs. There is consensus among bioanalytical chemists that intrabatch and interbatch accuracy is acceptable if the deviation of the mean from the nominal or spiked concentration is 15% or less, with more tolerance (20%) near the lower limit of quantification.[6]

Accuracy during actual sample analysis can be assessed by calculating the concentrations obtained for the standards back calculated from their observed peak heights and standard line parameters, and the concentrations of the control samples assayed with the samples. The back calculated concentrations of the standards and control concentrations would typically be collated at the conclusion of the analysis and the mean values calculated.[4]

V. PRECISION

Precision in analytical techniques is the variability in the concentrations obtained when the same sample is assayed a number of times. Precision in bioequivalence studies can be assessed from the data obtained from the same three runs used to determine accuracy in the validation process. The standard deviations of the measured concentrations are calculated at the same time the means are calculated, and the precision at each concentration is expressed as a percentage relative standard deviation (coefficient of variation). The individual runs yield intrabatch precision and the pooled results yield a measure of interbatch precision. The standards and controls processed during the analysis of study samples can be used to calculate the interbatch precision in addition to monitoring assay performance. These precision data may conveniently be summarized in the same tables used to present accuracy data.

In general, intrabatch measurements have less variability than interbatch measurements. The precision is usually better for chromatographic assays as concentration increases whereas in radioimmunoassays the precision is better at the concentrations at which 50% of the radioactive tracer is bound. There is a consensus among bioanalytical chemists[6] that relative standard deviations not exceeding 15% are generally acceptable, with up to 20% being acceptable near the lower limit of quantification for intrabatch and interbatch measurements.

The accuracy and precision determined during assay validation can be used to monitor assay performance during study sample analysis. Based on the observed accuracy and precision a confidence interval, e.g., at 99% confidence, can be constructed around the mean value in which a specified number of control samples must fall. Using this technique the acceptance of a run depends on criteria established for an individual method. A difficulty with this technique in bioequivalence studies is that acceptance criteria will be more severe for a precise assay than an imprecise one, and data which are acceptable for the purpose of establishing bioequivalence may be rejected. For very imprecise methods an upper limit to acceptable precision must be established to maintain acceptable standards. Plots of the control sample values obtained during sample study analysis are useful in monitoring assay performance by detecting systematic differences in the runs and observed trends could be indicative of an impending assay problem.[1,3]

VI. LIMITS OF QUANTIFICATION

During the development of an assay for a bioequivalence experiment, the range of expected concentrations can usually be obtained from pharmacokinetic and therapeutic studies described in the literature or from pilot studies. Upper and lower limits of quantification of the assay must be defined during the assay validation process.

The upper limit of quantification is rarely a problem in HPLC and GLC procedures because precision and accuracy are generally better at the higher concentrations, and there is less potential for interference by endogenous compounds. For this reason little attention needs to be given to the upper limit of quantification in chromatographic assays, with the highest concentration standard determining the upper limit of quantification. On the other hand, RIA assays have a limit on the upper range for acceptable quantification because of saturation of the antibody. This should be determined during assay validation although as a general rule the valid concentration is between 10 and 90% binding of the radioactive tracer drug to the antibody. With high concentration samples, however, there is the option of diluting them with blank matrix and then reassaying them.

The analytical procedure has a lower limit of quantification determined by the extraction efficiency, detection capabilities of the equipment used, and physicochemical properties of the analytes. The lower limit of quantification (LOQ) is of major concern, since this dictates the lowest concentrations which can be quantified and may place severe demands on the analytical method. In bioanalytical analysis the LOQ is defined as the lowest concentration that can be measured with a specified degree of accuracy and precision.[6] Sometimes this is referred to as the sensitivity of the assay, but the term sensitivity should not be used in this context unless it is clearly defined. This is because sensitivity can also be described as the smallest amount that can be detected at a signal-to-noise ratio of 2 to 4,[28,29] but this is better known as the lowest detectable amount or limit of detection (LOD). Although it is possible to show that a drug is present at the LOD, it may not be quantifiable with an acceptable degree of precision and accuracy. For example, in a published report[29] the LOQ defined in this way had a high error of 35%.

In reality, concentrations as low as the LOQ as defined in the above paragraph may not be required for certain drugs. For example, a 500-mg dose of a drug yields relatively high plasma concentrations and concentrations as low as the LOQ may not be needed in the assay. In these instances, it is required only that the lowest concentrations used in the standard line have acceptable accuracy and precision and the determination of the actual lower limit of quantitation is only of academic interest.

The LOQ required in bioequivalency testing depends on the individual drug, but generally the lower the dose, the lower the LOQ required in the assay. However, the plasma concentrations, for example, depend on pharmacokinetic parameters such as the volume of distribution, half-life, and metabolic pathway. The LOQ must be such that the elimination phase concentrations for 3 to 4 half-lives after the maximum concentration can be measured. This is adequate for calculation of the area under the curve and half-lives to be characterized.[4]

The LOQ may be determined by analyzing a series of replicate samples, usually five or six, of gradually lower concentrations until the accuracy and precision criteria are no longer met. In practice it is sufficient to demonstrate that adequate accuracy and precision are obtained at the lowest concentration of interest. This can be accomplished using the same experimental scheme used for the determination of accuracy and precision. The criteria for acceptable precision at the lower limit of quantitation is stated to be a 20% relative standard deviation and an accuracy within 20% of the nominal concentration.[6]

VII. SELECTIVITY

It must be demonstrated in a bioanalytical assay that analytes are being selectively quantified in a mixture which contains many other compounds. Potential sources of interference include (1) the large number of high and low molecular weight endogenous compounds always present in biological fluids; (2) metabolites of administered drugs; (3) unchanged coadministered drugs where more than one drug is administered in the bioequivalency study, e.g., triamterene and hydrochlorothiazide; and (4) other potential sources of interference such as anticoagulants, components in the analytical reagents, and plasticizers in storage tubes.[2]

Absence of interference from endogenous compounds in the biological matrix and reagents used in the assay procedure can be demonstrated during assay validation by processing serum or plasma (or other matrix) obtained from a number of drug-free volunteers through the complete assay procedure. A criterion that has been used for interference in chromatographic assays is that an interfering peak should have a height or area less than 20% of that of the concentration at the LOQ.[3] It has been suggested that at least six different blank samples of the matrix be examined,[6] and the author has seen validation protocols that require one of these samples to be severely hemolyzed in order to test for potential interference from red blood cell components. When using chromatographic methods, the analytical run used for selectivity testing should be much longer than that used for the assay of samples in order to detect any late-eluting peaks, particularly if the mobile phase in HPLC has weak eluting power or if low temperatures are used in GLC. Also in chromatographic assays it should be determined that there is no interference with the internal standard. Even if no interference from endogenous compounds is found during assay validation, a predose sample of each subject's serum should be obtained and processed — with and without any internal standard — along with the samples.

Interference by intact drugs other than the analytes of interest can readily be tested for, but it may be difficult to demonstrate a lack of interference by metabolites or drug degradation products since these may not be known or available as pure compounds. If such interference is likely, it is desirable during validation to examine samples drawn from a volunteer who had been administered the drug. In this way it might be possible to demonstrate lack of interference by observing the responses attributable to metabolites, by using a different chromatographic system or by using diode array detection for ultraviolet-absorbing compounds to test for peak purity. These methods may not prove that no interference is occurring but can increase confidence in the assay selectivity. Unlike bioanalytical assays for samples from clinical trials or therapeutic drug analysis, it is not necessary to check for interference by prescription drugs other than those being tested in the bioequivalence study, since volunteers taking prescription drugs are generally not acceptable for bioequivalence studies. It is useful, however, in the assay validation to test the potential interference for commonly used nonprescription compounds such as ibuprofen, aspirin and salicylic acid (metabolite of aspirin), acetaminophen, and caffeine.

It is more difficult to test for interferences in immunoassay methods because only numerical values are obtained in the raw data as opposed to tracings in chromatographic assays. The usual approach is to measure the "cross-reactivity" of potentially interfering compounds with the antibody by processing samples containing the suspected interfering substance with no analyte present, and expressing the interference as the concentration of the compound that displaces 50% of labeled analyte. The higher this value, the less interference is present. Lack of cross-reactivity is generally accepted when there is no immunologic response when the substance is present at 1000 times the lower limit of quantification.[1] Fortunately, in immunoassays the only interfering compounds are likely to be metabolites and degradation products, i.e., compounds with similar structure. When such interference is found, the interfering compounds may be removed by extraction prior to immunoassay. For example, clonidine may be separated from its metabolite hydroxyclonidine by ether extraction of alkalinized serum prior to radioimmunoassay.[30] Different lots of the blank matrix should be examined to determine what effect, if any, the matrix has on the immunologic response and nonspecific binding.[2]

VIII. CALIBRATION LINES, LINEARITY, AND DATA REDUCTION

Calibrators or spiked standards are processed along with controls and samples in each analytical run. It is generally anticipated that calibration lines for chromatographic assays will be linear, and those for immunoassays will not be linear with regard to primary instrument response and standard concentrations. However, data reduction in bioanalytical chemistry is not straightforward; and it has been pointed out that assay calibration has, in general, received inadequate attention by analytical laboratories.[4] The discussion of calibration lines, linearity, and data reduction for chromatographic and immunoassays will be presented separately.

A. CHROMATOGRAPHIC ASSAYS

In chromatographic assays the ratio of analyte peak height or area to that of the internal standard peak height or area is the dependent variable which is a function of the analyte concentration, the independent variable. A linear relationship between response and concentration is usually assumed; and the slope, intercept, and correlation coefficient (or its square, the coefficient of determination) of the regression line are calculated using the method of least squares. It is often stated incorrectly in this numerical analysis that a correlation coefficient with a value close to one proves a linear relationship between the response and concentration. It does show that the data fit to a linear model, but this was assumed in the least-squares calculation. A parabolic fit, for example, could also be fitted to the data, possibly obtaining a correlation coefficient closer to one. Demonstrating that the relationship between response and concentration is linear requires more data than obtained from analyzing a single calibration line.[31] However, it is not important that the calibration be linear, only that it fits the linear model within specified limits. After evaluation of the standard line, its shape and intercepts are used to calculate the concentrations of the unknowns.

There are no clear guidelines in the literature for evaluation of standard lines. The correlation coefficient is not suitable for this purpose, and other approaches are preferred.[31] After calculating the calibration line parameters the concentrations of the standards should be back calculated using the observed responses and the standard line parameters. The difference between each calculated and nominal concentration is the residual: this is often expressed as a percent of the nominal value. In a satisfactory standard line the relative residuals should be within specified limits. It is useful to view a plot of response vs. concentration to look for systematic deviations of points from the line and for the presence of outliers. Points should be eliminated from the calibration line only when there is good reason to do so such as outliers and processing errors; points should not be eliminated to force the control values into an acceptable range or to improve the correlation coefficient. Criteria for elimination of points in a standard line are difficult to formulate; thus it is best not to eliminate any points unless the deviation is obviously large. In the author's laboratory a combination of visual observation by an experienced chromatographer along with review of residuals is used to evaluate the points in the line. It has been suggested[3] that no points be eliminated unless the deviant values affect the slope and intercept, but no quantitative criteria are given. Also, it was also pointed out in the same reference that there is cause for concern when more than one or two points have to be eliminated from the standard line.

The standard lines in bioequivalency analyses may extend over a wide concentration range. When the assumed linear calibration line parameters are determined using the method of least squares, the higher concentrations play a greater role in determining the parameters of the calibration line than the lower concentrations. A consequence of this is that when the concentrations of the standards are back calculated using the standard line parameters, there may be a large discrepancy between the actual concentrations and the back calculated concentrations, particularly at the lowest concentrations. This discrepancy is due more to the intercept than the slope and results in a large error when low concentrations are measured. An example is shown in Table 4–1 for taxol.[32] The problem may be overcome in a number of ways. One method is to use the mean response factor of the calibrators, the response factor being the peak height ratio divided by the concentration. This is also shown in Table 4–1. The other method, more commonly used, is weighted linear regression analysis. It is assumed in least-squares analysis that there is no variance in the independent variable (concentration) and constant variance in the dependent variable (ratio). In reality, there is variance in the independent variable which may be considered to be negligibly small; and the variance in the dependent variable is generally proportional to the square of the concentration in bioanalytical assays. Thus, a weighting factor of $1/(\text{concentration})^2$ is appropriate.[33] The results of weighted regression on the taxol data are illustrated in Table 4–1. However, there is no consensus on what is the most appropriate weighting scheme; and 1/(concentration), $1/(\text{concentration})^2$, 1/(ratio), and $1/(\text{ratio})^2$ have been suggested.[1] However, there is usually some sacrifice in the accuracy at the high concentrations, where accuracy is greatest for chromatographic assays, when such weighting schemes are used.[1]

The calibration line in some chromatographic assays, e.g., electron capture detection[34] in a GLC assay, may exhibit significant obvious deviations from linearity. Nonlinear calibration lines can be detected from an examination of the response-concentration plot and the back calculated values of the standards. If the deviations from linearity are reproducible in a number of standard lines, then the response-concentration relationship for that assay cannot be considered linear. It is then appropriate to use a power equation or to divide the data into high and low standard curves.[4]

In summary, it appears to this author that the calibration lines in bioanalytical chemistry are an empirical fit of response to analyte concentration. In most chromatographic assays a weighted linear least squares is satisfactory. Otherwise, a nonlinear fit may be applied if the nonlinearity is reproducible in a given assay.

Table 4–1 **Back calculated concentrations of standards for various weighting schemes expressed as percent of nominal**

Nominal conc μg/ml	Peak height ratio	Concentrations (as percent of nominal) calculated by the method			
		(A) None	(B) 1/C	(C) $1/C^2$	(D) Mean RF
0.52	0.0056	442.3	114.0	100.0	74.7
1.04	0.0147	273.1	110.0	105.8	98.1
2.59	0.0322	149.4	85.3	85.7	86.3
25.9	0.4044	99.7	96.5	100.5	100.3
51.8	0.7923	94.1	94.0	98.2	106.1
104.0	1.599	92.6	94.7	99.0	106.7
166.0	2.865	103.0	106.0	110.2	119.8

Note: (A) = Linear regression, no weighting; (B) = linear regression, 1/concentration weighting; (C) = linear regression, $1/\text{concentration}^2$ weighting; and (D) = mean response factor.

B. IMMUNOASSAYS

In immunoassays the fractions of drug bound (or unbound) to the antibody are dependent on the analyte concentrations. For example, in radioimmunoassay a plot of bound or unbound radioactive analyte vs. concentration is not linear, except possibly over a very small range of concentrations. Numerical transformations of the raw data in many immunoassays yield a linear calibration line. The fraction bound (F), expressed as a percentage, is defined in Equation 4–1:

$$F = \frac{(B - NSB)}{(TB - NSB)} \times 100 \tag{4–1}$$

in which B = radioactivity bound for standard; NSB = nonspecific binding, i.e., binding when no antibody is present; and TB = radioactivity bound for 0 standard.

This relationship is linear over only a very small, often impractical, concentration; and interpolation of concentrations of unknowns from such plots is too subjective and gives no statistical analysis of the precision and accuracy of standard lines. This method was commonly used before the ready availability of computers. Such data can be linearized, however, by transforming the percent bound to its logit F, defined in Equation 4–2, and plotting logit F vs. the logarithm of concentration:

$$\text{logit } F = \ln\left(F/(100 - F)\right) \tag{4–2}$$

Although these calculations can easily be performed on a computer, logit-log graph paper is available and convenient for a rapid screening of the data. This logit-log calculation is objective, and calibration line parameters and statistics can be readily attained. Linearity is most satisfactory for values of F in the range 0.1 to 0.9. Sometimes, even with the logit transformation, curvature may still be obtained and a nonlinear fit of logit and natural logarithm (ln) concentration can be used. In reviewing standard lines in a bioequivalence study using a radioimmunoassay, it is a useful check of run-to-run consistency to calculate the concentration of analyte which produces 50% of the radioactive analyte to the antibody.

Other relationships such as four parameter equations can be used, particularly for enzyme immunoassays and related techniques. These fits are tedious to obtain in a laboratory which has developed the antibody and procedure, and are more often used with commercial kits for which the curve parameters are provided by the manufacturer.

IX. STABILITY

Drug and metabolites may undergo chemical degradation during a bioequivalence study. The administered dosage forms are current lots meeting content and purity specifications. Stability of the drug in stored stock or spiking solutions should be known. In the absence of such stability information fresh solutions should always be used.[2] Once the drug is administered, however, degradation may occur in the body during collection and processing of the blood, during storage, and during sample processing in the assay procedure. In the assay validation, it must be determined that the drug is stable during all these steps; and in addition, it should be determined that the assay will selectively measure the intact drug.

Most drug molecules are inherently stable, but there are some drugs that are so unstable that special precautions must be taken during blood collection and processing. For example, *p*-anisaldehyde has been added to hydralazine[35] and *N*-(4-dimethylamino)maleimide to captopril[36] to stabilize the drugs by derivatization. The derivative may also provide a means of enhancing detectability such as the adduct of *N*-(4-dimethylamino)maleimide with captopril which permits the use of electrochemical detection.

The mechanism of drug instability can be complex (captopril)[37] and subject to a number of factors including light (nifedipine),[38] acids and bases, and temperature (diltiazem).[39] The mechanism of drug degradation need not be known for bioequivalency testing, but stability during sample storage and analysis must be demonstrated.

The whole blood, plasma, serum, or urine is usually stored frozen at –20 or –70°C at which temperatures the drug may not undergo degradation; however, it is required to demonstrate stability during storage and during subsequent thawing and refreezing cycles.[1,2,6] Stability during short-term storage and during freezing and thawing cycles can be determined during validation. It would be more desirable to use actual subject samples for stability testing, but they are not generally available at the time the assay is developed and validated. Actual samples may contain unstable metabolites and conjugates which could degrade or revert to the parent compound. If samples are not to be assayed immediately after being drawn from the test subjects, it is necessary to demonstrate analyte integrity during storage. Matrix spiked with the analyte preferably at two different concentrations should be assayed immediately after preparation and when the study samples are analyzed.[1]

Assay procedures often involve solvent extraction of the drug and related compounds from the acidified or alkalinized biological matrix to which an internal standard has been added. The organic solvent extract is then evaporated with mild heating in a stream of gas, usually nitrogen. For chromatographic assays the residue is reconstituted in a small amount of a solvent (preferably the mobile phase in HPLC assays) and injected into the chromatographic system. The analytical run may be long, and samples may be sitting in an autoinjector for a number of hours. The stability of the analytes and internal standard in the final extracts must be demonstrated.[2] This can readily be accomplished by subjecting spiked samples to the total procedure and reinjecting extracts after an appropriate period of time. This process should be done early in the assay development so that appropriate steps could be taken to stabilize the samples if necessary. For example, taxol has been observed to hydrolyze during sample processing and particularly when the final solutions are waiting to be injected into the chromatographic system, unless the solutions were buffered at about pH 4.[32]

It would appear that the assay should be checked to determine whether degradation products would be detected, i.e., the assay is stability indicating, as is routinely done with dosage form or bulk powder analysis. However, most published validation protocols for assays of drugs in biological matrices do not explicitly demonstrate that the assay is stability indicating by showing that degradation products do not interfere. In a bioanalytical assay it may be difficult to detect small degradation peaks in the presence of the peaks arising from endogenous compounds extracted from the biological matrix. Rather, the evidence for stability is empirical, based on expecting a 100% assay (within experimental variability) result for a spiked sample. This is adequate for most bioanalytical purposes.

In addition to the stability of the analytes and internal standard, there could be stability concerns about other components of the assay such as reagents (e.g., ascorbic acid to be added as antioxidant during an assay) and, importantly, the activity of antisera stored for immunoassays. It is essential in such situations that the reagents be labeled with a realistic expiration date.

X. RECOVERY

Absolute recovery is defined as the amount (expressed as a percentage) of an analyte remaining after the sample has been prepared for analysis. Losses of analyte (and internal standard) during sample preparation can occur by incomplete extraction (partitioning between extraction solvent and aqueous sample), incomplete separation of the phase containing the analytes, incomplete redissolution of the sample from a dried down residue, nonspecific adsorption, and sublimation of volatile compounds. Variability in these losses during the analysis could lead to a loss of precision. Therefore, a quantitative determination of the recovery of the analytes and internal standard is performed during validation. This is readily accomplished by comparing instrument response (e.g., peak heights in a chromatographic assay) of processed samples compared to samples of the same concentration for the analytes and internal standard in the mobile phase injected directly into the system. This should be done at least in duplicate for three concentrations over the assay calibration range. A comparison of the slope of standard lines of samples injected directly compared to the slope of processed samples is also a method which can be used to assess absolute recovery. Absolute recovery of analytes and internal standard ideally should be 100%, but values of 50 to 90% have been stated to be satisfactory.[1] Since accuracy and precision of the method are measured independently of recovery experiments, absolute recovery may have no real value in evaluating a method;[4] however, high absolute recoveries or knowledge of where drug losses occur may contribute to the ruggedness of a method.

The term recovery is sometimes used in a relative sense, i.e., to describe the concentration of analyte obtained after spiked solutions are analyzed, expressed as a percentage of the nominal spiked concentration. This definition of recovery is, however, an expression of accuracy.[4] Also, relative recovery has been stated to be a comparison of the response of the drug in the matrix compared to the response in water.[1]

XI. REASSAYS

Data obtained from analytical runs which do not meet quality control criteria should not be used for any calculations such as pharmacokinetic parameters and stability assessment. For such runs it is appropriate to repeat the assay using fresh portions of standards, quality control samples, and study samples. The situation may occur where although the total run is deemed satisfactory some sample values may be suspect. This is inevitable when assaying a large number of samples for reasons such as (1) samples may have been lost due to processing accidents, (2) interference by extraneous peaks in chromatographic assays, and (3) human error such as omission of internal standard. Obviously, such samples should be reprocessed. Another reason for samples to be reassayed is that the measured concentrations fall outside the range of the calibrator concentrations. It has been stated[6] that no sample results should be considered valid if their concentrations are

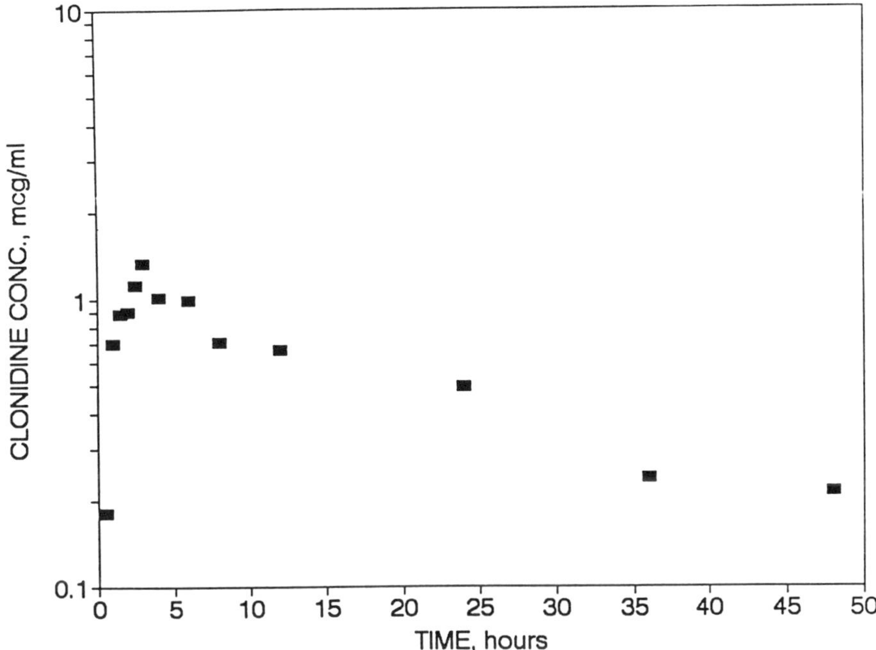

Figure 4–3 An example of a pharmacokinetic profile in which the points do not fall on a smooth curve. Data obtained in a radioimmunoassay for clonidine. (Unpublished data.)

outside the calibrator range. Generally, values below the LOQ are reported as zero. Samples having values above the highest calibrator should be appropriately diluted and reassayed, although it has been implied that extrapolation may be performed within specified limits.[2] A danger with extrapolation is that linearity is assumed but not usually demonstrated in bioanalytical assay methods. Extrapolation should never be used with immunoassay calibration lines.

Sample concentrations may be obtained which do not appear to fit the pharmacokinetic profile. Because of variability in the analytical method, a perfectly smooth profile will not always be obtained. An example is shown in Figure 4–3. Caution should be used in using reassayed values to smooth the pharmacokinetic profile;[6] and reassayed values should only be used when it is determined that the value is clearly an outlier by some statistical test (e.g., it is three standard deviations outside the "expected" value). It is desirable to perform the reassay at least in duplicate to avoid accepting a new value simply because it agrees with what has been anticipated.

It should be established *a priori* under what circumstances samples should be reassayed and when original or reassayed values are to be used. Whenever reassay values are used in the data in a study, the reasons for reassay should be justified in supporting documentation.

Bioequivalence studies submitted to the Health Protection Branch in Canada must include a reassay of 15% of randomly selected study samples as an additional quality control check. These are reported separately and are not included in the bioequivalency statistical calculations.[60]

XII. RUGGEDNESS

Ruggedness of an analytical method is the reproducibility of the method under different conditions.[1] The analytical procedure must be able to withstand minor changes in experimental conditions such as column changes (within the type used for assay development), ordinary room temperature changes, minor changes in mobile-phase composition, and changes of analyst; and to perform equally well with samples of the biological matrix from different sources. Because of differences in specificity and activity of antisera, the determination of ruggedness in immunoassays should include an assessment of the effect of changing batches of antiserum and radioactive analyte, if it is anticipated that different batches may be used.

An assessment of ruggedness should be made during validation and monitored during study sample analysis by observing any changes in instrument responses and trends in the results of quality control samples. In most bioequivalence studies the ruggedness of the method performance between laboratories is not an issue, as it is with compendial methods for dosage form analysis, since a bioequivalence study is a short-term relatively small study in which all the samples are analyzed within one laboratory. However, if a method has not been used for some time, a revalidation — not necessarily as extensive as the original — needs to be performed.

XIII. RECORD KEEPING AND DOCUMENTATION

Since bioequivalency experiments are performed in support of marketing approval applications, all experimentation and documentation must meet requirements of appropriate regulatory agencies. Standard operating procedures (SOPs) must be written for validation, sample storage, analytical procedures including acceptance criteria and data reduction, and review procedures before sample analysis is started. It should be documented that the SOPs are complied with during the performance of the study. Deviations to the SOPs must be explained and approved in writing. There must be complete instrument and equipment maintenance and calibration. All data, positive or negative, should be maintained and reported where appropriate. There should be an explanation why any data obtained are not used in the conclusions. Much of the analytical data obtained in bioequivalency studies is processed from collection of raw data to final calculations by computerized techniques. The computer systems must be demonstrated to be free from programming errors, operator errors must be readily detectable, and the system must be secure to prevent tampering and arbitrary manipulation of the data. Long-term data storage and integrity is assured.

REFERENCES

1. **Karnes, H. T., Shiu, G., and Shah, V. P.,** Validation of bioanalytical methods, *Pharm. Res.,* 8, 421, 1991.
2. **Buick, A. R., Doig, M. V., Jeal, S. C., Land, G. S., and McDowall, R. D.,** Method validation in the bioanalytical laboratory, *J. Pharm. Biomed. Anal.,* 8, 629, 1990.
3. **Causey, A. G., Hill, H. M., and Phillips, L. J.,** Evaluation of criteria for the acceptance of bioanalytical data, *J. Pharm. Biomed. Anal.,* 8, 625, 1990.
4. **Dighe, S. V. and Adams, W. P.,** in *Pharmaceutical Bioequivalence,* Welling, P. G., Tse, F. L. S., and Dighe, S. V., Eds., Marcel Dekker, New York, 1991, 347.
5. **Brooks, M. A. and Weinfeld, R. E.,** A validation process for data from the analysis of drugs in biological fluids, *Drug. Dev. Ind. Pharm.,* 11, 1703, 1985.
6. **Shah, V. P., Midha, K. K., Dighe, S., McGilveray, I. J., Skelly, J. P., Yacobi, A., Layloff, T., Viswanathan, C. T., Cook, C. E., McDowall, R. D., Pittman, K. A., and Spector, S.,** Analytical methods validation: bioavailability, bioequivalence, and pharmacokinetic studies, *J. Pharm. Sci.,* 81, 309, 1992.
7. **Snyder, L. R., Glajch, J. L., and Kirkland, J. J., Eds.,** *Practical HPLC Method Development,* John Wiley & Sons, New York, 1988.

8. **Carr, G. P. and Wahlich, J. C.,** A practical approach to method validation in pharmaceutical analysis, *J. Pharm. Biomed. Anal.,* 8, 613, 1990.
9. **Midha, K. K., McKay, G., Chakraborty, B. S., Young, M., Hawes, E. M., Hubbard, J. W., Cooper, J. K., and Korchinski, E. D.,** Bioequivalence of two thorazine tablet formulations using radioimmunoassay and gas chromatographic-mass spectrometric methods, *J. Pharm. Sci.,* 79, 196, 1990.
10. **Adamovics, J. A., Ed.,** *Chromatographic Analysis of Pharmaceuticals,* Chromatographic Science Series No. 52, Marcel Dekker, New York, 1990.
11. **Smith, R. V. and Stewart, J. T., Eds.,** *Textbook of Biopharmaceutical Analysis,* Lea & Febiger, Philadelphia, 1981, 50.
12. **Szepesi, G., Ed.,** *HPLC in Pharmaceutical Analysis,* Vol. 1, CRC Press, Boca Raton, FL, 1990.
13. **Kirschbaum, J. J. and Aszalos, A.,** in *Modern Analysis of Antibiotics, Drugs and the Pharmaceutical Sciences,* Marcel Dekker, New York, 1986, 239.
14. **Snyder, L. R. and Kirkland, J. J., Eds.,** *Introduction to Modern Liquid Chromatography,* Wiley Interscience, New York, 1979.
15. **Alexander, T. G.,** in *Modern Analysis of Antibiotics, Drugs and the Pharmaceutical Sciences,* Vol. 27, Marcel Decker, New York, 1986, 1.
16. **Jennings, W., Ed.,** *Analytical Gas Chromatography,* Academic Press, San Diego, 1987, 18; *Drugs and the Pharmaceutical Sciences,* Vol. 27, Marcel Dekker, New York, 1986.
17. **Smith, R. V. and Stewart, J. T., Eds.,** *Textbook of Biopharmaceutical Analysis,* Lea & Febiger, Philadelphia, 1981, 224.
18. **Dixon, D. E., Steiner, S. J., and Katz, S. E.,** in *Modern Analysis of Antibiotics, Drugs and the Pharmaceutical Sciences,* Vol. 27, Marcel Dekker, New York, 1986, 415.
19. **Breitig, D. and Voight, K. H.,** in *Treatise on Analytical Chemistry, Part I,* Vol. 14, 2nd ed., Elving, P. J., Ed., Wiley Interscience, New York, 1986, 285.
20. **McKay, G., Steeves, T., Cooper, J. K., Hawes, E. M., and Midha, K. K.,** Development and application of a radioimmunoassay for fluphenazine based on monoclonal antibodies and its comparison with alternate assay methods, *J. Pharm. Sci.,* 79, 240, 1990.
21. **Lo, E. S., Fein, M., Hunter, C., Suckow, R. F., and Cooper, T. B.,** A Highly Sensitive and Specific Radioimmunoassay for Quantitation of Plasma Fluphenazine, *J. Pharm. Sci.,* 77, 255, 1988.
22. **Eadon, G. A.** in *Treatise on Analytical Chemistry, Part I,* Vol. 11, 2nd ed., Winefordner, J. D., Ed., Wiley Interscience, New York, 1989, 1.
23. **Smith, R. V. and Stewart, J. T., Eds.,** *Textbook of Biopharmaceutical Analysis,* Lea & Febiger, Philadelphia, 1981, 249.
24. **Platt, T. B.,** in *Modern Analysis of Antibiotics, Drugs and the Pharmaceutical Sciences,* Vol. 27, Marcel Dekker, New York, 1986, 341.
25. **Gaffney, M.,** Variance components in comparative bioavailability studies, *J. Pharm. Sci.,* 81, 315, 1992.
26. U.S. Pharmacopeia National Formulary.
27. American Clinical Laboratory, 1991 Buyers' Guide, 1990.
28. **Rutledge, D. R. and Garrick, C.,** Determination of metoprolol and its alpha-hydroxide metabolite in serum by reversed-phase high-performance liquid chromatography, *J. Chromatogr. Sci.,* 27, 561, 1989.
29. **Bressolle, F., Bres, J., and Moulin, A.,** High-performance liquid chromatographic determination of 4-amino-5-chloro-*N*-[(1-ethylimidozolin-2-yl)methyl]-2-methoxybenzamide and its metabolite in biological fluids, applications in pharmacokinetic studies, *J. Pharm. Sci,* 79, 534, 1990.

30. **Arndts, D., Stahle, H., and Struck, C. J.,** A Newly Developed Precise and Sensitive Radioimmunoassay for Clonidine, *Arzneim. Forsch.,* 29, 532, 1979.
31. **Aarons, L., Toon, S., and Rowland, M.,** Validation of assay methodology used in pharmacokinetic studies, *J. Pharmacol. Methods,* 17, 337, 1987.
32. **Leslie, J., Kujawa, J., Eddington, N., Egorin, M., and Eiseman, J.,** *Pharm. Biomed. Anal.,* 11, 1349, 1993.
33. **Bolton, S., Ed.,** *Pharmaceutical Statistics, Drugs and the Pharmaceutical Sciences,* Vol. 44, 2nd ed., Marcel Dekker, New York, 1990, 234.
34. Electron Capture Handbook, Hewlett-Packard, 1971.
35. **Ludden, T. M., Rotenberg, K. S., Ludden, L. K., Shepherd, A. M. M., and Woodworth, J. R.,** Relative bioavailability of immediate- and sustained-release hydralazine formulations, *J. Pharm. Sci.,* 77, 1026, 1988.
36. **Shimada, K., Tanaka, M., Nambara, T., Imai, Y., Abe, K., and Yoshinaga, K.,** Determination of captopril in human blood by high-performance liquid chromatography with electrochemical detection, *J. Chromatogr.* 227, 445, 1982.
37. **Timmins, P., Jackson, I. M., and Wang, Y. J.,** Factors affecting captopril stability in aqueous solution, *Int. J. Pharm.,* 11, 329, 1982.
38. **Schmid, B. J., Perry, H. E., and Idle, J. R.,** Determination of nifedipine and its three principal metabolites in plasma and urine by automated electron-capture capillary gas chromatography, *J. Chromatogr.,* 425, 107, 1988.
39. **Bonnefous, J.-L., Boulieu, R., and Lahet, C.,** Stability of diltiazem and its metabolites in human blood samples, *J. Pharm. Sci.,* 81, 341, 1992.
40. **McGilveray, I. J.,** in *Pharmaceutical Bioequivalence,* Welling, P. G., Tse, F. L. S., and Dighe, S. V., Eds., Marcel Dekker, New York, 1991, 381.

Chapter 5

Pharmacodynamics and Bioequivalence

Nicholas H. G. Holford

CONTENTS

0-8493-6930-4/94/$0.00+$.50

I. INTRODUCTION

A. PHARMACOKINETICS AND PHARMACODYNAMICS

The study of drugs *in vivo* is conveniently divided into *pharmacokinetics* and *pharmacodynamics*. Pharmacokinetics includes the description of the relationship between dose and concentration while pharmacodynamics describes the relationship between concentration and effect. Using these definitions the distinction between pharmacokinetics and pharmacodynamics rests on the definition of concentration. There are two obvious sites which must be considered when defining concentration — the first is at the site of action of the drug (the effect compartment) and the second is that predicted by a pharmacokinetic model (usually the central compartment). For many practical purposes these may be indistinguishable, but it is important to realize that the effect compartment concentration can only be defined by observing a drug effect while the central compartment concentration can be defined without reference to a drug effect.

B. BIOAVAILABILITY AND BIOEQUIVALENCE

What has the distinction between pharmacokinetics and pharmacodynamics to do with *bioavailability* and *bioequivalence?* Bioavailability has a regulatory definition that includes both the extent and rate of drug absorption. The extent of bioavailability may be defined as the fraction of the administered dose which reaches the systemic circulation. The rate of bioavailability is most commonly described by the time to reach the maximum concentration after a dose. Both the rate and extent of bioavailability are defined in pharmacokinetic terms relating to amounts or concentrations in the body, i.e., bioavailability is a pharmacokinetic concept alone.

Bioequivalence is a more complex object, but with only three values — true, false, or undetermined. It can be applied to any pharmacokinetic or pharmacodynamic parameter which characterizes the concentrations or effects arising from a test preparation of a drug. A parameter is bioequivalent if the test preparation value lies within an equivalence interval defined in relation to a reference preparation. The probability that a parameter lies within the equivalence interval can be determined using a variety of statistical procedures (see Chapter 1) which hinge on the central tendency and variability of the parameter in the test and reference samples.

Three kinds of studies can be considered which shed different light on bioequivalence issues. These are therapeutic equivalence, pharmacokinetic equivalence, and pharmacodynamic equivalence. Each study provides a different set of parameters which can be used for an equivalence statement.

C. THERAPEUTIC EQUIVALENCE: THE GOLD STANDARD

There are several important reasons for asserting the bioequivalence of a formulation which have been discussed elsewhere in this volume (see Chapters 1 and 2). The gold standard for bioequivalence is to demonstrate that the intended therapeutic effect and adverse effects of the test formulation are equivalent to the reference formulation. A therapeutic trial could be mounted to compare the outcome when patients are treated with both formulations. There are important reasons why this approach is not used in the first instance. High among these is the ethical problem of using the test medicine for treatment when its equivalence is in doubt. In this setting there can be no benefit to the patient. At best the test preparation may be equivalent, but there is necessarily a risk that it might not be equivalent; and this is a risk that can be minimized by not exposing the patient to the test formulation without some supporting evidence, e.g., from a pharmacokinetic bioequivalence study. The therapeutic trial will also have difficulties in demonstrating equivalence with regard to uncommon adverse effects because of the large number of subjects that would need to be studied.

D. PHARMACOKINETIC EQUIVALENCE: A THEORETICALLY SOUND SUBSTITUTE

Presumptive evidence for therapeutic bioequivalence may be derived by demonstrating equivalence of formulation-dependent pharmacokinetic parameters. If the pharmacokinetics of the test formulation are similar to the reference, then it is highly likely that therapeutic bioequivalence will exist. The theoretical basis connecting a given time-concentration profile to the ensuing range of drug effects is very strong. There are limitations, however, if formulation-related factors such as packaging, tablet color, or manufacturer reputation may also influence the patient's response.

A different situation may exist if the test formulation is shown to be equivalent using the conventional 80 to 120% equivalence interval, but nevertheless is significantly different (e.g., the maximum concentration). When the drug response is related to concentration by a steep concentration-effect curve, there may appear to be a threshold concentration for response. In this case a 20% lower concentration arising from the test formulation may translate into a greater than 20% difference in a therapeutic response parameter.[1] Of course, this situation is only important when the conventional equivalence interval is determined without a rational basis in pharmacodynamics.

E. PHARMACODYNAMIC EQUIVALENCE: A THERAPEUTIC SURROGATE

It is sometimes possible to measure a drug effect which is a surrogate for the therapeutic effect, e.g., lowering of blood pressure is a surrogate for the desired therapeutic effect of reducing the risk of vascular events such as stroke and myocardial infarction associated with hypertension. The limitations of this approach arise in two main areas: the strength of the association between the surrogate effect and the therapeutic effect, and the difficulty of using pharmacodynamic parameters to assert equivalence. While decisions regarding the primary presumption of therapeutic effectiveness for a chemical entity are frequently based on surrogate markers, the use of a surrogate for an equivalence decision does not have the strength of one based on active drug concentration (itself a form of surrogate marker). This is because the surrogate effect will be only one of the effects of the drug — either beneficial or adverse — and its dynamic range may be quite different from that for an adverse effect.

II. PHARMACOKINETIC-PHARMACODYNAMIC MODELS

Models for describing the time course of drug effects have been described in detail elsewhere.[1,2] For the purposes of this discussion some central ideas will be reviewed with respect to those pharmacokinetic properties that are relevant to the assessment of bioequivalence in the absence of directly measured drug concentrations.

A. PHARMACOKINETIC MODELS

1. Noncompartmental

Noncompartmental models (sometimes wrongly described as model-independent methods) are largely based on the recirculatory model.[3] They provide a convenient tool for estimating the extent of bioavailability, F, through the area under the concentration curve, AUC_c, approach. The rate of bioavailability can also be described by the mean input time. Estimation of this parameter requires treatment with a preparation with defined input time in order to determine the mean disposition time of the drug.

The mean residence times (sum of mean input time and mean disposition time) could be compared for equivalence; however, because this parameter is derived from at least three functionally separate properties (volume of distribution, clearance, and input process), intersubject variability is usually too large to allow adequate sensitivity to conclude equivalence.

These noncompartmental parameters are of limited use in describing the time course of drug effect. In some instances it may be reasonable to use the AUC_c as a measure of drug exposure within some defined interval, and it may be possible to use this to estimate the parameters of a pharmacodynamic model. This is particularly appropriate when the time course of changes in drug effect are much slower than the time course of drug concentrations after each dose, e.g., the delayed effects which contribute to lowering of blood pressure after treatment with an angiotensin-converting enzyme (ACE) inhibitor require several days to be observed while ACE inhibitors commonly have half-lives of only a few hours. In the absence of drug concentration measurements, the AUC_c or (perhaps preferably) the average steady state concentration, $C_{ss,avg}$, can be predicted from a noncompartmental model using the dose rate and clearance/F as a parameter.

2. Compartmental

Compartmental models provide a well-understood basis for describing the processes of drug input and disposition. For bioequivalence assessment it is preferable to parameterize disposition in terms of clearance/F because this parameter is usually used to provide information about the extent of bioavailability. Bioavailability can be estimated without assuming constant clearance when two formulations are compared, but these approaches may be less robust.[4]

The choice of drug input model will necessarily be a simplification of the true input process, but first-order or zero-order input models can provide estimates for comparing rate of bioavailability that are less biased than the usual maximum measured value method. Compartmental models lend themselves readily to the efficient prediction of effect compartment concentrations.

3. Physiological

Models which incorporate organ blood flow and other physiological/anatomic features can provide valuable insight, but are generally impractical for bioequivalence evaluation because of the need to assume or measure many parameters related only to drug disposition.

Hybrid compartmental models which incorporate physiological features may be helpful in describing first-pass extraction and thus bioavailability; but at present these are likely to be limited to purely pharmacokinetic equivalence studies.

B. PHARMACOKINETIC-PHARMACODYNAMIC LINK MODELS

The link between concentration predicted from a pharmacokinetic model and the concentration at the site of the drug effect has been recognized as an essential step in recognizing a variety of phenomena that determine the time course of drug effect. In this context the pharmacokinetic model is one sufficient to account for the time course of measurable drug concentrations, but does not require that concentrations have actually been measured. For simplicity such concentrations will be referred to as C_{pk}.

1. The Instantaneous Link

An instantaneous link between concentration predicted by a pharmacokinetic model and the concentration at the site of action may be a reasonable description of events when there is no perceptible delay in onset of drug effect in relation to C_{pk}. This is the simplest way to link concentrations to effects because C_{pk} and the effect site concentration are always identical.

2. The Effect Compartment

An instantaneous link is often not realistic, however, because C_{pk} and the effect site concentration, C_e, are generally not identical. The effect compartment model[5] has been widely used to link C_{pk} to effects when the drug effects are delayed in relation to C_{pk} (hysteresis). If the concentration in a compartment linked by a first-order process to the site of C_{pk} is kinetically identical with the concentrations at the site of action of the drug, it is known as the effect compartment; and the concentrations are effect compartment concentrations, C_e. C_e is predicted by the solution to the differential equation:

$$\frac{dC_e}{dt} = K_{eq} \cdot \left(C_{pk} - C_e\right) \tag{5–1}$$

The only additional parameter required is an equilibrium rate constant, K_{eq}, which controls the exit rate of drug from the effect compartment.

The K_{eq} parameter can be estimated given a procedure for predicting C_{pk} as a continuous function of time (e.g., a compartmental model) or by interpolation between measured concentrations. A fully parametric approach would involve a parametric pharmacokinetic model and a parametric pharmacodynamic model. Methods for describing the kinetics of an effect compartment that do not rely on parametric pharmacokinetic and pharmacodynamic models have recently been reviewed.[6] While these semiparametric methods can be useful for exploring the shape of the concentration-effect relationship, they appear to be of limited use for bioequivalence studies because K_{eq} is the only parameter that can be derived to compare test and reference formulations.

C. PHARMACODYNAMIC MODELS

The relationship between drug concentration, C_e, at the effect site and the consequent effect of the drug, E, can usually be described by one of three models.

1. Sigmoid E_{max}

$$E = E_0 + \frac{E_{max} \cdot C_e^N}{EC_{50}^N + C_e^N} \tag{5–2}$$

where E_0 is the response in the absence of drug, E_{max} is the maximum effect produced by the drug and EC_{50} is the concentration producing 50% of E_{max}. The steepness of the curve, particularly around the EC_{50}, is controlled by the Hill coefficient, N. Values of N greater than 1 give rise to an S-shaped curve, hence, the name sigmoid E_{max} model.

2. E_{max}

$$E = E_0 + \frac{E_{max} \cdot C_e}{EC_{50} + C_e} \tag{5–3}$$

A simpler form of the sigmoid E_{max} model is obtained when the Hill coefficient is equal to 1. This model is identical to that describing receptor/binding site interactions with a drug or ligand and has a firm theoretical basis in the law of mass action.

3. Linear

$$E = E_0 + S \cdot C_e \tag{5–4}$$

When concentrations are much less than the EC_{50}, the E_{max} model can be simplified further to define a linear relationship between effect and concentration. The parameter S is the slope of the line.

D. PHYSIOLOGICAL MEDIATOR KINETICS

The ability to predict the time course of drug action at the effect site using pharmacokinetic, link, and pharmacodynamic models is not necessarily sufficient to describe the observed drug response. Most observed drug responses are based on the measurement of some physiological function that is modified by the action of the drug at its effect site. The time course of the physiological response will add a further delay to the expression of the drug effect. Often this can be thought of in terms of the half-life of a physiological mediator for which synthesis or elimination is changed by the drug.[7]

For example, the drop in blood pressure produced by an angiotensin-converting enzyme (ACE) inhibitor can only be observed after the synthesis of angiotensin II has been inhibited and the concentration of angiotensin II at its vascular receptor has been reduced by its removal. In this case, the time course of angiotensin II changes are sufficiently rapid that the observed response may appear to be instantaneously related to the ACE inhibitor concentration in plasma. The longer term changes in blood pressure which are a consequence of changes in sodium clearance will, however, take a week or longer to reach equilibrium[8] so that plasma concentrations will be clearly separated from this effect.

III. PHARMACODYNAMIC ASSAY

Because of the central role of concentration in both pharmacokinetics and pharmacodynamics, the limitations of attempting to predict concentration using measurements of drug effects need to be discussed.

A. *EX VIVO* PHARMACODYNAMIC ASSAY

1. Calibration Model

The first problem to be overcome is to define a suitable calibration curve model. Physicochemical analytical techniques can usually be based on a linear relationship between concentration and the assay output, e.g., absorbance from a spectrophotometer. Receptor/binding site-blocking assays will inevitably be nonlinear. The linearizing transformations that are often applied to ligand-binding curves introduce biases into the predicted concentration unless a suitable, usually nonlinear, model for the error (weighting function) is also used. Nevertheless, if the need for a nonlinear error model is recognized, it will usually be easier to implement a model for the ligand-binding curve as a nonlinear regression problem. *Bioassay of drug concentrations usually requires a nonlinear model and nonlinear regression.*

2. Specificity

The second problem introduced by a bioassay procedure is lack of specificity. It is essential that bioavailability is estimated from a specific measurement of the drug. Nearly all drugs that are readily absorbed from the gastrointestinal tract (GI) will undergo some degree of biotransformation. The metabolite that is formed will necessarily be structurally similar to the parent compound and be a highly probable candidate for interaction with a ligand-binding site. It is usually the rule that not all drug metabolites have been characterized, and in the early stages of drug development (when bioavailability studies are often needed most) even major metabolites may not have been identified. In the situation where a bioassay must be performed to try and measure the parent species, it is even more likely that metabolites will not be known and the specificity of the *ex vivo* bioassay cannot be verified. *When bioassay is needed, the specificity of the measurement will always be in doubt and bioavailability of the parent compound will usually be overestimated.*

3. Sensitivity

Binding assays will have a limited dynamic range requiring dilution of samples containing concentrations which displace greater than ca. 80% of the measurable ligand. Attention must then be paid to the nature of the error introduced into the assay by the dilution and other processing steps.

B. *IN VIVO* PHARMACODYNAMIC ASSAY

In vivo bioassays can be performed in two ways. A *homo*assay uses drug effects measured in the same individual during exposure to the dose for which bioavailability is being studied. A *hetero*assay involves the administration of a sample obtained from an individual participating in the bioavailability study to a second individual who is used to determine the effect arising from that particular sample. This *meta*-assay process will then depend on knowing the bioavailability in the second individual — a potentially recursive process eventually requiring a call to GOD.[9] This difficulty may be overcome by parenteral administration usually to a small animal species.

1. Calibration Model

The calibration curve model is more difficult to define when it is based on measurements of drug effects *in vivo*. A calibration curve is defined in terms of effect site concentration and the measurable drug effect. The problem of predicting the effect site concentration is dealt with below, but information about the calibration curve model (or pharmacodynamic model) is necessarily dependent on the assumptions made to predict effect site concentration. Unlike the *ex vivo* assay system, it is not possible to study the response to each concentration independently of previous responses. The notional calibration curve may change as time passes, as a consequence of physiological homeostatic responses, which may manifest as tolerance to the drug effect (i.e., diminished drug effects at the same concentration at later times). These problems can be formidable to resolve even when drug concentrations can be measured directly. It would seem to be highly unlikely that they can even be detected in the situation where the effect is being used to deduce the drug concentration itself by the use of a homoassay. Heteroassays will usually involve replication of a calibration curve using known doses bracketing the unknown sample. This can be used as a check on the shape and the stationarity of the calibration curve. *The stationarity of the calibration curve will usually be in doubt when in vivo homobioassay is attempted.*

2. Specificity

The specificity of the drug effect as a measure of the drug concentration will be in doubt for reasons similar to those described above for *ex vivo* bioassays. However, the situation may be less severe when the measured effect is based on activity as an agonist because biotransformation is more likely to produce an inactive compound. These inactive compounds using an agonist system may be detected by an *ex vivo* assay based on ligand binding.

3. Sensitivity

Because of the generally nonlinear relationship between concentration and effect, the bioassay has poor sensitivity when the effect is greater than 80% of the maximum. A relatively large change in concentration will produce a relatively small change in effect, e.g., concentrations in the range of 4 times the EC_{50} to 10 times the EC_{50} (a 250% change) will have effects differing by less than 10%. Unlike the *in vitro* bioassay it is not possible to dilute the sample into a more sensitive range. If the concentration-effect curve is steep, e.g., the Hill coefficient of a sigmoid E_{max} model is 5 or greater, the assay will be insensitive both at low and high concentrations and very sensitive in the middle.

The problem of sensitivity and relatively narrow dynamic range is potentially important when an adverse drug effect has a different dynamic range from the effect used in the bioassay. The peak concentration from a test product could be twice as high as the reference and be associated with a high risk of an adverse effect. If the peak concentrations of both products produce bioassay effects that are greater than 80% of the maximum, it could be relatively easy to conclude equivalence for the peak bioassay effect when the peak concentration-related adverse effects of the two products are very different.

4. Effect Site Concentration

Calibration curves (pharmacodynamic models) are implicitly independent of time. The equilibration of drug between the systemic circulation and the site of action will be a time-dependent process. The systemic circulation concentration will not be proportional to the effect site concentration until equilibration has been achieved. The effect site concentration predicted from the calibration curve at any time (even at equilibrium) can be produced by a limitless set of systemic circulation concentration profiles. *In the absence of prior information about the systemic concentration profile it is impossible to predict the systemic concentrations from effects without assuming instantaneous equilibration.* This is a major limitation of bioassay methods which are to be used to define the rate of drug input.

5. Physiological Links

The action of a drug *in vivo* always requires the involvement of a chain of physiological processes before an observable response can be measured. The information about systemic concentrations of a drug as reflected in the observed drug response will therefore change depending on the time scale of the observations. Delayed drug effects due to modifications in physiological processes produce similar problems to those mentioned earlier under the heading of effect site concentration.

IV. BIOEQUIVALENCE

A. BIOAVAILABILITY

Bioavailability is purely a pharmacokinetic concept. It has nothing to do with drug effect. Its determination rests only on the ability to describe the rate and extent of absorption of a drug into the systemic circulation.

1. Extent

In terms of linear pharmacokinetic models, the extent can be computed from the integral of the concentrations predicted in the compartment representing the systemic circulation — the area under the curve or AUC approach. For drugs with nonlinear pharmacokinetics, it may be necessary to estimate the extent of bioavailability more directly by integrating the instantaneous input rate into the systemic circulation which usually requires a model for first-pass extraction. Bioavailability is estimated from measurements which are able to predict the integral of systemic concentrations (or input rates). Most commonly this is done using blood samples (usually venous but sometimes arterial) which can be used to measure the concentration in a compartment closely linked to the systemic circulation. If linear pharmacokinetics can be assumed, it is possible to obtain a measure of extent of absorption that is directly proportional to the true extent by collecting the drug that has been eliminated, e.g., in the urine. Absolute bioavailability can then be estimated by comparison with the amount eliminated after a parenteral dose.

2. Rate

Rate of bioavailability is always defined in terms of a description of a time-concentration profile. The usual approach is to estimate the time of maximum concentration from the time of the sample with the highest measured concentration. Except by chance this will never be the actual time of the maximum. The time of the maximum can be estimated with less bias by interpolation of the measured concentrations or by using an explicit model for concentration.

These methods for estimating bioavailability all require the ability to measure the drug in an accessible biological fluid. It is conceivable that bioavailability is to be studied in humans in the absence of a suitable analytical procedure, but this is very unlikely given the current state of technology and widespread expertise. However, should such a situation arise, then drug concentrations could be measured by a form of bioassay that relies on measuring drug effects. It may be feasible to measure an effect *ex vivo,* and radio-receptor assays or radioimmunoassay can be thought of in this category. In this instance, the drug effect is the ability to block binding to a receptor or binding site. Although such techniques are usually considered part of the class of conventional analytical methods, such as HPLC, they possess properties similar to those discussed earlier (Section III).

3. Area under the Effect Curve

It may be thought that the extent of absorption may be estimated from the area under the effect curve (AUC_e) because this is a time-independent parameter and the integral of the time-effect profile will reflect systemic exposure. Indeed it will, but the AUC_e will be proportional to systemic bioavailability only if there is a linear relationship between systemic concentration and observed effect, i.e., a linear pharmacodynamic model. Extent of bioavailability *can* be calculated from nonlinear drug effects, but only after a suitable calibration curve has been used to transform the measured effects into the equivalent systemic concentrations and bioavailability parameters calculated from the predicted concentrations.

B. NONSYSTEMICALLY EFFECTIVE MEDICINES

The evaluation of bioequivalence for nonsystemically effective medicines poses difficulties for establishing pharmacokinetic equivalence. The dose of these medicines is usually small because their effects are limited to a specific region or organ of the body, and the distribution volume required to achieve an effective concentration is smaller. Because the dose is small, it may be technically difficult to measure systemic concentrations adequately. However, even if analytical difficulties can be overcome, there are more fundamental issues to be addressed.

The pharmacokinetics of distribution from the site of application to the effect site will determine the intensity and time course of the desired local effect. Local adverse effects will be determined by the same processes, but systemic adverse effects will be reflected in the time course of concentrations in the systemic circulation.

Apart from the medicine itself, which necessarily will be the same in the test and reference products, there may be several other components which may vary among formulations and have an important effect on the kinetics of absorption. While these will also be present in systemically effective formulations, their influence on bioavailability can be adequately assessed using a systemic pharmacokinetic equivalence study. It is, of course, possible that a nonmedicine component of a systemically effective medicine could give rise to adverse effects. These adverse effects can only be detected by a therapeutic equivalence study.

Systemic effects will usually be considered adverse effects and be relatively infrequent in the reference product. As indicated earlier therapeutic equivalence, i.e., a clinical trial, will be fraught with difficulty in establishing equivalence of the incidence of adverse effects. The combination of a pharmacodynamic equivalence based on effects at the site of application and a systemic pharmacokinetic equivalence study would appear to be a realistic alternative to a therapeutic equivalence trial.

1. Skin

The rate and extent of absorption of a medicine from a topical preparation into the skin from stratum corneum to systemic circulation will be determined by formulation-dependent factors that may modify skin permeability and blood flow. Systemic effects (such as adrenocortical suppression from topical glucocorticoids) are well known; but apart from unusual uses (such as extensive application under occlusion), the equivalence of such effects will be difficult to assert. A systemic pharmacokinetic equivalence study of a corticosteroid would provide valuable reassurance about equivalence of adverse effects if concentrations can be measured after application of a typical dose.

2. Lung

Topical application to the lungs, e.g., bronchodilators or antiallergic agents, may provide an opportunity to establish systemic pharmacokinetic equivalence. The extent of absorption of the medicine via the respiratory tract compared with the alimentary tract may be an important determinant of the desired therapeutic effect. Differences in design of an inhaler, for example, may deliver different droplet sizes or dispersion patterns even though the device may appear to be physically similar. These determinants of delivery may influence the extent of pulmonary deposition and thus therapeutic effect. It is possible that systemic pharmacokinetic equivalence criteria may be met while clinically relevant effects are not equivalent. Thus a pharmacodynamic equivalence criterion is also required using an effect such as peak expiratory flow rate.

The recent demonstration of a systemic concentration-effect relationship after pulmonary inhalation of terbutaline, a β-agonist bronchodilator, throws light on the correlation between the time course of effect site and plasma concentrations for β-agonists.[10] If confirmed for another agent in this class, this kind of observation would provide strong support for basing equivalence of these agents on a systemic pharmacokinetic study. Systemic pharmacokinetic equivalence would be a valuable prerequisite for these agents in any event because most potentially serious adverse effects (hypokalemia, tachycardia, arrhythmias) are consequent on systemic exposure. It might even be argued that the rationale for a systemic pharmacokinetic equivalence study is more strongly based for inhaled β-agonists than for other systemically administered drugs which have not had their concentration-effect relationships elucidated.

Pharmacokinetic interactions, apparently at the site of absorption in the lung, have been demonstrated for nedocromil sodium, an anti-inflammatory agent administered by dry powder inhalation.[11] The ability to use systemic concentrations as a marker of the rate of absorption from the lung, presumably close to the site of action, indicates that a pharmacokinetic equivalence study might be sufficient for agents in this class.

3. Eye

Ophthalmic application of medicines is used for local benefit, but in many cases it must be assumed that rapid absorption into the systemic circulation will follow. The use of systemic pharmacokinetic equivalence would appear to be appropriate for ophthalmic formulations of β adrenoceptor blocking agents that have readily detectable systemic adverse effects.[12] If a reliable association can be demonstrated between the time course of systemic concentrations and the local (therapeutic or surrogate) effect, e.g., reduction in intraocular pressure, then a systemic pharmacokinetic equivalence study with a limited pharmacodynamic (surrogate effect) demonstration of equivalence may be sufficient. The lowering of intraocular pressure in the contralateral untreated eye[12] and the ability to measure timolol concentrations typical of those after ophthalmic application[13] imply that serious attention be paid to the use of a systemic pharmacokinetic equivalence study for beta blockers that enter the systemic circulation.

4. Gastrointestinal Tract

As for other topical sites of application, equivalence of systemic adverse effects is difficult to conclude on the basis of equivalence of a clinical effect. If a systemic pharmacokinetic equivalence study is feasible, then this should be required if systemic effects are potentially serious. For example, the long-term systemic consequences of the use of bismuth salts are still controversial. If a test formulation had a clearly greater systemic extent of absorption, then it should not be considered equivalent. Effectiveness in healing peptic disease is an inadequate criterion for concluding equivalence because it cannot exclude the risk of systemic adverse effects.

V. ROLE OF PHARMACODYNAMICS IN DEFINING EQUIVALENCE CRITERIA

The most important role of pharmacodynamics in bioequivalence evaluation is not as a substitute for therapeutic or pharmacokinetic equivalence studies but as a rational basis for defining equivalence criteria.

In the simplest case equivalence criteria are defined by upper and lower bounds for an equivalence interval. There will also be an associated statistical criterion based on the probability of rejecting an equivalence hypothesis. Statistical aspects of equivalence determination are discussed elsewhere (see Chapter 1).

The traditional equivalence interval of 80 to 120% for differences or 80 to 125% for ratios of test and reference parameters is an arbitrary construction. It is widely accepted and has an intuitively reasonable quality to it. The intuitive assumption is that the therapeutic effectiveness of the formulation will be defined by this interval. That this assumption is incorrect is discussed below. Pharmacodynamic theory can provide some insight into rational deviations from the traditional standard.[16]

A. DIFFERENT PARAMETER, DIFFERENT INTERVAL?

The therapeutic benefits of allopurinol in the management of hyperuricemia are a consequence of the inhibition of xanthine oxidase and the subsequent decrease in uric acid synthesis. In the management of tophaceous gout, the benefit of decreased uric acid synthesis takes several weeks to become evident as urate deposits in the tissues are mobilized and urate is eliminated. It would seem highly unreasonable that the peak extent of inhibition of xanthine oxidase after each dose would be closely related to the eventual outcome. More likely it is more closely related to the average extent of inhibition of urate production over the steady-state dosing interval. If an allopurinol test formulation meets the 80 to 120% equivalence criterion using oxypurinol (the active metabolite) AUC_c, then it would be reasonable to suppose that the consequent therapeutic effects would also be within this interval (but see comments below on symmetrical equivalence intervals). The rate of bioavailability is irrelevant given the lack of adverse effects associated with the concentration profile within a dosing interval.

On the other hand, even though effects may be delayed the pattern of a concentration profile within a dosing interval may be important. It is well known that aminoglycosides administered intermittently are less likely to produce renal damage than a continuous infusion producing the same AUC_c.[15] In this instance, the mechanism of renal damage depends on saturable transport into the renal cortex. The transport mechanism is therefore less efficient at high concentrations after intermittent doses, and less cortical drug accumulation occurs.

B. ASYMMETRICAL PHARMACOKINETIC INTERVALS

Symmetrical equivalence intervals for pharmacokinetic parameters would appear to be irrational for drugs with pharmacodynamics that are known to be nonlinear. If the underlying goal of a pharmacokinetic equivalence interval is to predict a symmetrical therapeutic equivalence interval, the nonlinear relationship between concentration and therapeutic effect should be recognized. For example, if the reference preparation produces a peak concentration at the EC_{50}, the pharmacokinetic equivalence interval required to match an 80 to 120% pharmacodynamic interval for the resulting effect would be 67 to 150% (E_{max} model).

It should be noted that if a surrogate effect is proposed to substitute for a pharmacokinetic interval (e.g., C_{max}) that would be acceptable at 80 to 120%, then the peak effect should have an interval of 89 to 109% (under the same assumptions as the preceding example).

C. PREDICTIONS OF PHARMACODYNAMIC EQUIVALENCE

If a test preparation is not equivalent on one or more pharmacokinetic parameters, it is useful to consider the consequences of these differences by determining whether a predicted pharmacodynamic parameter might support equivalence.

If the therapeutic effect can be related to the cumulative response to the instantaneous action of the drug, the pattern of the concentration profile will have a marked influence. Equivalent AUCs for two preparations are insufficient to establish equivalence. On the other hand, differences in rate of bioavailability may be detectable on pharmacokinetic grounds, but have little relevance for cumulative drug effect. For example, the therapeutic benefit of diuretics is clearly more closely linked to cumulative sodium (and water) excretion than an instantaneous action on inhibiting sodium reabsorption. The pharmacodynamic parameters of sodium excretion have been established for many diuretic agents, especially the loop diuretics. The cumulative sodium excretion can be predicted for each of the individuals in a pharmacokinetic equivalence study using a typical set of pharmacodynamic parameters taken from the literature and the measured drug concentrations.[17]

Another example is offered by ACE inhibitors such as enalapril. Peak concentrations after each dose differing by a factor of 10 or more will produce less than a 10% difference in ACE inhibition because the concentrations are typically many times the EC_{50}. Like diuretics, a major part of the response to ACE inhibition can be connected to a cumulative action on sodium balance.[8] The use of a predicted ACE inhibition time course and derivation of parameters such as AUC_e after a dose would appear to offer a more rational basis for determining equivalence than one based on measures of the systemic concentration of the active species alone.

By establishing equivalence for a predicted pharmacodynamic parameter, the clinical significance of accepting a wider equivalence interval for pharmacokinetic parameters can be evaluated.

D. PRODRUGS AND METABOLITES

When a drug is administered in an inactive form and/or is converted to one or more metabolites, new issues must be addressed when defining a pharmacokinetic equivalence study. In many cases high-performance liquid chromatography (HPLC) allows the measurement of additional species with little extra effort so that two or more concentration time profiles are available for bioequivalence analysis.

1. Single Active Species

It would seem that first priority should be accorded to the active species. The active species may be in the administered formulation or be formed *in vivo* (prodrug). If all other measurable species are known to be inactive, there does not appear to be any rational basis for considering them when evaluating equivalence.

The proliferation of parameters resulting from the addition of each measurable species to the active species parameter list can only increase the risk of deeming a test formulation nonequivalent without any rational benefit derived from a noninformative measurement. A recent review of pharmacokinetic equivalence studies[18] has shown that the variability in C_{max} of active metabolites is less than that for the parent compound (although this is offset by greater variability in AUC_c). This could lead to the pharmacokinetics of an active metabolite being equivalent, but the formulation being denied approval because of functionally irrelevant differences in the rate of absorption of the parent prodrug.

2. Multiple Active Species

Activity may reside in more than one identifiable species —usually as an active moiety in promoting the therapeutic effect — but antagonistic activity is theoretically possible. The relative efficacy and potency of each active species should be considered when evaluating equivalence. A metabolite with concentrations that are similar to those of an active parent but with a potency of only 5% can presumably be ignored for the purposes of equivalence. Using knowledge of the pharmacodynamics of each active moiety, the predicted time-effect profile of the combination could be predicted in each individual and the equivalence of the derived pharmacodynamic parameters could be used in conjunction with the pharmacokinetics of the most active species to determine bioequivalence for the product.

VI. CONCLUSION

Pharmacodynamic equivalence based on a single marker of effect is inferior to pharmacokinetic equivalence based on systemic concentrations because equivalent concentrations are compatible with equivalent therapeutic and adverse effects; on the other hand, equivalence using a single, usually surrogate, effect is a poor predictor of other effects with different concentration-effect relationships. A combination of a pharmacodynamic equivalence criterion and a systemic pharmacokinetic equivalence criterion is needed to establish equivalence for nonsystemically active drugs with potentially serious adverse effects.

Pharmacodynamics can be used to conduct bioassays if a chemical procedure for measuring concentration is impractical. Although specificity and sensitivity may be a problem for a bioassay procedure, the predicted concentrations could be used to evaluate pharmacokinetic equivalence.

The key role of pharmacodynamics in bioequivalence decision making is in providing a rational basis for defining pharmacokinetic equivalence criteria. The weaknesses of traditional equivalence criteria are exposed by simple predictions of the effects associated with an equivalence interval. The inclusion of an overt pharmacodynamic rationale into existing guidelines would require an understanding of the basic and clinical pharmacology of a drug as well as the ability to make parametric model-dependent predictions based on the well-established links between dose, concentration, and effect. Surely the time, effort, and money that go into pharmaceutical development and the training of regulators can rise above the simplistic approaches inherent in the AUC, T_{max}, and C_{max} approach to the evaluation of bioequivalence.

REFERENCES

1. **Forgue, S. T. and Colburn, W. A.,** Pharmacodynamic models in bioequivalence, in *Pharmaceutical Bioequivalence,* Welling, P. G., Tse, F. L. S., and Dighe, S. V., Eds., Marcel Dekker, New York, 1991, chap. 11.
2. **Van Boxtel, C., Holford, N. H. G., and Danhof M., Eds.,** *The In Vivo Study of Drug Action,* Elsevier, Amsterdam, 1992.
3. **Weiss, M.,** Recirculatory models: a rigorous basis for a pharmacokinetic theory, in *Topics in Pharmaceutical Sciences,* Breimer, D. D., Ed., F. I. P., The Hague, 1989, chap. 29.
4. **Holford, N. H. G., Ambros, R. J., and Stoeckel, K.,** Models for describing absorption rate and estimating extent of bioavailability, *J. Pharmacokinet. Biopharm.,* 20, 421, 1992.
5. **Holford, N. H. G. and Sheiner, L. B.,** Understanding the concentration-effect relationship, *Clin. Pharmacokinet.,* 6, 429, 1981.
6. **Verotta, D. and Sheiner, L. B.,** Semiparametric models of the time course of drug action, in *The In Vivo Study of Drug Action,* Van Boxtel, C., Holford, N. H. G., and Danhof M., Eds., Elsevier, Amsterdam, 1992, chap. 5.
7. **Holford, N. H. G.,** Parametric models of the time course of drug action, in *The In Vivo Study of Drug Action,* Van Boxtel, C., Holford, N. H. G., and Danhof, M., Eds., Elsevier, Amsterdam, 1992, chap. 4.
8. **Holford, N. H. G.,** Relevance of pharmacodynamic principles to therapeutics, *Ann. Acad. Med. (Singapore),* 20, 26, 1991.
9. **Hofstadter, D. R.,** *Goedel, Escher, Bach: An Eternal Golden Braid,* Penguin, U.K., 1980, 119.
10. **Engel, T., Scharling, B., Skovsted, B., and Heinig, J. H.,** Effects, side effects and plasma concentrations of terbutaline in adult asthmatics after inhaling from a dry powder inhaler device at different inhalation flows and volumes, *Br. J. Clin. Pharmacol.,* 33, 439, 1992.
11. **Summers, Q. A., Singh, S., Honeywell, R. G., Renwick, A. G., and Holgate, S. T.,** The effect of respiratory manoeuvres and pharmacological agents on the pharmacokinetics of nedocromil sodium after inhalation, *Br. J. Clin. Pharmacol.,* 33, 431, 1992.
12. **Bauer, K., Brunner-Ferber, F., Distlerath, L. M., Lippa, E. A., Binkowitz, B., Till, P., and Kaik, G.,** Assessment of systemic effects of different ophthalmic β-blockers in healthy volunteers, *Clin. Pharmacol. Ther.,* 49, 658, 1991.
13. **Novack, G. T.,** Ophthalmic beta-blockers since timolol, *Surv. Ophthalmol.,* 31, 307, 1987.
14. **Kaila, T., Huupponen, R., Karhuvaara, S., Havula, P., Scheinin, M., Iisalo, E., and Salminen, L.,** β-Blocking effects of timolol at low plasma concentrations, *Clin. Pharmacol. Ther.,* 49, 53, 1991.
15. **Reiner, N. E., Bloxham, D. D., and Thompson, W. L.,** Nephrotoxicity of gentamicin and tobramycin given once daily or continuously in dogs, *J. Antimicrob. Chemother.,* 4, 85, 1978.
16. **Olson, S. C., Eldon, M. A., Toothaker, R. D., Ferry, J. J., and Colburn, W. A.,** Controversy II: bioequivalence as an indicator of therapeutic equivalence: modeling the theoretic influence of bioinequivalence on single-dose drug effect, *J. Clin. Pharmacol.,* 27, 342, 1987.
17. **Holford, N. H. G.,** *MKMODEL,* Biosoft, Cambridge, U.K., 1991.
18. **Chen, M.-L. and Jackson, A.,** The role of metabolites in bioequivalency assessment. I. Linear pharmacokinetics without first-pass effect, *Pharm. Res.,* 8, 25, 1991.

Chapter 6

In Vivo and *In Vitro* Correlations: Scientific and Regulatory Perspectives

Vinod P. Shah and Roger L. Williams

CONTENTS

I. INTRODUCTION

Over the last two decades, the *in vitro* dissolution (release) test has emerged as the single most important and useful quality control procedure to assure product quality and performance, once the bioavailability and/or bioequivalence of the dosage form has been established. The value of an *in vitro* dissolution test to assess drug quality is increased when differences in the dissolution rate can be correlated with known differences in *in vivo* product performance. With such data, the specifications of an *in vitro* test can be shown to be related to *in vivo* performance limits of a specific formulation. A product with poor *in vitro* performance will thus be likely to fail an *in vivo* test. *In vitro* experiments can serve as indicators of bioavailability only when appropriate *in vivo/in vitro* correlations exist.

For immediate-release (IR) products, useful correlations may sometimes be developed for several dosage forms, i.e., a correlation or association is applicable irrespective of formulation differences. For controlled-release (CR) products, the correlation is generally formulation specific. For IR products, generally one or in some instances two time points form the basis for an *in vitro* specification, while for CR products three to four time points are generally required. For both IR and CR products, the dissolution test is generally considered a quality control test to assure batch-to-batch drug release uniformity. Dissolution is also sometimes employed as a surrogate marker to assure *in vivo* bioavailability or bioequivalence.

Science and regulatory issues relative to *in vivo/in vitro* correlations have been topics of several national and international conferences and publications.[1-6] These conferences

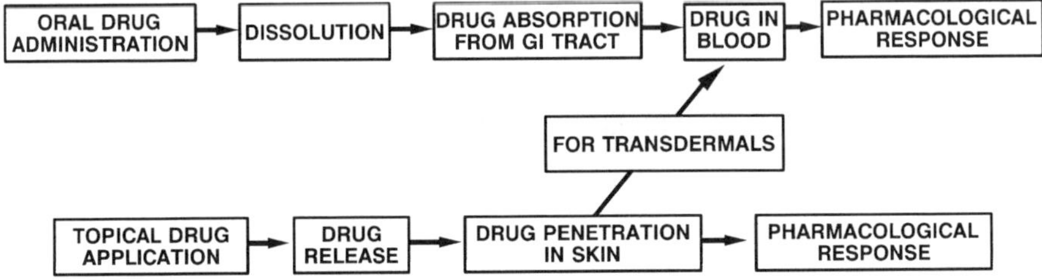

Figure 6–1 Sequence of steps after administration of oral drugs and application of topical drugs.

have considered correlation definitions, means of achieving specific correlations, and utility of such correlations. This chapter will focus on general approaches and utility of *in vivo/in vitro* correlations and associations. *In vitro* tests must be validated by an *in vivo* correlation/association to be a meaningful quality control tool and to be useful as a surrogate marker for *in vivo* performance.

II. BACKGROUND

The sequence of steps resulting in entry of drug into the body after oral or topical (dermal and transdermal) drug administration is shown in Figure 6–1. For most oral solid dosage forms to be bioavailable and therapeutically effective, the drug must undergo dissolution or be solubilized in the aqueous environment of the gastrointestinal (GI) tract for absorption to occur. Drug absorption and thus bioavailability are governed to a large extent by factors related to drug product dissolution and gastrointestinal permeability of the drug.[3] For topical drug products, efficacy is dependent on complex drug release characteristics and factors influencing drug permeability.

The dissolution characteristics of an oral or topical product may be assessed by an *in vitro* test procedure. Characteristics of the drug, the formulation, and the test system will determine the *in vitro* dissolution results. Various physical and chemical properties of the drug, inactive ingredients in the formulation, and manufacturing parameters influence the *in vitro* dissolution of a drug product. The dissolution rate of a drug product is also a function of the dynamics of the test system and thus varies according to the dissolution equipment and methods employed. Various conditions of the dissolution test — such as apparatus type and geometry, rate of agitation, composition of dissolution medium (pH, type, and concentration of the buffer), and temperature — significantly affect *in vitro* dissolution.

Two general relationships can be defined between *in vitro* dissolution and *in vivo* bioavailability as follows: (1) *in vivo/in vitro* correlations; and (2) *in vivo/in vitro* associations. In the former, one or more *in vivo* parameters are correlated with one or more *in vitro* release (dissolution) parameters of the product. This relationship necessarily requires formulations that differ in *in vivo* as well as *in vitro* performance characteristics. In the latter, *in vivo* and *in vitro* performance parameters of different formulations coincide but a correlation does not exist. Situations also exist where no correlation or association is possible between *in vitro* and *in vivo* data.

III. METHODOLOGY

A. *IN VIVO* METHODS

The *in vivo* parameters essential for correlation and/or association with *in vitro* data are obtained from bioavailability and/or bioequivalence studies in humans. These studies result in plasma or urine concentration-time profiles, from which selected parameters of interest are calculated. These parameters can include model-independent parameters such as AUC, C_{max}, and T_{max} for plasma or ARE (amount remaining to be eliminated) plots for urine; or model-dependent parameters such as rate of absorption (k_a). In some instances, plasma *in vivo* dissolution parameters are obtained by using statistical moments and deconvolution methods.[7-8]

B. *IN VITRO* METHODOLOGY

In vitro parameters for correlation and/or association with *in vivo* performance parameters are obtained from *in vitro* dissolution test procedures that yield dissolution profiles. From these profiles, the following parameters may be calculated: dissolution (release) rate, amount of drug dissolved at a given time, time required to achieve a certain percentage of drug dissolved, or mathematical equation that describes the dissolution curve.

Extensive research over the last two decades has shown that dissolution test conditions should be mild enough to discriminate between different formulations of the same drug that manifest different bioavailability parameters. Dissolution conditions can also be developed to detect manufacturing changes. For immediate-release products, the agitation speed should generally be 50 to 100 rpm using the U.S. Pharmacopeia (USP) basket method and 50 to 75 rpm with the USP paddle method.[9,10] Higher agitation may not be predictive of formulation or process changes. The dissolution medium should be physiologically meaningful, should be as simple as possible, and generally should be aqueous. The most common dissolution media are water, simulated gastric fluid (pH 1.2, 0.1 *N* HCl) or intestinal fluid (pH 6.8 or 7.4) without enzymes, and buffers with a pH range of 4.5 to 7.5. The volume of the medium is generally between 500 and 1000 ml and is maintained at 37°C during a study. Basic criteria are that the test should be simple, reliable, reproducible, discriminating, flexible, and capable of automation.

For products with poor solubility in commonly used aqueous media, dissolution testing in aqueous media containing surfactants such as sodium lauryl sulfate (SLS) has been utilized.[11] Use of organic solvents is discouraged because they lack physiological relevance. The dissolution profile of water-insoluble drug products should be determined with gradually increasing concentration of the surfactant (e.g., 0.1, 0.25, 1, and 2% SLS) under mild agitation conditions. This procedure has been successfully utilized for dissolution testing of drug products such as griseofulvin, carbamazepine, cortisone acetate, prazosin, and other drug products.[11]

IV. *IN VIVO/IN VITRO* CORRELATIONS: ORAL DOSE FORMULATIONS

Correlations or associations between *in vivo* and *in vitro* parameters are based on observed *in vivo* pharmacokinetic performance of several formulations. These parameters are not subject to experimental manipulation and thus are invariant. In contrast, the *in vitro* dissolution performance of a formulation is variable and can be manipulated to facilitate the correlation or association. *In vitro* parameters may be changed by altering test conditions such as stirring rate, dissolution media, and apparatus geometry to achieve the most appropriate *in vivo/in vitro* correlation. Achievement of a useful correlation is highly dependent on the success in obtaining formulations with varying *in vivo* performance characteristics. When the products differ in some *in vivo* bioavailability or bioequivalence performance parameter, the *in vitro* test conditions should be modified to obtain the most discriminating *in vivo/in vitro* relationship. When no differences are observed with *in vivo* parameters, the *in vitro* conditions should be adjusted to obtain similar *in vitro* parameters to achieve an *in vivo/in vitro* association. For adequate *in vivo/ in vitro* correlations, at least three formulations of the same drug demonstrating a range in absorption are needed. With only two products with differing performance characteristics, only a rank order relationship is possible. Reasonable *in vivo/in vitro* correlations

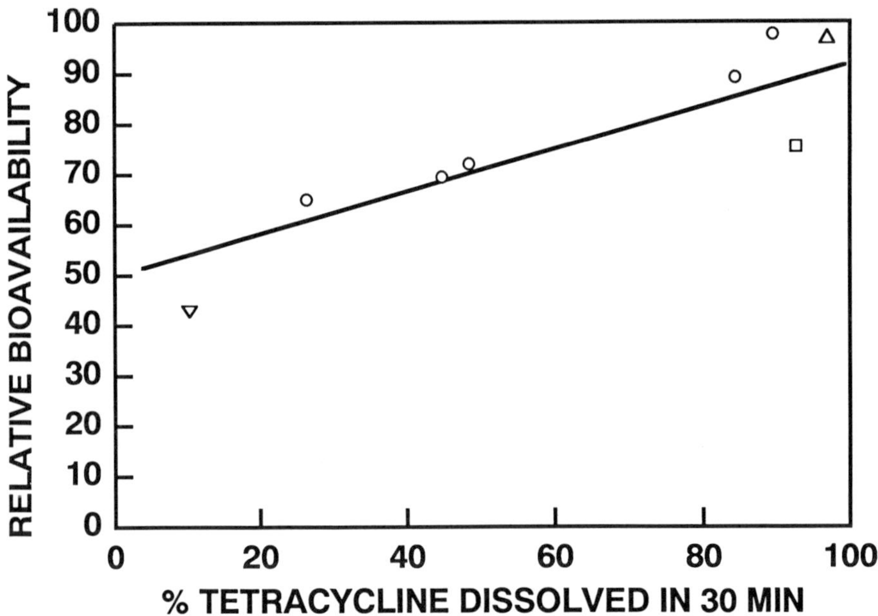

Figure 6–2 *In vivo/in vitro* correlation for tetracycline hydrochloride capsules. (△) Innovator drug product, (○) generic drug products, (□) generic drug product with borderline bioavailability, and (▽) generic product K which had poor bioavailability and was bioequivalent.

have been demonstrated for aspirin, digoxin, digitoxin, prednisone, phenytoin, warfarin, and tetracycline.

Several approaches can be utilized in analyzing and evaluating *in vivo* and *in vitro* data. Generally, the *in vivo* parameter is plotted on the y axis and the corresponding *in vitro* dissolution parameter is plotted on the x axis. Parameters such as AUC, C_{max}, k_a, relative bioavailability of two formulations, A_e, or even a pharmacological response parameter can be plotted against a dissolution parameter of the product. Examples of this general approach are described below.

A. IMMEDIATE-RELEASE PRODUCTS

1. Tetracycline

The Food and Drug Administration (FDA) has studied seven generic and one innovator formulation of tetracycline hydrochloride capsules *in vivo*. These studies documented that four of the seven products were not bioequivalent to the reference product. Products were selected for investigation based on preliminary *in vitro* characteristics, using the basket method at 50 rpm in water. After preliminary evaluation of the *in vivo* and *in vitro* data, the *in vitro* tests were repeated under modified conditions to improve the observed *in vivo/in vitro* correlation. A good correlation was observed for relative bioavailability (y axis) vs. amount of drug dissolved in 30 min (x axis), with Product K showing both poor dissolution and poor bioavailability (Figure 6–2).[12] Following these investigations, product K was reformulated to improve its *in vitro* dissolution characteristics. Repeat bioequivalence testing on the reformulated product indicated improvement in its relative bioavailability as assessed by AUC. The other three products noted in Figure 6–2 manifesting both poor dissolution and unacceptable bioequivalence are no longer marketed.

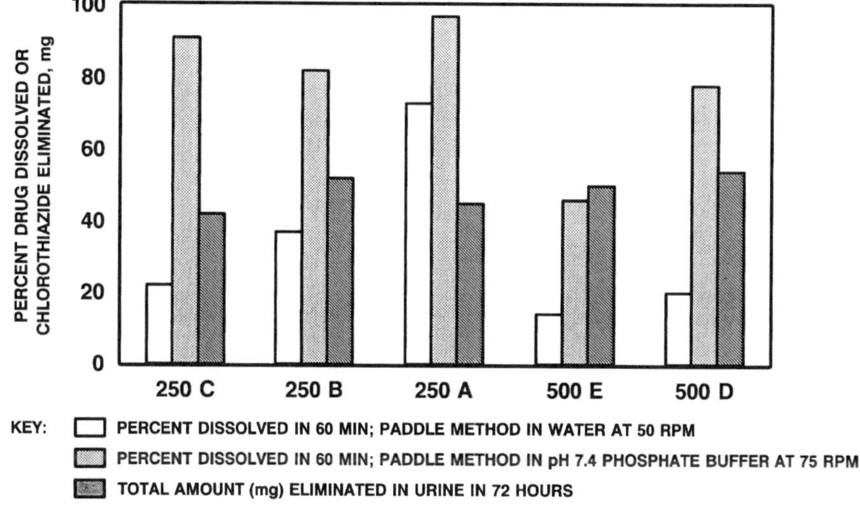

Figure 6–3 *In vivo/in vitro* association for chlorothiazide tablets.

2. Chlorothiazide

FDA has conducted studies in healthy subjects of five chlorothiazide products with significantly different *in vitro* dissolution profiles, using the USP paddle method with water at 50 rpm. The amount of drug eliminated in urine, A_e, was used to estimate extent of bioavailability. The results of these *in vivo/in vitro* studies indicated that the amount of chlorothiazide excreted in the urine in 72 h did not significantly differ between the five formulations and did not correlate significantly with the amount of drug dissolved *in vitro* in 60 min (Figure 6–3). For this drug, the *in vitro* procedures were thus overly discriminating. Because the *in vivo* performance of the product was invariable, *in vitro* conditions were changed (basket method, 75 rpm, pH 7.5 buffer) to achieve *in vitro* profiles that were as invariant as the *in vivo* results (Figure 6–3),[13] resulting in an *in vivo/in vitro* association.

3. Carbamazepine

In this study also performed in healthy subjects, the FDA evaluated three generic and one innovator carbamazepine products with differing in *in vitro* release profiles (Figure 6–4). The fastest dissolving product also demonstrated the highest rate, and extent of absorption as estimated by C_{max} and AUC. The more slowly dissolving products showed equivalently lower C_{max} and AUC. In these studies, the *in vivo* performance of the four carbamazepine products thus correlated well with their *in vitro* performance.[14] Both C_{max} of the four products, when plotted vs. amount of drug dissolved in 15 min, or their AUC, when plotted against amount of the drug dissolved in 60 min, yielded a good *in vivo/in vitro* correlation. Based on these data, a two-time point dissolution specification (15 and 60 min) has been recommended for this drug to provide better control on *in vitro* release and product performance.

4. Additional Drugs

The different release profiles of prompt and extended phenytoin products have been correlated with T_{max} and C_{max} (Figure 6–5).[15] Using mild *in vitro* dissolution test conditions, an *in vivo/in vitro* correlation has also been demonstrated for seven marketed brands of trisulfapyrimidine suspensions (Figure 6–6).[16] In general, data summarizing *in vivo/in vitro* correlations or associations for immediate-release formulations have been the subject of numerous reviews.[1,2,5]

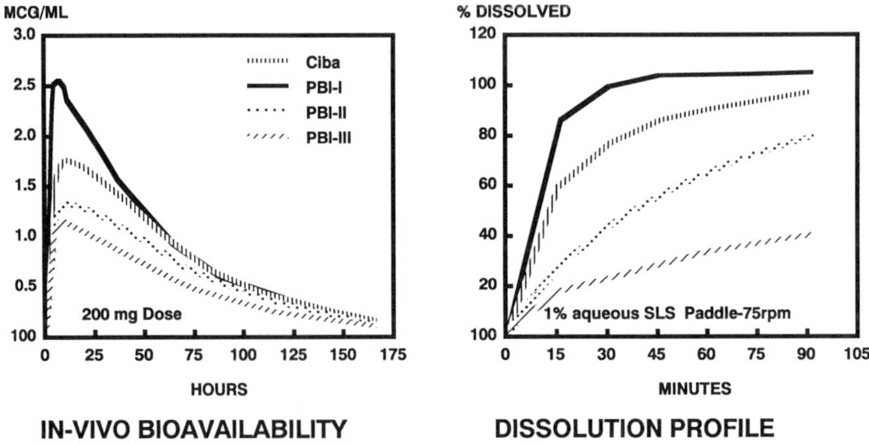

Figure 6–4 Bioavailability and dissolution profile for four carbamazepine tablets.

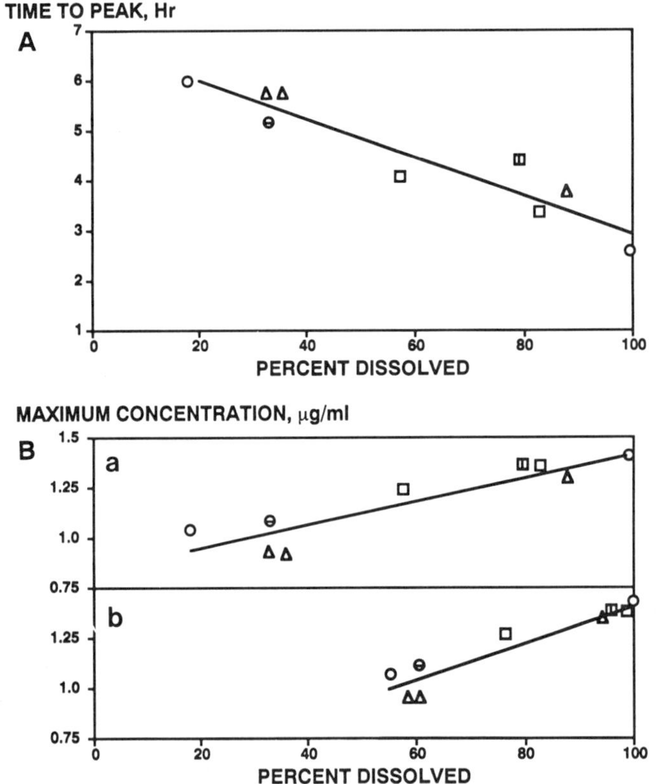

Figure 6–5 *In vivo/in vitro* correlation for phenytoin products. **(A)** *In vitro/in vivo* correlation between T_{max} and percent drug dissolved in 30 m by basket method at 50 rpm (slope = 0.038, r = 0.944, $p < 0.001$). **(B)** *In vitro/in vivo* correlation between C_{max} and percent drug dissolved in 30 min (slope = 0.06, r = 0.902, $p < 0.001$) (a); 60 min (slope = 0.10, r = 0.940, $p < 0.001$) (b).

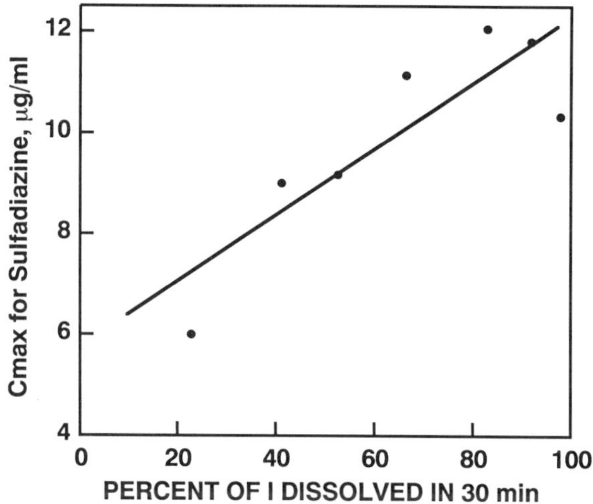

Figure 6–6 *In vivo/in vitro* correlation for trisulfapyrimidine suspensions.

These examples of *in vivo/in vitro* correlation using different formulations suggest that for immediate-release products, *in vitro* dissolution methods may be developed to allow correlation with observed *in vivo* performance parameters. If successful, this documentation supports the application of *in vitro* dissolution methodology as a quality control test procedure. Dissolution of most immediate-release drug products has been characterized by a single time point, e.g., 75 to 85% drug dissolved in 30 to 60 min. While a single point standard probably may be adequate as a general quality control method for some drugs, for certain drugs such as carbamazepine a multipoint dissolution test may be better.

B. CONTROLLED-RELEASE OR EXTENDED-RELEASE PRODUCTS

Different principles are employed in the manufacture of controlled-release (CR) preparations that complicate the development of *in vivo/in vitro* correlations across product lines. Because of the use of different technologies to control drug release in CR preparations, *in vivo/in vitro* correlations are thus formulation specific. Despite this general limitation, formulations for a specific product can nonetheless be prepared that exhibit different release properties by varying critical formulation, manufacturing, and processing variables. *In vivo* performance of these formulations, using a specific mechanism of drug release, can then be established to form the basis for an *in vivo/in vitro* correlation in the same way that different IR formulations can be studied.

Three different levels of *in vivo/in vitro* correlations are described in USP XXII for CR preparations.[8] The level is based on how well the dissolution profile reflects the blood level profile of the controlled-release product.

- A Level A correlation is a point-to-point correlation between *in vitro* and *in vivo* dissolution where both curves may be superimposed on one another, perhaps after suitable mathematical adjustment. The *in vivo* dissolution curve is obtained by deconvolution of plasma concentration time data.
- In a Level B correlation, mean *in vitro* dissolution time is compared to mean *in vivo* residence time or mean *in vivo* dissolution time, using principles of statistical moment analysis. This is a single point correlation.
- In a Level C correlation, mean *in vitro* dissolution time is correlated with a single *in vivo* pharmacokinetic parameter such as AUC or C_{max}. This is also a one-point correlation.

Although a Level A correlation is most desirable, in practice this level of correlation is usually possible only when *in vitro* and *in vivo* release characteristics of the product are independent of *in vitro* test and *in vivo* gastrointestinal conditions. Under these circumstances, the drug may be released from the formulation in solution; and a high degree of correlation between *in vitro* release and *in vivo* performance is possible. For such optimal formulations, products with different release characteristics should demonstrate a good correlation between *in vitro* and *in vivo* performance.

With controlled-release preparations, *in vitro* release profiles should be studied in several media with a range of pH values and also under several conditions of agitation. Studies with quinidine gluconate demonstrate the inadequacy of determining a release profile for a formulation under single test conditions. Two quinidine gluconate products with similar *in vitro* release profiles over 8 h in acid media demonstrated different *in vivo* performance. Modification of the *in vitro* methodology after these preliminary studies permitted differentiation of the *in vitro* performance of the quinidine gluconate products in pH 5.4 acetate buffer, with good correspondence to their *in vivo* performance (Figure 6–7).[17] The less bioavailable product was subsequently reformulated to match the *in vitro* release of the more bioavailable product. *In vivo* studies thereafter documented bioequivalence between the two formulations. Given that only two formulations were tested in these studies, the data in Figure 6–7 represents a rank order relationship and not a correlation. Several Level A correlations have been reported, particularly for osmotic delivery systems. In one example, chlorpheniramine maleate formulations with different *in vitro* release profiles were prepared by varying the amount of the release-controlling cellulosic polymer. Subsequent *in vivo* studies demonstrated a Level A correlation between the absorption profile obtained by deconvolution and the *in vitro* release profile.[18]

V. *IN VIVO/IN VITRO* CORRELATIONS: TOPICAL DRUG PRODUCTS

For topical glucocorticoids such as hydrocortisone and β-methasone valerate, a rank order relationship has been observed between *in vitro* release rate and skin-blanching response.[19,20] In these examples, the *in vitro* release rate was determined using a diffusion cell system, a cellulose acetate/nitrate synthetic membrane, and an appropriate receptor medium. The *in vivo* studies assessed the degree of vasoconstriction 2 h after 16 h of drug application.

For transdermal drug products, *in vivo/in vitro* correlations have been difficult to develop. To obtain a true *in vivo/in vitro* correlation, products with differing *in vivo* performance are needed, which in turn should have different *in vitro* release characteristics. The availability of transdermal formulations with different release characteristics might occur with the availability of several multisource versions of a reference product. The only multisource products available to date are nitroglycerin and nicotine patches, and these formulations exhibit nearly the same *in vivo* characteristics. A simple and reproducible *in vitro* release method has been developed for transdermal patches that utilizes a modified paddle system, where the patch is held in position between a watch glass, and a Teflon mesh.[21] The *in vitro* release profile using this procedure for two fluocinolone acetonide transdermal patches was shown to have rank order relationship with the *in vivo* absorption rate in animals.[22] In another set of experiments, the *in vitro* release profile of estradiol patches demonstrated a rank order relationship with *in vitro* drug penetration/absorption, using cadaver skin in a Franz diffusion cell system.[23]

VI. *IN VIVO/IN VITRO* CORRELATIONS: REGULATORY ISSUES

A modern approach for the development of a pharmaceutical formulation should be to prepare several formulations of a new dosage form that are likely to perform differently *in vivo*. Depending on the formulation, *in vivo* performance may be particularly sensitive to critical manufacturing and process variables. These formulations are then screened for

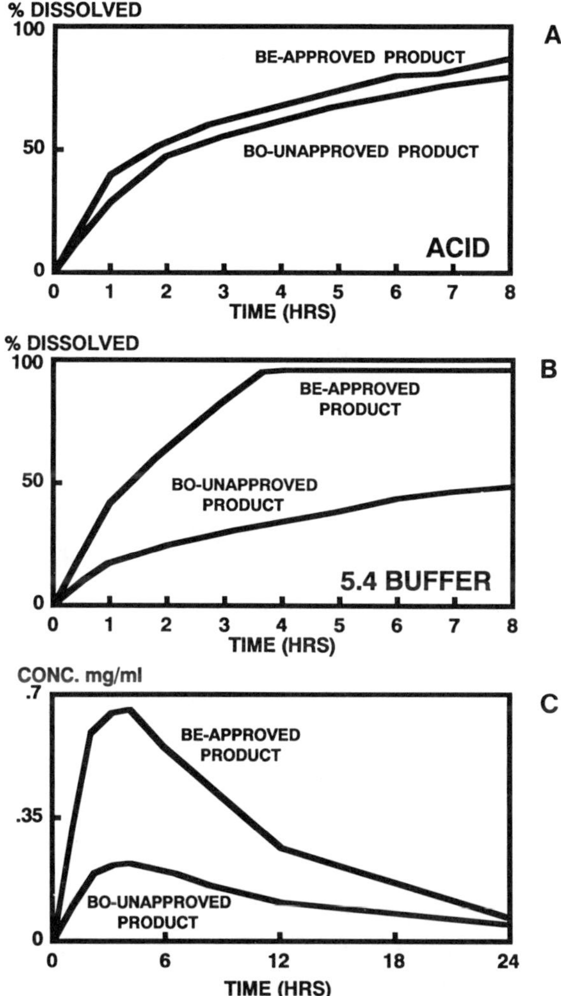

Figure 6–7 *In vitro* dissolution profiles **(A, B)** and *in vivo* **(C)** bioavailability for quinidine gluconate tablets.

in vitro release characteristics. *In vitro* conditions should then be developed to discriminate among the different formulations. Further *in vivo* bioavailability studies may be needed to better establish the range of *in vivo* pharmacokinetic or pharmacodynamic parameters and to confirm that the associated *in vitro* data are sufficiently discriminating. This iterative process may require several cycles to achieve a meaningful *in vitro* dissolution test.

A discriminating *in vitro* dissolution test for any drug product can be used:

- To serve as a quality control procedure to assure batch-to-batch drug release uniformity
- To assess the likelihood that scaleup of batches, change in site of manufacture, and minor changes in formulation and manufacturing equipment will impact on product performance
- To provide a tool in product development to design and selection of appropriate test formulations
- To help minimize requirements for *in vivo* experiments
- To facilitate development of product specifications based on *in vivo* data

For these various reasons, a well-established and discriminating *in vitro* dissolution method that can predict the *in vivo* performance of the product is highly desirable. *In vitro* release product specifications should be established whenever possible based on *in vivo-in vitro* correlation.

In vitro dissolution data are routinely utilized to assure equivalence between the bioequivalence or pilot batch and the scaleup batch; and to confirm continuing bioequivalence when postapproval manufacturing process and formulation changes occur. Dissolution data in these instances are used as a surrogate marker for *in vivo* bioequivalence and assumes at a minimum the existence of an *in vivo/in vitro* correlation. Even when available, these correlations generally utilize mean data and do not address *in vivo* variability in drug release and absorption. Furthermore, even a good *in vivo/in vitro* correlation does not guarantee *in vivo* bioequivalence between two formulations as determined by modern confidence interval methods of analysis. An important regulatory issue therefore relates to the question of whether *in vitro* dissolution can ever be used as a measure of *in vivo* bioequivalence. Pending further studies to answer this question definitively, a prudent regulatory conclusion at this time is that it cannot.

VII. CONCLUSION

In vivo/in vitro correlations are important to achieve a meaningful and predictive *in vitro* dissolution specification. For immediate-release (IR) products, a single *in vivo/in vitro* correlation or association may be predictive of the *in vivo* performance of several formulations. For controlled-release (CR) formulations, the *in vivo/in vitro* correlation must be developed for each formulation. The suitability of *in vitro* dissolution as a surrogate marker for bioequivalence has not been established.

REFERENCES

1. **Abdou, H. M.,** Correlation of *in vitro* rate of dissolution with *in vivo* bioavailability, in dissolution, bioavailability and bioequivalence, Abdou, H. M., Ed., Edison Mack Publishing, Easton, PA, 1989, 491.
2. **Dakkuri, A. and Shah, A.,** Correlation of *in vitro* rate of dissolution with *in vivo* bioavailability: an overview, *Pharm. Technol.,* 6, 67, 1982.
3. **Wagner, J.,** Biopharmacokinetics, rate of dissolution *in vitro* and *in vivo.* VI. Correlation of *in vivo* and *in vitro* —theoretical and practical considerations, *Drug Intell. Clin. Pharm.,* 4, 160, 1970.
4. Workshop report: *In vitro* and *in vivo* testing and correlation for oral controlled/ modified-release dosage forms, Skelly, J. P., Amidon, G. L., Barr, W. H., Benet, L. Z., Carter, J. E., Robinson, J. R., Shah, V. P., and Yacobi, A., *Pharm. Res.,* 7, 975, 1990.
5. **Banakar, U.,** Dissolution and bioavailability, in *Pharmaceutical Dissolution Testing,* Marcel Dekker, New York 1992, 347.
6. International Open Conference on Dissolution, Bioavailability and Bioequivalence, cosponsored by U.S. Food and Drug Administration (FDA), Canadian Health Protection Branch (HPB), and the U.S. Pharmacopeial Convention (USP), Toronto, Canada, June 16–18, 1992.
7. **Riegelman, S. and Collier, P.,** The application of statistical moments theory to the evaluation of *in vivo* dissolution time and absorption time, *J. Pharmacokinet. Biopharm.,* 8, 509, 1980.
8. USP Subcommittee on Biopharmaceutics, *In vitro/in vivo* correlation for extended release oral dosage forms, *Pharmacopeial Forum,* July-August, 4160, 1988.
9. **Levy, G.,** Comparison of dissolution and absorption rates of different commercial aspirin tablets, *J. Pharm. Sci.,* 50, 388, 1961.

10. **Shah, V. P., Gurbarg, M., Noory, A., Dighe, S., and Skelly, J. P.,** Influence of higher rates of agitation on release patterns of immediate-release drug products, *J. Pharm. Sci.,* 81, 500, 1992.
11. **Shah, V. P., Koneckney, J. J., Everett, R., McCullough, P., Noorizadeh, A. C., and Skelly, J. P.,** *In vitro* dissolution profile of water insoluble drug dosage forms in the presence of surfactants, *Pharm. Res.,* 6, 612, 1989.
12. **Shah, V. P., Hunt, J. P., Fairweather, W. R., Prasad, V. K., and Knapp, G.,** Influence of dioctyl sodium sulfosuccinate on the absorption of tetracycline, *Biopharm. Drug Dispos.,* 7, 27, 1986.
13. **Shah, V. P., Knight, P., Prasad, V. K., and Cabana, B. E.,** Thiazides IV: comparison of dissolution with bioavailability of chlorothiazide tablets, *J. Pharm. Sci.,* 71, 822, 1982.
14. **Meyer, M. C., Straughn, A. B., Jarvi, E. J., Wood, G. C., Pelsor, F. R., and Shah, V. P.,** The bioequivalence of carbamazepine tablets with a history of clinical failure, *Pharm. Res.,* 9, 1612, 1992.
15. **Shah, V. P., Prasad, V. K., Alston, T., Cabana, B. E., Gural, R. P., and Meyer, M. C.,** Phenytoin 1: *in-vitro/in-vivo* correlation for 100 mg phenytoin sodium capsules, *J. Pharm. Sci.,* 72, 306, 1983.
16. **Mathur, L., Colaizzi, J., Jaffe, J., Poust, R., and Shah, V. P.,** *In-vivo-in-vitro* correlation for trisulfapyrimidine suspensions, *J. Pharm. Sci.,* 72, 1072, 1983.
17. **Prasad, V. K., Shah, V. P., Knight, P., Malinowski, H., Cabana, B. E., and Meyer, M. C.,** Importance of media selection in establishment of *in-vitro-in-vivo* relationships for quinidine gluconate, *Int. J. Pharm.,* 13, 1, 1983.
18. **Mojaverian, P., Rodwanski, E., Ching-Chung, L., Cho, P., Vadino, W. A., and Rosen, J. M.,** Correlation of *in-vitro* release rate and *in-vivo* absorption characteristics of four chlorpheniramine maleate extended release formulations, *Pharm. Res.,* 9, 450, 1992.
19. **Caron, D., Roussel-Queille, C., Shah, V. P., and Schaefer, H.,** Correlation between the drug penetration and the blanching effect of topically applied hydrocortisone creams in human beings, *J. Am. Acad. Dermatol.,* 23, 458, 1990.
20. **Shah, V. P., Elkins, J., and Skelly, J. P.,** Relationship between *in-vivo* skin blanching and *in-vitro* release rate for betamethasone valerate creams, *J. Pharm. Sci.,* 81, 104, 1992.
21. **Shah, V. P., Tymes, N. W., Yamomoto, L. A., and Skelly, J. P.,** *In vitro* dissolution profile of transdermal nitroglycerin patches using paddle method, *Int. J. Pharm.,* 32, 243, 1986.
22. **Uchiyama, M.,** personal communication, NIHS, Tokyo, Japan 1989.
23. **Brain, K. R., Hadgraft, J., James, V. J., Shah, V. P., Walters, K., and Watkinson, A. C.,** *In vitro* assessment of skin permeation from a transdermal system for the delivery of oestradiol, *Int. J. Pharm.,* 89, R13, 1993.

Chapter 7

Stereochemical Considerations in Bioavailability Studies

William R. Ravis and Joel S. Owen

CONTENTS

I. INTRODUCTION

Bioavailability assessment of new drug products and formulations requires monitoring drug concentration in the plasma or urine to establish the time course of drug in the body. Recognizing that many existing as well as future drug products are administered as racemates, the usefulness of pharmacokinetic and bioavailability studies performed with nonstereospecific assays may be questionable. In many cases, the stereoisomers of the racemate have markedly different pharmacological and toxicological activities. For this reason, deriving a racemate pharmacokinetic profile based on an assay which is unable to distinguish between stereoisomers may greatly compromise its therapeutic significance.

The additional expense required to perform and evaluate bioavailability and pharmacokinetic studies of the separate stereoisomers for a racemic product has forced the drug industry to reconsider their research and marketing strategies for future drugs and for those already in the development process. Decisions about whether a product should be promoted as a racemate or as an individual isomer require considerable pharmacokinetic and pharmacodynamic information early in the development of a drug. In addition, for racemic multisource drug products, stereospecific bioavailability determinations must be considered. The added expense of proving isomer bioequivalence will be reflected in the eventual product cost.

0-8493-6930-4/94/$0.00+$.50

No single statement or guideline can be applied to all products since the impact of stereoisomerism on drug therapy and toxicity is drug specific. Even within a drug class or a series of derivatives, the stereoselectivity of absorption, disposition, and pharmacodynamics may vastly differ.

Chemical synthesis often results in the formation of an optically inactive racemate which contains an equal amount of two stereoisomers. Approximately 60% of clinically used drugs are optically active. Nearly four fifths of all chiral pharmaceuticals are marketed as racemates that may contain isomers which differ in activity. The more active stereoisomer is termed the "eutomer" and the less active form the "distomer". The distomer is often incorrectly viewed as a passive component of the racemate with little pharmacological or pharmacokinetic significance. However, in some cases, the distomer may act as an agonist or antagonist at the receptor site or compete for drug metabolizing enzymes and binding sites. In other cases, the two stereoisomers may have different pharmacological effects, and administration of a racemate would represent a combination drug product (e.g., indacrinone[1]).

Pairs of stereoisomers with one chiral site that exist as mirror images which cannot be superimposed are called enantiomers. The addition of another chiral site or the inversion of a chiral site for a molecule with more than one chiral center results in multiple pairs of stereoisomers called diastereoisomers. Pairs of these stereoisomers are not mirror images and are not superimposable. Most racemic products are composed of enantiomers. Since enantiomers share similar chemical and physical characteristics while diastereoisomers do not, the distinction between these types of stereoisomers is important in predicting stereoselectivity in absorption and disposition.

Macromolecules in the body involved with drug distribution and elimination can recognize stereoisomeric differences. Slight spatial differences between stereoisomers can markedly influence the degree to which isomers associate and interact with receptors, proteins, and enzymes. Enantiomers may display stereoselective absorption and disposition when these processes are highly structurally, and thus stereochemically specific. Since enantiomers have similar partitioning and solubilities in achiral environments, passive drug absorption and tissue partitioning are expected to be nonstereoselective.

The presence of two or more chiral sites in diastereoisomers results in not only stereospecificity in macromolecule interactions, but also differences in isomer partitioning and solubility. While there are limited examples of stereoselective bioavailability and pharmacokinetics of diastereoisomers, this group of stereoisomers has the greatest potential for displaying substantial stereospecificity.

During product development of a racemic drug, pharmacological testing and evaluation may reveal potency differences for pairs of stereoisomers. The potency ratio, or eudismic ratio, is the ratio of eutomer affinity for the binding site to distomer affinity for the binding site.[2] Significant variations in effective and lethal doses of the isomers reveal both their pharmacokinetic and pharmacodynamic differences. For example, all or most of the anti-inflammatory activities of 2-aryl propionic acid (nonsteroidal anti-inflammatory drugs [NSAIDs]) reside in the S-isomer.[3] Another example of pharmacodynamic differences between isomers is quinidine and its diastereoisomer quinine. Although quinidine is the more active diastereoisomer as an antiarrhythmic and antimalarial, quinine has been selected to treat malaria based on its lower potential to lead to cardiodepressant effects.[4] For most pairs of stereoisomers, differences in potency and pharmacological profile reflect receptor, or pharmacodynamic, differences more so than pharmacokinetic factors.

II. PHARMACODYNAMIC ASPECTS

Possibly the greatest impact of spatial differences between stereoisomers is on the pharmacodynamics of a drug product. The effect of small spatial differences between enantiomers appears to be most clearly demonstrated in the mechanism of drug action.

It has been suggested that the more potent or active the eutomer, the lower the activity of the distomer (Pfeiffer's rule).[5] Thus, the better the fit of the eutomer to the target receptor, the poorer will be the fit of the distomer. Several reviews of pharmacodynamic and toxicological differences between stereoisomeric pairs have been conducted by Drayer,[6] Jamali et al.,[7] and Smith.[8]

Stereoselectivity in therapeutic effect is noted across many classes of drugs. α-Dextropropoxyphene has analgesic properties while α-levopropoxyphene has little analgesic activity and is marketed as an antitussive agent.[9] The *l*-isomer of pentazocine is several times more potent as an analgesic than the *d*-isomer.[10] Early in the development of racemic-dopa it was recognized that the side effects associated with its administration could be avoided by administering only L-dopa.[11] The R(–)-enantiomer of indacrinone appears to be an effective diuretic while the S(+)-isomer enhances uric acid secretion with little diuretic activity.[1] As noted for several NSAIDs, the anti-inflammatory and analgesic activities of ketorolac appear to reside in the S-stereoisomer. By animal anti-inflammatory evaluations, S-ketorolac is over 50 times more effective than the R-isomer and has twice the activity of the racemate.[12] Stereoselective activity is also observed with antibiotics. For example, the minimum inhibitory concentration of R-moxalactam is approximately 50% that of S-moxalactam.[13]

Numerous cardiovascular drugs classified as beta blockers, antiarrhythmics, and calcium channel blockers are marketed as racemates with one of the stereoisomers being principally responsible for their desired therapeutic effects. For example, the R- and S-isomers of disopyramide have different antiarrhythmic activities. After administration of the racemate, the antiarrhythmic response is believed by some investigators to be due primarily to the S-stereoisomer.[14,15] Other studies[16] have suggested that the R-isomer is an effective antiarrhythmic agent and is preferred to the administration of S- or racemic disopyramide since the anticholinergic side effects are due to the S-isomer. At equivalent doses, R-propranolol has much less effect on sinus rate and ventricular rate in atrial flutter and fibrillation than R,S-propranolol.[17] This suggests that beta-blocking activity of propranolol resides in the S-isomer. R-Propranolol appears to have antiarrhythmic activities; however, these actions are possibly by other mechanisms than beta blockade. Similarly, the beta-blocking effects of sotalol and metoprolol are related to primarily one of their stereoisomers.[18,19] For sotalol, while beta-blocking activity is predominately in the S-isomer, both isomers display electrophysiological actions as reflected in their repolarization effects.[19]

Examination of graded pharmacological effect as a function of plasma concentration for individual stereoisomers can reveal pharmacodynamic selectivity. With increasing plasma concentrations of both S- and R-ketamine, a graded decrease in median electroencephalogram (EEG) frequency is noted. However, at equivalent plasma concentrations, S-ketamine is several times more effective in producing these EEG changes.[20] The S-isomer of verapamil is primarily responsible for the negative dromotropic effects noted after the administration of the racemate. Based on percentage prolongation in PR interval vs. plasma concentration, the EC_{50} (plasma concentration producing 50% effect) and E_{max} (maximum effect attributable to the drug) show distinct pharmacodynamic differences between the two stereoisomers (see Figure 7–1).[21] The E_{max} of both isomers are similar while the EC_{50} of S-verapamil is one tenth that of the R-isomer.[22] The EC_{50} of the racemate has a value between that of the two stereoisomers. Based on free plasma concentrations of warfarin, S-warfarin can produce a 50% inhibition of synthesis of prothrombin-activity complex at a concentration one fifth that required by R-warfarin.[23]

III. PHARMACOKINETIC-BIOAVAILABILITY ASPECTS

The time course of stereoisomer effects is affected by their pharmacokinetic disposition and bioavailability. Many enantiomeric pairs show differences in kinetic disposition between isomers. Some of these are collected in Table 7–1.

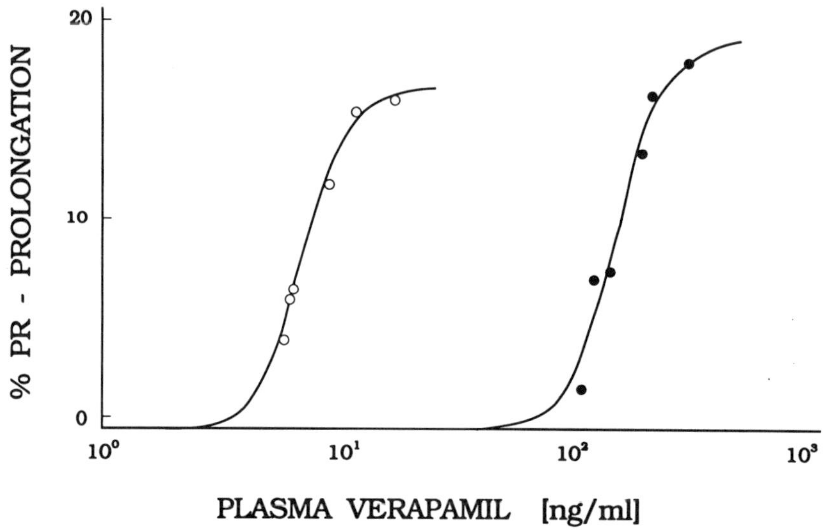

Figure 7–1 Relationship between plasma verapamil concentration and PR interval prolongation in a representative subject following intravenous administration of 50-mg d-verapamil (●) and 5-mg l-verapamil (○). (From Echizen, H. et al., *Am. Heart J.*, 109(2), 210, 1985. With permission.)

A. STEREOISOMER ABSORPTION AND DISSOLUTION

Sources of stereoselective absorption would include diastereoisomer- or enantiomer-specific membrane transport, presystemic metabolism and degradation, and dissolution. Stereoisomer-specific aspects of presystemic biotransformation will be addressed in a later section.

One of the most obvious potential sources of stereospecific bioavailability is the preferential gastrointestinal (GI) absorption of one stereoisomer over the other. The rate of passive absorption across the intestinal epithelium is governed by the concentration gradient and the partitioning of drug into and across the lipidlike cell membrane of the epithelium. Since enantiomers have similar lipid solubility and partitioning, pairs of enantiomers are expected to display equal passive absorption rates across the gastrointestinal membrane. Phospholipids of membranes may show little if any ability to recognize the subtle stereochemical differences between enantiomers.[36] However, diastereoisomers due to their differences in lipophilicity could have stereospecificity in passive absorption.

The stereoselective gastrointestinal absorption of the specific isomers of amino acids and sugars is a consequence of their carrier-mediated transport. Stereoisomers which possess structural similarities to endogenous substrates and nutrients may also demonstrate differences in absorption rates. Stereoisomers that undergo carrier-mediated absorption may share and compete for the same transport systems. For other pairs, one stereoisomer may not be sterically acceptable and is absorbed by only passive absorption. Only a limited number of examples of stereoselective drug absorption have been reported. Utilizing the rat small intestine, L-dopa is absorbed by a saturable carrier transport mechanism at a rate 4 to 5 times greater than the D-isomer.[37] The absorption and/or uptake of L-dopa is decreased by L-leucine and D,L-phenylalanine. While the rate of absorption of the two isomers appear different, D-dopa is still completely absorbed in man.[38] Both isomers of methotrexate are poorly absorbed by passive absorption, but only L-methotrexate is absorbed by active transport. Following oral doses of the separate isomers of methotrexate, the oral availability of the D-isomer based on AUCs and urinary results is only a small percentage (2.5%) of that of L-isomer.[39] Unlike L-dopa, differences in gastrointestinal

Table 7–1 **Pharmacokinetic parameters of stereoisomers**

Drug	Total clearance			Volume of distribution			Elimination half-life (h)			Ref.
	R	S	R:S ratio	R	S	R:S ratio	R	S	R:S ratio	
Atenolol	—	—	—	0.790 (l/kg)	0.879	0.900	6.08	6.13	0.99	24
Disopyramide	111 (ml/min)	111	1	48 (l)	50	0.96	5.2	5.5	0.95	25
Ibuprofen	68 (ml/min)	74	0.92	9.9 (l)	10.5	0.94	2	1.7	1.18	26
Indoprofen	48.8 (ml/min)	32.2	1.52	12.6 (l)	8.97	1.40	3.12	3.35	0.93	27
Prenylamine	2.7 (l/min)	12.4	0.22	—	—	—	13.7	17.4	0.79	28
Propranolol	1210 (ml/min)	1030	1.17	4.8 (l/kg)	4.1	1.17	3.6	3.5	1.03	29, 30
Terbutaline (+,–,+:–)[a]	0.186 (l/h/kg)	0.125	0.149	1.90 (l/kg)	1.76	1.08	12.7	15.3	0.83	31
Tocainide	2.62 (ml/min/kg)	1.70	1.54	2.52 (l/kg)	2.47	1.02	11.7	17.1	0.68	32
Verapamil	10.24 (ml/min/kg)	18.1	0.57	2.74 (l/kg)	6.42	0.43	4.08	4.81	0.85	33
Warfarin	3.5 (ml/h/kg)	4.9	0.71	0.154 (l/kg)	0.16	0.96	35	24	1.46	34, 35

[a] Absolute configuration not known to authors.

absorption between stereoisomers of methotrexate appear to have greater impact on their comparative extents of oral absorption. This is probably due to the great dependence of methotrexate on carrier-mediated absorption in the presence of a minimal passive absorption component.

Several amino-β-lactam antibiotics with an α-amino side chain have been noted to be absorbed across the gastrointestinal membrane by dipeptide carrier systems.[40] β-Lactam derivatives containing L-amino acids are expected to be more rapidly absorbed by dipeptide transport systems than D-amino acid isomers. The stereoisomers of cephalexin are believed to be actively transported by the gastrointestinal brush border. Tamai et al.[41] concluded that L-cephalexin has a higher affinity for the dipeptide carrier than D-cephalexin. This was based on studies examining competitive mucosal uptake between the two isomers. However, after separate administration of the isomers to rats, L-cephalexin had poor systemic bioavailability and D-cephalexin appeared to be well absorbed. This can be explained by the fact that L-cephalexin is rapidly degraded by intestinal homogenates while the D-isomer is not. Thus, the stereospecific intestinal hydrolysis of L-cephalexin results in its low bioavailability despite its better intestinal uptake and absorption.

Presently, few investigations of selective gastrointestinal absorption of stereoisomers have been performed or reported. Unfortunately, differences in membrane absorption are difficult to evaluate from bioavailability studies in the presence of other factors, especially presystemic metabolism. As with L-dopa in man and cephalexin in rats, demonstrated differences in gastrointestinal membrane transfer may not be the predominate factor dictating systemic bioavailability.

While the potential for stereoisomer specific dissolution from solid dosage forms exists, little evidence is currently available to support stereospecific dissolution study requirements. Crystalline forms composed of both stereoisomers as in a racemic powder can differ from the crystalline forms found for the separate isomers.[42] This represents a source of differences in rates of dissolution between a racemate and the individual isomers. Ignoring crystalline forms, enantiomers are expected to have the same rates of dissolution and solubilities from dosage forms containing achiral components and in dissolution environments which are also achiral. This would not be true if pairs of diastereoisomers are compared. Numerous formulation adjuncts including cellulose derivatives (methylcellulose and cellulose acetate phthalate), cyclodextrins, and starch are themselves chiral. For this reason, differences in strength of attractions and interactions between these components and isomers could potentially yield selectivity in dissolution. Stereoselectivity in component interactions might be expected to have greater dissolution consequences when stereoisomers must diffuse through chiral components during their dissolution than when simple component dissolution and erosion controls drug release. In a formulation of hydroxypropyl methylcellulose and propranolol, slightly greater (8 to 10%) dissolution was noted for the R-isomer of propranolol than the S-isomer.[43] However, differences appear variable in that selectivity was noted in only four of six dissolution experiments. Until more information is available, it cannot be assumed that stereoisomers will display the same dissolution rates from racemate formulations.

B. STEREOSELECTIVE DISPOSITION

In bioavailability studies, the rate and completeness of drug absorption are compared and evaluated from parameters such as AUC, peak time, maximum plasma concentration (C_{max}), and amount of drug excreted unchanged. These observed values are not only a function of input rate and extent of absorption, but also the disposition characteristics of the drug. Due to differences in clearance (renal or hepatic) between two enantiomers, the extent of absorption of total enantiomers following administration of the racemate may not be simply compared in all cases by examining the ratio of their AUC values. There is considerable information illustrating that stereoisomers may differ in the rate and degree to which they are eliminated by clearing organs as well as the degree to which they distribute throughout body tissues. An appreciation for the magnitude of these differences is important in investigating the pharmacokinetics and bioavailability of racemate products. The discussion which follows is an overview of stereoselectivity in enantiomer distribution and elimination.

The extent of stereoisomer binding and uptake by intravascular and extravascular sites is reflected in the overall pharmacokinetic profile for the isomer. Only the free or unbound isomers are susceptible to elimination and distribution to receptors. Stereoselectivity is noted in plasma protein binding, tissue binding, and cellular uptake. Differences in stereoisomer distribution are expected when uptake and binding is related to structurally specific interactions with macromolecules and less expected when simple partitioning is responsible.

Human serum albumin (HSA) and α_i-acid glycoprotein (AGP) are capable of discriminating between stereoisomer pairs. The selective properties of these macromolecules allow their use as stationary phases in commercially available chiral columns for high-performance liquid chromatography (HPLC) applications. Interactions between an enantiomer and a plasma protein results in a diastereoisomeric complex. The warfarin (site 1) and the indole:benzodiazepine (site 2) binding centers of HSA are reported to display selective binding toward stereoisomeric pairs. Affinity constants may be similar or markedly different (30-fold for oxazepam hemisuccinate) for isomeric pairs.[44] While HSA is thought to display greater stereoselectivity than AGP, there are examples of isomer-specific binding to both plasma proteins. Binding of R-propranolol to HSA is 39% compared to 35% for the S-isomer; whereas S-propranolol binds (87%) to a greater extent to AGP than the R-isomer (84%).[45] Overall plasma binding of stereoisomers reflects the stereospecific binding of basic drugs to AGP and acidic drugs to HSA. Ratios of fractions free for acidic stereoisomer pairs may be as great as 3 for indacrinone[6] and 1.7 for basic drugs such as verapamil.[6]

Before stereoselectivity in elimination and tissue distribution can be properly interpreted, plasma protein binding differences of the isomers should be considered. Table 7-2 gives a summary of fraction-free values for pairs of stereoisomers.

The rate of organ clearance will be proportional to the fraction free for enantiomers which are considered to have low hepatic and/or renal extraction. For these isomers, the ratio of systemic clearance would be expected to equal the ratio of the free fractions if both stereoisomers have the same intrinsic clearance. The R:S ratio of total body clearance of moxalactam is 1.67[59] and the ratio of fractions free for R:S is 1.42.[60] This may suggest that the major contributing factor for the observed difference in clearance is stereoselectivity in plasma protein binding. On the other hand, the R:S ratio for warfarin clearance is 0.95; however, the same ratio for the fractions free is 1.64.[61] In this case, the differences in plasma protein binding hides apparent differences in intrinsic clearance. Comparison of intrinsic clearance (Cl/ff) between stereoisomers should be performed before true stereoselectivity in clearance can be concluded. For warfarin, the intrinsic clearance of R-warfarin is 52.8 ml/min/kg and S-warfarin is 90.9 ml/min/kg for an R:S ratio of intrinsic clearances of 0.58.[61]

While more difficult to accurately evaluate, the greater fraction free for one stereoisomer may explain its larger volume of distribution when compared to the other. The 18% larger volume of distribution of R-propranolol can be interpreted as a consequence of the higher fraction free for the R-isomer (20.3%) relative to the S-isomer (18.9%).[30,45] The R-isomer of warfarin has a volume of distribution approximately 80% greater than the S-isomer.[61] This also appears to result from fraction-free differences in that R-warfarin has a fraction free 64% greater than S-warfarin. The larger volume of distribution and greater clearance of R-disopyramide appears to be due to its lower plasma protein binding.[62,25]

For reasons discussed above, stereospecific drug distribution is difficult to evaluate from convenient pharmacokinetic studies, and thus studies of tissue to plasma isomer partitioning may be particularly useful to explore distribution differences between stereoisomers.

Table 7–2 **Plasma protein binding of stereoisomers**

	Fraction free(%)			
	(+)	(–)	+:– ratio	Ref.
Acids				
Acenocoumerol	1.61	1.45	1.11	46
Ibuprofen	0.77	0.45	1.71	47
Indacrinone	0.3	0.9	0.33	9
Mephobarbital	66	53	1.25	48
Moxalactam	47	32	1.47	49
Pentobarbital	36.6	26.5	1.38	50
Phenprocoumon	1.07	0.9	1.19	51
Bases				
Amphetamine	84	84	1.0	52
Disopyramide	7.5	12.5	0.6	53
Fenfluramine	2.8	2.9	0.97	54
Methadone	9.2	12.4	0.74	55
Mexiletine	28.3	19.8	1.43	56
Propoxyphene	1.8	1.8	1.0	9
Propranolol	20.3	17.6	1.15	30, 45
	12	11	1.1	57
Quinidine	8.9	9.5	0.94	58
Terbutaline	20	20	1.0	31
Tocainide	83–89	86–91		32
Verapamil	6.4	11	0.58	21, 33

Several studies in animals have demonstrated differences in tissue partitioning between pairs of stereoisomers. For low doses of propranolol in rats, the S-isomer has an apparent volume of distribution greater than that of the R-isomer.[63] Comparing areas under the tissue vs. plasma concentration curves demonstrated preferential uptake of S-propranolol in heart and brain tissue and of R-propranolol in lung tissue. Timolol also displays greater uptake and persistence of the S-isomer in rat heart, lung, and brain tissue when compared to the R-isomer.[64] The uptake of timolol is inhibited by S-propranolol, but not R-propranolol, suggesting stereospecific binding of these betablockers to several tissues.[64]

Unfortunately, a large percentage of pharmacokinetic and tissue distribution studies of stereoisomers have not included plasma protein-binding studies, thus limiting interpretation of selective distribution as well as clearance. Tocainide isomers have been reported to display little plasma protein binding in humans.[32] Stereospecific salivary secretion of tocainide has been suggested based on the higher saliva to plasma concentration ratios for the R-isomer (3.7) compared to the S-isomers (2.1).[65] In this case, since plasma protein binding is similar, stereoselective distribution may be considered. Day et al.[66] noted that the active S-isomer of ibuprofen had synovial fluid concentration approximately twice that of the inactive R-isomer. However, in this example, the apparent selective distribution of the S-isomer is probably a consequence of the 7% higher fraction free for this S-isomer.[67] For tiaprofenic acid, synovial concentrations are similar for the two isomers.[68]

C. STEREOSELECTIVE BIOTRANSFORMATION

While drug receptors are probably the most discriminating source of stereoselectivity, the subtle conformation variations of enantiomers are also likely to result in differences in drug metabolism. Biotransformation systems such as mixed-function oxidases, esterases, glucuronyl transferases, glutathione transferases, and others have shown varying degrees of enantiomer selectivity. Comparisons of stereoisomer biotransformation and its therapeutic implications have been documented and reviewed in the literature.[3,69,70] In some cases, the less active isomer may be primarily responsible for the therapeutic effects of the racemate due to the rapid removal of the active isomer by hepatic clearance.

Substantial differences in clearance between stereoisomers which are primarily metabolized illustrate the high selectivity of biotransformation pathways. For extensive metabolizers of mephenytoin, the oral clearance of the S-isomer is approximately 170-fold greater than the R-isomer.[71] This clearance difference results in R-mephenytoin having a half-life 30 times greater than that of S-mephenytoin. Metabolic stereoselectivity is not apparent in poor metabolizers of mephenytoin where the clearance and half-lives of the two isomers are similar. In young men, R-mephobarbital clearance following oral administration is more than 100 times greater than that of the S-isomer.[72] The half-life of the slowly cleared S-isomer is 50.5 h compared to only 3.1 h for the R-isomer. In young females, the clearance difference is only 50-fold. This pronounced selectivity in biotransformation is also noted for another barbiturate, hexobarbital. A ninefold difference in clearance between stereoisomers is observed in young adults while in elderly subjects the clearance differences are five-fold.[73]

For racemates which have a high hepatic extraction ratio, large differences in hepatic clearance will produce even larger variations in plasma concentration for the isomers following oral administration. These will be examined under the topic of pharmacokinetic and bioavailability evaluations of racemates.

The above examples demonstrate marked differences in stereoisomer biotransformation as well as the importance of intersubject variability in the magnitude of these differences. However, this should not be expected for all stereoisomers since in many cases the clearance and metabolic differences may not be nearly as great. For racemate drugs such as pentobarbital,[50] misonidazole,[74] and mexiletine,[56] there are not more than 20% differences between the clearances of the two enantiomers. As previously discussed, these smaller variations in clearance may result from plasma protein binding differences.

Metabolic patterns for stereoisomers are not necessarily similar and are also reflected in intrinsic hepatic clearance differences. S-warfarin is predominately oxidized to 7-hydroxy-S-warfarin whereas the R-isomer is eliminated by ketone oxidation and reduction to the metabolites, 6-hydroxy- and 8-hydroxy-warfarin.[61] Both isomers of verapamil are approximately equally metabolized by N-dealkylation; however, O-demethylation occurs considerably faster to S-verapamil compared to the R-isomer.[75,76] It is suspected that stereoselectivity in biotransformation results not only from differences in the degree of interaction between isomers and the same enzymes, but also from the possibility that different isoenzymes are involved with the biotransformation of each isomer. This concept is supported by evidence that inducers and inhibitors of drug metabolism may alter each stereoisomer biotransformation to a different degree. Phenytoin therapy increases the clearance of (+)-misonidazole by 55% and the (–)-isomer by only 33%.[74] Ticrynafen prolongs the half-life of S-warfarin from 28 to 88 h while no change in half-life of R-warfarin is observed.[77] In this case, the apparent change in the half-life of racemic warfarin was from 48 to 74 h.

D. STEREOISOMER CONVERSION

Except for a few drugs, spontaneous inversion of enantiomers in solution generally does not occur due to the high energetic barriers to inversion. Metabolic interconversion is found for many but not all of the 2-arylpropionate nonsteroidal anti-inflammatory drugs. While *in vitro* prostaglandin synthetase inhibition is related to the S-isomer, administration of separate isomers or racemates produce similar *in vivo* activities. The conversion of the inactive R-isomer occurs through an isomer thioester formation by acyl CoA synthetase followed by the action of a nonstereospecific racemase to convert the R- to the S-isomer.[78] The conversion of S- to R-isomer is not possible due to the inability of the S-isomer to form the thioester. There appears to be significant R- to S-isomer conversion for the NSAIDs, ibuprofen,[26] fenoprofen,[79] benoxaprofen,[80] and limited conversion for flurbiprofen,[81] indoprofen,[27] flunoxaprofen,[82] and tiaprofenic acid.[68] Conversion of R-ibuprofen to S-ibuprofen has been estimated as 60% in humans.[26] Since the R-isomer of NSAIDs may be considered inactive, it is possible that equal therapeutic effects can be obtained by administering only the S-isomer at lower doses than that which is required for total doses of the racemate. Lower total doses of NSAIDs displaying R- to S-isomer conversion could lower the incidence of side effects such as GI upset.

One interesting aspect to NSAID inversion is evidence that this isomeric change may occur in the GI tract. Based on AUC values for different routes of administration (oral, i.v., i.p.), benoxaprofen R- to S-isomer conversion appears to be greatest in the GI tract and not in the liver of the rat.[80] Also, for ketoprofen in rats, the AUC ratio for S:R is similar for the i.p. and i.v. routes whereas the oral route yields an S:R ratio 3 times that of the other two routes.[83] Based on this information, the R- to S-isomer conversion in the rat would appear to occur in the GI tract as well as in the liver. Since ketoprofen does not show significant inversion in humans, there are questions as to the significance of presystemic GI inversion in humans. Due to the saturable nature of gastrointestinal biotransformation, GI stereoisomeric conversion of drugs such as NSAIDs represents a potential source of bioavailability differences among solid dosage forms. Evidence for significant concerns in humans has been presented by Jamali et al.,[84] and will be discussed later in the context of ibuprofen.

E. STEREOSELECTIVE RENAL EXCRETION

Glomerular filtration of free stereoisomer in the plasma is expected to be the same for each isomer. However, the active secretion and reabsorption of drug in the kidney tubules may display stereoselectivity. Calculations of intrinsic renal clearance as renal clearance divided by fraction free can be applied toward identifying differences in active excretion of stereoisomers. The (+)-isomer of terbutaline displays a 30% greater renal clearance than its (–)-isomer.[31] Since the isomers have equal as well as low plasma protein binding (20%), stereoselectivity in renal clearance and tubular secretion was suggested. The unbound renal clearance of l-pindolol is slightly but significantly greater than d-pindolol.[85] The stereoisomers quinine and quinidine are both approximately 88% plasma protein bound; however, the renal clearance of quinidine is 4 times that of quinine. These two stereoisomers are diastereoisomers and therefore are expected to display greater differences in pharmacokinetics.

F. PHARMACOKINETIC INTERACTIONS BETWEEN STEREOISOMERS

The similarity in structural and chemical features of stereoisomers suggests a strong potential for them to interact and alter the pharmacokinetics as well as pharmacodynamics of each other. Competition between stereoisomers for plasma protein and tissue-binding sites and drug biotransformation enzymes is expected. There are a few examples suggesting potential pharmacokinetic interactions between stereoisomers. Enantiomers of disopyramide appear to have similar clearance, volume of distribution, and half-life when administered separately.[25] However, if the racemate is dosed intravenously, the R-isomer displays 50 to 100% greater total body and renal clearances and volumes of distribution. These differences in pharmacokinetics appear to result from displacement of R-disopyramide by the S-isomer from plasma protein as well as dose dependency in the kinetics of this drug. In addition, the clearance and volume of distribution of R-ibuprofen is slightly increased after dosing the racemate compared to single R-isomer dosing.[26] While this requires further study, plasma protein displacement of R-ibuprofen by S-ibuprofen may be the reason.

As presented in the next section, interpretation of racemate bioavailability reflects a composite of absorption and disposition features of the stereoisomers. However, should the stereoisomers produce a pharmacokinetic interaction the interpretation of bioavailability and pharmacokinetic results may become even more perplexing. The magnitude of these interactions probably will show evidence of dose dependency. Being unable to predict the impact of the isomer-isomer interactions on standard bioavailability and pharmacokinetic parameters can make the relevance of racemate results even more questionable.

G. STEREOSELECTIVE HEPATIC FIRST-PASS BIOTRANSFORMATION

Several drug classes including beta blockers and calcium channel blockers are administered orally as racemates and have low oral bioavailability due to hepatic first-pass biotransformation. While the high hepatic clearance and extraction of one or both stereoisomers results in the loss of a significant portion of the oral dose, the stereoisomers may not necessarily be effected to the same degree. Should the stereoisomers have different pharmacological characteristics, a route of administration effect will be observed for the racemate.

If both stereoisomers have very high hepatic extraction following intravenous doses, they will have similar total body clearance which will approach hepatic plasma or blood flow. Differences in intrinsic hepatic clearance may not be evident from clearances obtained after intravenous dosing due to flow limitations on clearance. However, after oral administration, intrinsic clearance differences may lead to large variations in the systemic availability between the stereoisomers. The pharmacokinetics and bioavailability of propranolol isomers appear to follow this relationship (see Figure 7–2).[86] The active S-isomer is primarily responsible for the therapeutic activity of the racemate. The systemic clearance measured after i.v. dosing is approximately 17% greater for the S-isomer compared to the R-isomer.[87] The stereoisomer systemic clearances are both similar to blood flow with values of 1.21 and 1.03 l/min for the R- and S-isomer, respectively. This similarity in propranolol clearance results in both the stereoisomers having superimposable plasma concentration profiles following an intravenous dose. However, determination of the S:R ratio for plasma concentrations after oral administration yields ratios ranging from 0.99 to 2.04, illustrating that the active to inactive isomer plasma concentration ratio is increased after oral dosing.[86] Apparent oral clearance (Cl/F) following oral administration of the inactive R-isomer is 40% greater than that of the active isomer. This represents a larger first-pass metabolic loss of the inactive isomer than the active form. The S- and R-isomers of nitrendipine also display only a slight difference (7%) in total body clearance after i.v. dosing.[88] However, following oral administration of nitrendipine, the S-isomer has oral availability of 13.4% while the R-isomer is 7.9% available. Thus, the S-isomer of nitrendipine has approximately 75% greater bioavailability than the R-isomer.[88]

In the case of verapamil, a greater difference in the systemic and oral clearances of the stereoisomers is observed. S-verapamil, which is considered the most active isomer, has an 80% greater systemic clearance than R-verapamil after i.v. dosing.[33] For verapamil, the difference between the plasma concentrations for the stereoisomers seen after intravenous dosing is further amplified after oral administration. The dissimilarity in the systemic clearances of the two isomers of acenocoumarol also results in a stereoselective first-pass effect. The more rapidly cleared S-isomer displays a 30% loss during first-pass while the R-isomer has a small 3% loss. This first-pass extraction difference in part contributes to an apparent oral clearance of S-acenocoumarol which is more than 13 times that of the R-isomer.[46]

H. PHARMACOKINETIC AND BIOAVAILABILITY EVALUATIONS OF RACEMATES AND STEREOISOMERS

The vast majority of bioavailability and pharmacokinetic information for racemic drug mixtures found in the literature has been derived from nonstereoselective plasma analysis methods. This has led many reviewers to conclude that such pharmacokinetic and pharmacodynamic information is inaccurate and perhaps nonsensical.[89] From the above

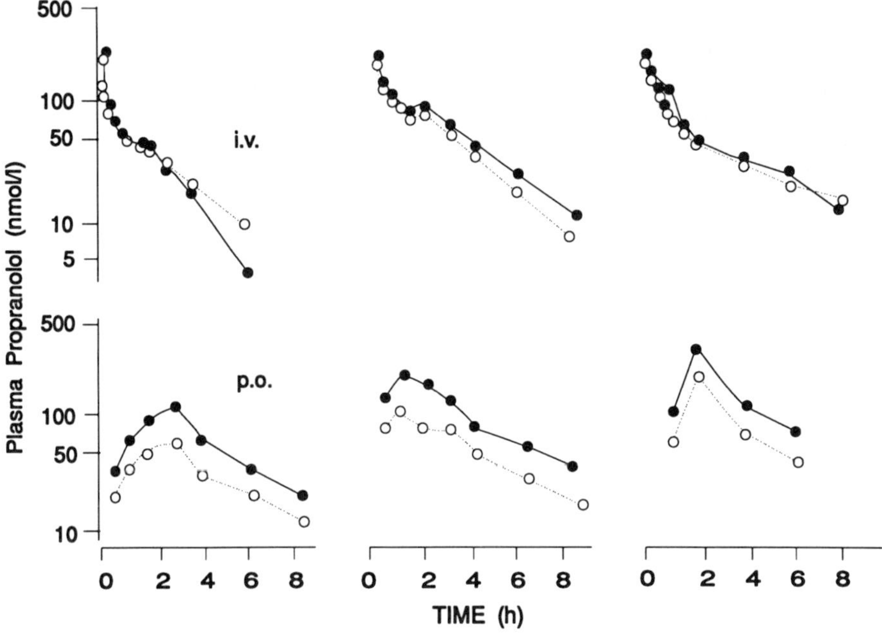

Figure 7–2 Plasma concentrations of (+)– and (–)–propranolol obtained in three subjects after administration of racemic (±)-propranolol; 40-mg propranolol was given orally and 5 mg, intravenously. ○(+)-propranolol, ●(–)-propranolol. (From Von Bahr, C., Hermansson, J., and Tawara, K., *Br. J. Clin. Pharmacol.,* 14, 79, 1982. With permission.)

discussion, it appears that the small spatial aspects of enantiomers can result in substantial differences between their absorption, distribution, and elimination. Stereospecific assays are more expensive and in some cases not available to determine the pharmacokinetic profile of both enantiomer components. However, the clinical significance of pharmacokinetic and pharmacodynamic results, in which the stereoisomers are indistinguishable, would appear to be questionable. In several cases, the inactive stereoisomer may comprise the greater percentage of the measured plasma concentration. If the active isomer appears as a constant percentage of the total plasma concentration, interpretation of nonstereospecific results would perhaps have some validity. However, ratios of active to inactive isomer in the plasma may vary from subject to subject and perhaps even between formulations of the same racemic product.

A better understanding of when stereoselective pharmacokinetic and bioavailability investigations are needed or not needed can be obtained by exploring the relationships that exist between the separate pharmacokinetic parameters of enantiomers and racemates. Awareness of the contributions of the separate isomers to the plasma concentration profile of the racemate can provide insight toward better design and evaluation of bioavailability and pharmacokinetic studies. Comparative bioavailability studies of racemic drugs based on nonstereospecific assays have been and may continue to be acceptable. It should be recognized that the parameters of clearance, extent of absorption, volume of distribution, and half-life for a racemate are complex collections and composites of those of each stereoisomer. Assay of a racemate by nonspecific methods effectively results in the summation of the individual stereoisomer plasma concentrations. Due to possible differences in the rates of absorption and elimination, the concentration ratio of the stereoisomers may vary throughout the plasma concentration profile. For this reason, parameters of rate and extent of absorption, total and renal clearance, volume of distribution, and the fraction free for total drug will be time dependent.[90]

I. SINGLE-DOSE PHARMACOKINETICS AND BIOAVAILABILITY

The clearance after intravenous dosing of a racemate (CL_{RS}) reflects contributions of the individual isomer clearances (CL_R and CL_S). CL_{RS} is estimated from the area under the curve for the racemate (AUC_{RS}):

$$CL_{RS} = \frac{Dose_{RS}}{AUC_{RS}} \tag{7–1}$$

Since the dose contains equal proportions of both isomers of equal molecular weight and the AUC_{RS} is the sum of the AUCs for each stereoisomer, AUC_{RS} is described by Equation (7–2):

$$AUC_{RS} = AUC_R + AUC_S = \frac{0.5\ Dose_{RS}}{CL_R} + \frac{0.5\ Dose_{RS}}{CL_S} \tag{7–2}$$

Substituting AUC_{RS} into Equation 7–1 and rearranging provides an expression for CL_{RS} in terms of the individual clearances:

$$CL_{RS} = \frac{CL_R CL_S 2}{CL_R + CL_S} \tag{7–3}$$

This result has also been reported by Tucker and Lennard.[2] If one stereoisomer has a clearance substantially greater than that of the other, the CL_{RS} will be approximately twice that of the more slowly cleared isomer. For example, if $CL_R \gg CL_S$, then CL_{RS} approaches 2 CL_S.

To illustrate this relationship with Equation 7–3, the R- and S-isomers of moxalactam have total body clearances of 69.6 and 41.6 ml/min/m^2, respectively. The racemate, by Equation 7–3, would have a predicted clearance of 52.1 ml/min/m^2 which is close to the observed value for the racemate of 51.2 ml/min/m^2.[59] For verapamil, the isomers have clearances of 10.2 and 18.1 ml/min/kg, and the racemate is 14.3 ml/min/kg.[33] Equation 7–3 would estimate clearance as 13.1 ml/min/kg. These clearance predictions assume that there is no interaction between the isomers such as competition for plasma-binding sites or eliminating enzyme or transport mechanisms. Thus, these interpretations would not be valid for a drug such as disopyramide which exhibits plasma protein-binding competition. They would, however, be useful in identifying enantiomer-enantiomer interactions when the predictions for racemate clearance do not agree with the observed racemate clearance.

The extent of absorption of a racemate when given orally or by any other nonintravenous route reflects the extent of absorption of each isomer. In this case, the AUC_{RS} is not only a function of the separate extents of absorption (F_R and F_S) but also the total body clearances. The apparent total body clearance following oral administration (CL_{RS} oral) can be derived based on Equation 7–2 and considering the separate extents of absorption:

$$CL_{RS}oral = \frac{CL_R CL_S 2}{CL_R F_S + CL_S F_R} = CL_{RS}/F_{RS} \tag{7–4}$$

It then follows that the extent of absorption of the racemate, as determined from AUCs following oral and intravenous dosing to the same subject at the same dose, is

$$F_{RS} = \frac{F_S CL_R + F_R CL_S}{CL_R + CL_S} = \frac{AUC_{RS}\text{oral}}{AUC_{RS}\text{iv}} \qquad \textbf{(7–5)}$$

This equation applies if the pharmacokinetics are linear and there is no interaction between isomers. As suggested by Equation 7–5, the F_{RS} is not a simple sum or average of the fractions absorbed for each stereoisomer. Using the systemic clearances of 10.2 and 18.1 ml/min/kg for the R- and S-isomers of verapamil as well as an F_R of 0.5 and an F_S of 0.2, Equation 7–5 predicts an F_{RS} of 0.39. This is quite similar to the 0.4 observed for racemic verapamil.[91]

Should the systemic clearances of both isomers be the same, then F_{RS} will equal the average of the extents of absorption for each isomer.

$$F_{RS} = \frac{F_S + F_R}{2} \quad \text{if } CL_S = CL_R \qquad \textbf{(7–6)}$$

However, even in this special case, differences in the saturable first-pass features of the stereoisomers would disrupt this calculation. As discussed previously, enantiomers displaying high extraction ratios may have similar clearances after intravenous dosing. After oral dosing, the metabolic intrinsic differences will reveal themselves. This can result in F_S and F_R being markedly different despite similarities in CL_R and CL_S.

In a comparative bioavailability study between two formulations (A and B) of a racemate, the relative extent of absorption (F_{rel}) is calculated:

$$F_{rel} = \frac{F^A_{RS}}{F^B_{RS}} = \frac{AUC^A_S + AUC^A_R}{AUC^B_S + AUC^B_R} = \frac{AUC^A_{RS}}{AUC^B_{RS}} \qquad \textbf{(7–7)}$$

$$F_{rel} = \frac{AUC^A_{RS}}{AUC^B_{RS}} = \frac{AUC^A_R}{AUC^B_R} = \frac{AUC^A_S}{AUC^B_S} \quad \text{(if } AUC_R/AUC_S \text{ is constant for A and B)} \qquad \textbf{(7–8)}$$

$$F_{rel} = \frac{CL_R F^A_S + CL_S F^A_R}{CL_R F^B_S + CL_S F^B_R} \qquad \textbf{(7–9)}$$

By inspection of Equation 7–7, if the ratio of AUC_S:AUC_R is the same for both formulations, the F_{rel} determined from total AUC (AUC_{RS}) or the ratio of the AUCs for either stereoisomer will yield the same estimate of F_{rel} (Equation 7–8). On this basis, nonspecific assay results could be used to compare extents of absorption between two racemate products. In this case, the extent of absorption of the racemate would approximate that of the active stereoisomer. To validate the use of nonstereospecific methods for bioequivalence appraisals, proof of no formulation, rate of absorption, or extent of absorption effects on AUC ratios of stereoisomers should be established. Racemate products with demonstrated differences in isomer ratio would be candidates for stereospecific bioavailability evaluations. This will be discussed later with ibuprofen and verapamil products.

Other parameters such as volume of distribution for a racemic drug cannot be as easily related to those of its stereoisomers. Generally, the racemate volume of distribution will be between that of the individual isomers. For example, R- and S-verapamil have a volume of distribution of 2.74 and 6.42 l/kg, respectively. That of the racemate is 3.40 l/kg which falls between its stereoisomers.[33]

The most commonly reported pharmacokinetic parameter is half-life. Half-life is a measure of drug persistence in the body and is useful in predicting the time to steady state and the degree of drug accumulation following multiple dosing. Since bioavailability evaluations require the estimate of the AUC to infinity, half-life has a significant impact on predicting the AUC contribution from the last observed plasma concentration to infinity. If — as in the case of some NSAIDs and propranolol —the half-lives of the stereoisomers are nearly the same, then the half-life of the racemate will be approximately equal to that of the individual stereoisomers. This again assumes no pharmacokinetic interaction between the stereoisomers. If one isomer is converted to the other whether metabolically or spontaneously, the two isomers will appear to have the same half-life. Ibuprofen isomers have similar half-lives with 2.0 ± 0.5 h for the R-isomer and 1.7 ± 0.4 h for the active S-isomer.[26]

When stereoisomers have different half-lives, as mentioned previously for several drugs including mephenytoin, the observed terminal half-life will be that of the stereoisomer with the longest half-life. Knowledge of this phenomenon for particular drugs is necessary to ensure accurate calculation of AUC for the racemate drug. A time period of at least 4 to 5 half-lives for the more rapidly eliminated stereoisomer is required before the half-life of the slowly eliminated isomer and racemate can be assessed. This situation is similar to that which must be considered to obtain half-lives of drugs displaying multiexponential decay in plasma concentrations. While exhibiting some intersubject variability, the half-life of R-warfarin (20 to 70 h) was found by Breckenridge et al.[34] to be significantly longer than that of S-warfarin (18 to 34 h). The appropriate half-life of the racemate would be that of R-warfarin (20 to 70 h). In extensive metabolizers of mephenytoin, the R-isomer has a half-life of 76 h and the S-isomer has one only of 2.1 h due to the S-isomer clearance being approximately 170 times that of the R-isomer. A few hours after mephenytoin administration to these subjects, the S-isomer would be not detectable in plasma and the apparent half-life for a nonspecific assay would yield the 76-h half-life of S-isomer.

It is possible that the multicompartment features noted after intravenous administration of a racemate may be an artifact of the kinetics of the stereoisomers.[92] In a situation where one isomer has a much smaller volume of distribution and greater clearance than the other, two stereoisomers which display one-compartment features may provide an apparent multicompartment profile for the racemate.[90]

The peak concentration and time of peak are reflections of bioavailability differences between formulated products and are critically evaluated to prove or disprove bioequivalency. In the simplest case of a drug described by a one-compartment model, the time of peak is a function of the absorption rate, the absorption lag time, and the drug disposition half-life. In the case where the half-lives of stereoisomers are similar, differences in time of peak between stereoisomers would reflect their differences in absorption rate and lag time. Should both stereoisomers have equal peak times, then the racemate time of peak will be the same. If the absorption rate constants or elimination half-lives of the isomers are different, then the peak time will not be the same and the peak time of the racemate will appear as that of the isomer with the highest peak concentration value. For these same reasons, two peaks could be noted. In the case where the peak concentration of the inactive stereoisomer is manyfold greater than the active form, the clinical significance of the peak concentration and time of peak would be questionable.

J. MULTIPLE-DOSE PHARMACOKINETICS AND BIOAVAILABILITY

Assessment of bioavailability and pharmacokinetics at steady state reveals the pharmacokinetic and absorption differences between stereoisomers. The average steady-state plasma concentration (Css) is proportional to the AUCs and inversely proportional to the clearances of each stereoisomer. AUCs at steady state are compared to establish extent of absorption differences between formulations of the same drug at the same dose. The AUC_{RS} at steady state would be expected to equal that predicted by Equation 7–2. Recognizing that Css for the racemate ($C_{RS}ss$) equals the AUC_{RS} divided by the dosing interval (τ), $C_{RS}ss$ is predicted as:

$$C_{RS}ss_{(IV)} = \frac{0.5\ Dose_{RS}\left(CL_R + CL_S\right)}{\left(CL_R CL_S\right)\tau} = C_R ss_{(IV)} + C_S ss_{(IV)} \tag{7–10}$$

$$C_{RS}ss_{(oral)} = \frac{0.5\ Dose_{RS}\left(CL_R F_S + CL_S F_R\right)}{\left(CL_R CL_S\right)\tau} = C_R ss_{(oral)} + C_S ss_{(oral)} \tag{7–11}$$

Obtaining F_{RS} for the racemate by dividing AUCs at steady state for the oral by the intravenous route will yield the same estimate of F_{RS} found in Equation 7–5. Estimations of F_{rel} from multiple-dosing results would also follow the relationships described in Equations 7–7 through 7–9. For this reason, multiple-dose bioequivalency studies of stereoisomers would involve the same assumptions and conditions as those of single-dose studies.

When differences exist in half-lives, the time to steady state or any fraction of steady state will not be the same for the stereoisomers. As observed for tocainide during a continuous infusion, the mean ratio of S- to R-isomer changes from 1 to 1.7 over 48 h of infusion.[93] The steady-state ratio displayed considerable intersubject variations with values ranging from 1.3 to 4. R-tocainide is the active stereoisomer, and at steady state the percentage of total drug which is active ranged from 20 to 44%. In multiple-dose bioequivalency evaluations by nonstereospecific methods, the time required for each isomer to reach steady state must be considered.

IV. STEREOSELECTIVE BIOAVAILABILITY: EXAMPLES

The consequences of nonstereospecific drug assays on interpreting therapeutic implications of bioavailability and pharmacokinetic information has become a concern to both the drug industry and government. It is generally agreed that requirements for stereospecific bioavailability and pharmacokinetic data will be on a case-by-case basis. Substantially more studies are needed to identify for which racemate products full stereoselective information will be essential. Presented below are two interesting racemate products which illustrate the possible importance of stereoisomer-specific evaluations.

A. VERAPAMIL

The stereoisomers of verapamil display considerable differences in both pharmacokinetics and pharmacodynamics and have been the subject of several investigations.[21,33,94] The primary A-V conduction effects reside in the S-isomer which is believed to be tenfold more potent than the R-isomer. The active S-isomer has a fraction free about twice that of the R-isomer which accounts for the larger volume of distribution of the S-isomer. The apparent intrinsic clearance of the S-isomer is approximately 2.5 times the R-isomer. The combined effects of intrinsic clearance, protein binding, and blood flow result in the S-isomer having a total body clearance about 80% greater than the inactive R-isomer. The S-isomer appears to be more blood flow limited than the R-isomer.

Following intravenous single and multiple dosing, it is expected that the S-isomer will have plasma concentrations approximately 50 to 60% that of the inactive R-isomer. Thus, only 35% of total concentrations would be the active stereoisomer. The greater intrinsic clearance of the S-isomer results in its greater first-pass loss and lower bioavailability of S-verapamil (20%) compared to R-verapamil (50%). After oral administration, S-verapamil is 18 to 20% of the total verapamil plasma concentration. The S:R ratio for steady-state plasma concentrations would be expected to average 0.5 to 0.6 for intravenous dosing and 0.20 to 0.25 following oral doses. Consequentially, total plasma concentrations which are primarily the inactive R-isomer may have limited therapeutic importance especially if the S:R ratio varies across subject populations. For these reasons, the relationship between percentage change in prolongation (PR) interval and log plasma concentration is different between the intravenous and oral routes.[22]

How useful total plasma concentrations are in evaluating verapamil bioavailability and pharmacokinetics, considering that plasma concentrations are predominantly the inactive R-isomer, would appear to raise concerns. Interpretations based on plasma concentration results of total isomer would be of less concern should the stereoisomer ratio appear constant throughout patient populations and oral formulations. In bioavailability studies, intersubject variability is controlled by the crossover design and thus would not be viewed as invalidating results. If presystemic biotransformation is nonsaturable and not dose dependent for both isomers, then formulation differences should not affect plasma concentration ratios or evaluations by achiral assays. In the absence of dose-dependent presystemic biotransformation, the fractions of the dose of each stereoisomer reaching the systemic circulation are not a function of oral dose and would not be expected to be influenced by rates of release from dosage forms. However, formulation effects on stereoisomer plasma concentration ratios might be expected if the nonlinearity and saturability of presystemic metabolism are different for the isomers. In these cases, the rate of overall drug delivery to the liver may produce time and dose-dependent effects on the plasma concentration ratios of stereoisomers. For this situation, nonstereospecific assay results would appear to be inappropriate for bioequivalency determinations.

The bioavailability of verapamil determined by chiral and achiral assay methods has been reported.[95] An achiral assay revealed no difference between two sustained release preparations, Calan SR and Verapamil CR, when taken without food. However, stereospecific assay demonstrated differences in AUCs and peak concentrations for S-verapamil between the sustained-release products. When the products were taken with food, evaluations based on either separate stereoisomers or the total drug showed no differences between products. Whether this is a consequence of stereoselective nonlinearity in first-pass metabolism requires further study. In this same study, an immediate-release verapamil product displayed different stereoisomer plasma concentration ratios than the sustained-release products.

Propranolol bioavailability appears to be dose dependent with increased bioavailability at higher oral doses due to saturation of first-pass biotransformation.[63] It has been suggested that if this nonlinearity in first-pass loss is stereospecific in humans, then the dose and rate of absorption of total drug from propranolol dosage forms may influence the ratio of stereoisomers in plasma. Again, potential formulation effects on chiral vs. achiral bioavailability assessment of high hepatic extraction drugs such as verapamil and propranolol appear to require particular attention.

B. IBUPROFEN

The 2-arylpropionic acid NSAIDs, with the exception of naproxen, are available as racemates. *In vivo* inversion of the inactive R-isomer to the therapeutically active S-isomer via coenzyme A thioester formation is noted for several of these, including ibuprofen. Following oral administration, approximately 60% of the R-isomer is converted to S-ibuprofen.[26] When conversion is only in one direction, the fraction converted can be estimated from AUC values obtained after the administration of the separate stereoisomers as shown for ibuprofen below:[26]

$$\text{Fraction inverted} = \frac{(\text{AUC}_\text{S}\text{ following R})/(\text{Dose}_\text{R})}{(\text{AUC}_\text{S}\text{ following S})/(\text{Dose}_\text{S})} \qquad \textbf{(7–12)}$$

While interconversion itself does not imply a need for stereoselective bioequivalency studies, there is some suggestion that the NSAID interconversion is presystemic and the extent of this conversion is formulation dependent. Jamali et al.[96] noted that for humans the conversion of R- to S-ibuprofen is not dependent on the dosage given (50- to 1200-mg doses), but is directly related to the residence time in the intestine. The latter conclusion was based on increased S:R AUC ratios for a tablet formulation compared to those of liquid formulations.

A previous study reported on the stereospecific bioavailability of four racemic ibuprofen tablet products.[84] Two formulations displayed apparently slower oral absorption than the others based on time of peak for S-ibuprofen. The more slowly absorbed formulations had times to peak of 2.75 and 2.83 h compared to 1.44 and 1.42 h for the other two. The ratio of AUCs for S:R was significantly greater for the more slowly absorbed products (1.68 and 1.94) than the products with shorter peak times (1.47 and 1.60). It could be interpreted that the rate of absorption, perhaps limited by solid dosage form dissolution, influences the percentage of the R-isomer converted to S-isomer by presystemic biotransformation. The gastrointestinal wall may be a site of this conversion. Should this GI pathway be saturable, rapid dissolution would overwhelm the inversion enzymes leading to a lower percentage conversion of R to S. In this study, bioequivalence based on total isomer concentration was not compared.

Further investigations are required to confirm the relationship of product influences on isomer ratios. Other studies have shown bioinequivalence between ibuprofen products based on stereoselective assay of the S-isomer (see Figure 7–3).[97,98] In one study, oral products were found to be bioequivalent based on standard achiral drug assay but the AUC for S-ibuprofen was significantly different between products by chiral assay.[98] The overall clinical significance of these observations and the possibility of these differences being detected by nonspecific methods, still need to be answered. Central to understanding the mechanism of ibuprofen formulation effects is the role of its presystemic inversion. Proof of presystemic GI and/or hepatic inversion of NSAIDs such as ibuprofen in humans has not been clearly identified. Presystemic inversion would generally imply a route of administration effect on isomer plasma concentration ratios. In a study where racemate ibuprofen was administered both intravenously and orally to obtain systemic extent of absorption, the extent of absorption was approximately one for both isomers.[99] If presystemic R- to S-isomer conversion is significant for ibuprofen, the extent of absorption of the S-isomer should be greater than one and the R-isomer less than one. These apparent inconsistencies in conclusions require additional study.

V. SUMMARY

Stereoisomer pharmacokinetic differences which display themselves after the isomers reach the systemic circulation should not alone have an impact on bioavailability comparisons of pharmaceutical equivalents. This is true provided intersubject variation is accounted for by crossover design and attempts are made to appropriately obtain complete AUCs. In cases where stereoselective passage across GI membrane is suspected, the uneven distribution and capacity of drug transport systems in the GI tract may reveal dissolution effects on the bioavailability of stereoisomers. Any source of nonlinear or saturable presystemic biotransformation or inversion which does not affect each isomer equally represents a need for stereospecific bioavailability determination. These specific absorption and disposition characteristics may yield differences in systemic availability and plasma concentration ratios of stereoisomers as a function of the drug release rate from the oral dosage forms. Unfortunately, extensive and accurate stereoselective pharmacokinetic and clinical information concerning the effects of racemate dosage and route of administration are required to properly determine whether these presystemic effects are

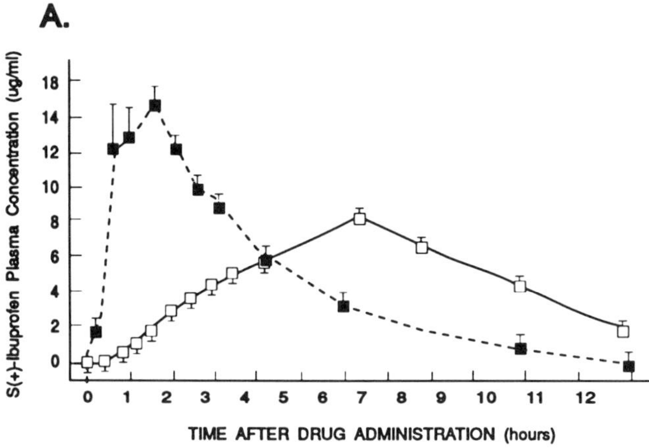

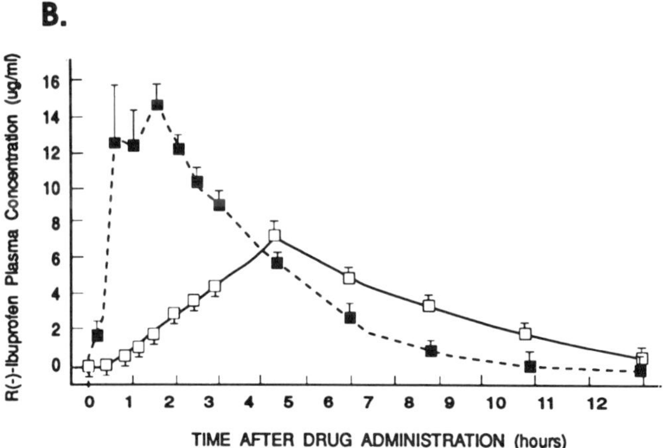

Figure 7–3 Average ibuprofen enantiomer concentration-time data from 11 subjects. (A) shows (S)-ibuprofen data and (B) shows (R)-ibuprofen data. Error bars indicate the standard errors of the mean values. Key: (■) Tablet A, (□) tablet B. (From Cox, S. R. et al., *Biopharm. Drug Dispos.,* 9, 539, 1988. With permission of John Wiley & Sons.)

of clinical significance. Considering the large number of racemate products, there is a deficiency in stereoselective information needed to clearly identify which racemates should be evaluated by chiral approaches.

As presented in this chapter, the pharmacokinetic and pharmacodynamic features of two stereoisomers administered in a racemate should not be considered to be the same. From many examples in the literature, the pharmacological activities and profiles of stereoisomers may be markedly different. In some cases, the risk-benefit aspects of a drug can be improved by providing the drug as a single stereoisomer product. Pharmacokinetic and thereby biopharmaceutical results based on nonstereospecific analysis methods could yield confusing and misleading disposition and absorption information on racemic products. It is recognized that racemates have been safely administered for years and are less expensive to develop. However, an appreciation of the influence of their stereoisomeric features on pharmacokinetic and bioavailability data is necessary to identify situations in which stereoselective approaches are required. While nonspecific data evaluation of many racemates may be suitable for properly designed comparative bioavailability studies, plasma concentration data from these studies may not always be extrapolated toward predicting or interpreting clinical effects.

REFERENCES

1. **Vlasses, P. H., Irvin, J. D., Huber, P. B., Lee, R. B., Ferguson, R. K., Schrogie, J. J., Zacchei, A. G., Davies, R. O., and Abrams, W. B.,** Pharmacology of enantiomers and (–) *p*-OH metabolite of indacrinone, *Clin. Pharmacol. Ther.,* 29, 798, 1981.
2. **Tucker, G. T. and Lennard, M. S.,** Enantiomer specific pharmacokinetics, *Pharm. Ther.,* 45, 309, 1990.
3. **Caldwell, J. C., Winter, S. M., and Hutt, A. J.,** The pharmacological and toxicological significance of the stereochemistry of drug disposition, *Xenobiotica,* 18, 59, 1988.
4. **White, N. J., Looareesuman, S., and Warrell, D. A.,** Quinine and quinidine: a comparison of EKG effects during the treatment of malaria, *J. Cardiovasc. Pharmacol.,* 5, 173, 1983.
5. **Pfeiffer, C. C.,** Optical isomerism and pharmacological action, a generalization, *Science,* 124, 29, 1956.
6. **Drayer, D. E.,** Problems in therapeutic drug monitoring: the dilemma of enantiomeric drugs in man, *Ther. Drug Monit.,* 10, 1, 1988.
7. **Jamali, F., Mehvar, R., and Pasutto, F. M.,** Enantioselective aspects of drug action and disposition: therapeutic pitfalls, *J. Pharm. Sci.,* 78, 695, 1989.
8. **Smith, D. F.,** *CRC Handbook of Stereoisomers: Drugs in Psychopharmacology,* CRC Press, Boca Raton, FL, 1984.
9. **Drayer, D. E.,** Pharmacodynamic and pharmacokinetic differences between drug enantiomers in humans: an overview, *Clin. Pharmacol. Ther.,* 40, 125, 1986.
10. **Forrest, W. H., Jr., Beer, E. G., Bellville, J. W., Ciliberti, B. J., Miller, E. V., and Paddock, R.,** Analgesic and other effects of the *d*- and *l*-isomers of pentazocine, *Clin. Pharmacol. Ther.,* 10, 468, 1969.
11. **Cotzias, G. C., Papavasiliou, P. S., and Gellene, R.,** Modification of parkinsonism: chronic treatment with L-dopa, *N. Engl. J. Med.,* 280, 337, 1969.
12. **Guzman, A., Yuste, F., Toscano, R. A., Young, J. M., Van Horn, A. R., and Muchowski, J. M.,** Absolute configuration of (–)-5-benzoyl-1,2-dihydro-3H-pyrrolo[1,2-a]pyrrole-1-carboxylic acid, the active enantiomer of ketorolac, *J. Med. Chem.,* 29, 589, 1986.
13. **Wise, R., Wills, P. J., and Bedford, K. A.,** Epimers of moxalactam: *in vitro* comparison of activity and stability, *Antimicrob. Agents Chemother.,* 20, 30, 1981.
14. **Lima, J. J., Boudoulas, H., and Shields, B. J.,** Stereoselective pharmacokinetics of disopyramide enantiomers in man, *Drug Metab. Dispos.,* 13, 572, 1985.
15. **Morady, F., Scheinman, M. M., and Desai, J.,** Disopyramide, *Ann. Intern. Med.,* 96, 337, 1982.
16. **Le Corre, P., Gibassier, D., Descaves, C., Sado, P., Daubert, J. C., and Le Verge, R.,** Clinical pharmacokinetics of levorotatory and racemic disopyramide, at steady state, following oral administration in patients with ventricular arrhythmias, *J. Clin. Pharmacol.,* 29, 1089, 1989.
17. **Howitt, G., Husaini, M., Rowlands, D. J., Logan, W. F. W. E., Shanks, R. G., and Evans, M. G.,** The effect of the dextro isomer of propranolol on sinus rate and cardiac arrhythmias, *Am. Heart J.,* 76, 736, 1968.
18. **Lennard, M. S., Tucker, G. T., Silas, J. H., Freestone, S., Ramsey, L. E., and Woods, H.,** Differential stereoselective metabolism of metoprolol in extensive and poor debrisoquine metabolizers, *Clin. Pharmacol. Ther.,* 34, 732, 1983.

19. **Johnston, G. D., Finch, M. B., McNeil, J. A., and Shanks, R. G.,** A comparison of the cardiovascular effects of (+) -sotalol and (±) -sotalol following intravenous administration in normal volunteers, *Br. J. Clin. Pharmacol.,* 20, 507, 1985.
20. **Schuttler, J., Stanski, D. R., White, P. F., Trevor, A. J., Horai, Y., Verotta, D., and Sheiner, L. B.,** Pharmacodynamic modeling of the EEG effects of ketamine and its enantiomers in man, *J. Pharmacokinet. Biopharm.,* 15, 241, 1987.
21. **Echizen, H., Brecht, T., Niedergesass, S., Vogelgesang, B., and Eichelbaum, M.,** The effect of dextro-, levo-, and racemic verapamil on the atrioventricular conduction in humans, *Am. Heart J.,* 109 (2), 210, 1985.
22. **Echizen, H., Vogelgesang, B., and Eichelbaum, M.,** Effects of *d, l*-verapamil on atrioventricular conduction in relation to its stereoselective first-pass metabolism, *Clin. Pharmacol. Ther.,* 38, 71, 1985.
23. **Wingard, L. B., O'Reilly, R. A., and Levy, G.,** Pharmacokinetics of warfarin enantiomers: a search for intrasubject correlations, *Clin. Pharmacol. Ther.,* 23, 212, 1978.
24. **Mehvar, R., Gross, M. E., and Kreamer, R. N.,** Pharmacokinetics of atenolol enantiomers in humans and rats, *J. Pharm. Sci.,* 79, 881, 1990.
25. **Giacomini, K. M., Nelson, W. L., Pershe, R. A., Valdivieso, L., Turner-Tamiyasu, K., and Blaschke, T. F.,** *In vivo* interaction of the enantiomers of disopyramide in human subjects, *J. Pharmacokinet. Biopharm.,* 14, 335, 1986.
26. **Lee, E. J. D., Williams, K., Day, R., Graham, G., and Champion, D.,** Stereoselective disposition of ibuprofen enantiomers in man, *Br. J. Clin. Pharmacol.,* 19, 669, 1985.
27. **Bjorkman, S.,** Stereoselective disposition of indoprofen in surgical patients, *Br. J. Clin. Pharmacol.,* 20, 463, 1985.
28. **Gietl, Y., Spahn, H., Knauf, H., and Mutschler, E.,** Single- and multiple-dose pharmacokinetics of R-(–)- and S-(+)-prenylamine in man, *Eur. J. Clin. Pharmacol.,* 38, 587, 1990.
29. **Olanoff, L. S., Walle, T., Walle, U. K., Cowart, T. D., and Gaffney, T. E.,** Stereoselective clearance and distribution of intravenous propranolol, *Clin. Pharmacol. Ther.,* 35, 755, 1984.
30. **Walle, T., Webb, J. G., Bagwell, E. E., Walle, U. K., Daniell, H. B., and Gaffney, T. E.,** Stereoselective delivery and actions of beta receptor antagonists, *Biochem. Pharmacol.,* 37, 115, 1988.
31. **Borgstrom, L., Nyberg, L., Jonsson, S., Lindberg, C., and Paulson, J.,** Pharmacokinetics evaluation in man of terbutaline given as separate enantiomers and as the racemate, *Br. J. Clin. Pharmacol.,* 27, 49, 1989.
32. **Sedman, A. J., Bloedow, D. C., and Gal, J.,** Serum binding of tocainide and its enantiomers in human subjects, *Res. Commun. Chem. Pathol. Pharmacol.,* 38, 165, 1982.
33. **Eichelbaum, M., Mikus, G., and Vogelgesang, B.,** Pharmacokinetics of (+)-, (–)- and (±)-verapamil after intravenous administration, *Br. J. Clin. Pharmacol.,* 17, 453, 1984.
34. **Breckenridge, A. M., Orme, M., Wesseling, H., Lewis, R. J., and Gibbons, R.,** Pharmacokinetics and pharmacodynamics of the enantiomers of warfarin in man, *Clin. Pharmacol. Ther.,* 15, 424, 1974.
35. **Yacobi, A. and Levy, G.,** Protein binding of warfarin enantiomers in serum of humans and rats, *J. Pharmacokinet. Biopharm.,* 5, 123, 1977.
36. **Arnett, E. M., Gold, J. M., Harvey, N., Johnson, E. A., and Whitesell, L. G.,** Stereoselective recognition in phospholipid monolayers, *Adv. Biol. Med.,* 238, 21, 1988.
37. **Wade, D. N., Mearrick, P. T., and Morris, J. L.,** Active transport of L-dopa in the intestine, *Nature (London),* 242, 463, 1973.

38. **Williams, K. and Lee, E.,** Importance of drug enantiomers in clinical pharmacology, *Drugs,* 30, 333, 1985.
39. **Hendel, J. and Brodthagen, H.,** Entero-hepatic cycling of methotrexate estimated by use of the D-isomer as a reference marker, *Eur. J. Clin. Pharmacol.,* 26, 103, 1984.
40. **Nakashima, E., Tsuji, A., Mizuo, H., and Yamana, T.,** Kinetics and mechanism of *in vitro* uptake of amino-β-lactam antibiotics by rat small intestine and relation to the intact-peptide transport system, *Biochem. Pharmacol.,* 33, 3345, 1984.
41. **Tamai, I., Ling, H., Timbul, S., Nishikido, J., and Tsuji, A.,** Stereospecific absorption and degradation of cephalexin, *J. Pharm. Pharmacol.,* 40, 320, 1988.
42. **Hague, D. and Smith, R. L.,** Enigmatic properties of (±) -thalidomide; an example of a stable racemic compound, *Br. J. Clin. Pharmacol.,* 26, 632, 1988.
43. **Duddu, S. P., Vakilynejad, M., Jamali, F., and Grant, D. J. W.,** Interaction of a chiral drug with a chiral excipient: stereoselective dissolution of propranolol HCl from matrices containing hydroxypropyl methylcellulose, presented at ACCP 20th Annual Meet., Atlanta, GA, October 1991.
44. **Müller, W. E. and Wollert, U.,** High stereospecificity of the benzodiazepine binding site of human serum albumin, *Mol. Pharmacol.,* 11, 52, 1975.
45. **Walle, U. K., Walle, T., Bai, S. A., and Orlanoff, L. S.,** Stereoselective binding of propranolol to human plasma, α_1-acid glycoprotein, and albumin, *Clin. Pharmacol. Ther.,* 34, 718, 1983.
46. **Gill, T. S., Hopkins, K. J., and Rowland, M.,** Stereospecific assay of nicoumalone: application to pharmacokinetics studies in man, *Br. J. Clin. Pharmacol.,* 25, 591, 1988.
47. **Gilman, A. G., Rall, T. W., Nies, A. S., and Taylor, P.,** *The Pharmacological Basis of Therapeutics,* 8th ed., 1990, 1655.
48. **Buch, H., Knabe, J., Buzello, W., and Rummel, W.,** Stereospecificity of anesthetic activity, distribution, inactivation and protein binding of the optical antipodes of two *N*-methylated barbiturates, *J. Pharmacol. Exp. Ther.,* 175, 709, 1970.
49. **Yamada, H., Ichihashi, T., Hirano, K., and Kinoshita, H.,** Plasma protein binding and urinary excretion of R- and S-epimers of an arylmalonylamino 1-oxacephem I: in humans, *J. Pharm. Sci.,* 70, 112, 1981.
50. **Cook, C. E., Seltzman, T., Tallent, C. R., Lorenzo, B., and Drayer, D. E.,** Pharmacokinetics of pentobarbital enantiomers as determined by enantioselective radioimmunoassay after administration of racemate to humans and rabbits, *J. Pharmacol. Exp. Ther.,* 241, 779, 1987.
51. **Schmidt, W. and Jahnchen, E.,** Species-dependent stereospecific serum protein binding of the oral anticoagulant drug phenprocoumon, *Experientia,* 34, 1323, 1978.
52. **Wan, S., Matin, S. B., and Azarnoff, D. L.,** Kinetics, salivary excretion of amphetamine isomers, and effect of urinary pH, *Clin. Pharmacol. Ther.,* 23, 585, 1978.
53. **Le Corre, P. G., Bibassier, D., Sado, P., and Le Verge, R.,** Stereoselective metabolism and pharmacokinetics of disopyramide enantiomers in humans, *Drug Metab. Dispos.,* 16, 858, 1988.
54. **Caccia, S., Ballabio, M., and De Ponte, P.,** Pharmacokinetics of fenfluramine enantiomers in man, *Eur. J. Drug Metab. Pharmacokinet.,* 4, 129, 1979.
55. **Romach, M., Piafsky, K. M., and Abel, J. G.,** Methadone binding to orosomucoid (alpha 1-acid glycoprotein): determinant of free fraction in plasma, *Clin. Pharmacol. Ther.,* 29, 211, 1981.
56. **McErlane, K. M., Igwemezie, L., and Kerr, C. R.,** Stereoselective serum protein binding of mexiletine enantiomers in man, *Res. Commun. Chem. Pathol. Pharmacol.,* 56, 141, 1987.
57. **Albani, F., Riva, R., Contin, M., and Baruzzi, A.,** Stereoselective binding of propranolol enantiomers to human alpha$_1$-acid glycoprotein and human plasma, *Br. J. Clin. Pharmacol.,* 18, 244, 1984.

58. **Notterman, D., Drayer, D., Metakis, L., and Reidenberg, M. M.,** Stereoselective renal tubular secretion of quinidine and quinine, *Clin. Pharmacol. Ther.,* 40, 511, 1986.
59. **Nahata, M. C., Durrell, D. E., and Barson, W. J.,** Moxalactam epimer kinetics in children, *Clin. Pharmacol. Ther.,* 31, 528, 1982.
60. **Morse, G., Janicke, D., Cafarell, R., Piontek, K., Apicella, M., Jusko, W. J., and Walshe, J.,** Moxalactam epimer disposition in patients undergoing continuous ambulatory peritoneal dialysis, *Clin. Pharmacol. Ther.,* 38, 150, 1985.
61. **Toon, S., Low, L. K., Gibaldi, M., Trager, W. F., O'Reilly, R. A., Motley, C. H., and Goulart, M. A.,** The warfarin-sulfinpyrazone interaction: stereochemical considerations, *Clin. Pharmacol. Ther.,* 39, 15, 1986.
62. **Takahashi, H., Ogata, H., Shimizu, M., Hashimoto, K., Mashuhara, K., Kashiwada, K., and Someya, K.,** Comparative pharmacokinetics of unbound disopyramide enantiomers following oral administration of racemic disopyramide in humans, *J. Pharm. Sci.,* 80, 709, 1991.
63. **Lemmer, B. and Bathe, K.,** Stereospecific and circadian-phase-dependent kinetic behavior of *d, l*-, and *d*-propranolol in plasma, heart, and brain of light-dark-synchronized rats, *J. Cardiovasc. Pharmacol.,* 4, 635, 1982.
64. **Tocco, D. J., Hooke, K. F., Deluna, F. A., and Duncan, E. W.,** Stereospecific binding of timolol, a beta-adrenergic blocking agent, *Drug Metab. Dispos.,* 4, 323, 1976.
65. **Pillai, G. K., Axelson, J. E., Kerr, C. R., and McErlane, K. M.,** Stereoselective salivary excretion of tocainide enantiomers in man, *Res. Commun. Chem. Pathol. Pharmacol.,* 43, 209, 1984.
66. **Day, R. O., Williams, K. M., Graham, G. G., Lee, E. J., Knihinicki, R. D., and Champion, G. D.,** Stereoselective disposition of ibuprofen enantiomers in synovial fluid, *Clin. Pharmacol. Ther.,* 43, 480, 1988.
67. **Hansen, T., Day, R., Williams, K., Lee, E., Knihinicki, R., and Duffield, A.,** The assay and *in vitro* binding of the enantiomers of ibuprofen, *Clin. Exp. Physiol. Pharmacol.,* 9 (Suppl.), 82, 1985.
68. **Singh, N. N., Jamali, F., Pasutto, F. M., Russell, A. S., Coutts, R. T., and Drader, K. S.,** Pharmacokinetics of the enantiomers of tiaprofenic acid in humans, *J. Pharm. Sci.,* 75, 439, 1986.
69. **Jenner, P. and Testa, B.,** The influence of stereochemical factors on drug disposition, *Drug Metab. Rev.,* 2, 117, 1973.
70. **Testa, B.,** Mechanisms of chiral recognition in xenobiotic metabolism and drug-receptor interactions, *Chirality,* 1, 7, 1989.
71. **Wedlund, P. J., Aslanian, W. S., Jacqz, E., McAllister, C. B., Branch, R. A., and Wilkinson, G. R.,** Phenotypic differences in mephenytoin pharmacokinetics in normal subjects, *J. Pharmacol. Exp. Ther.,* 234, 662, 1985.
72. **Hooper, W. D. and Qing, M. S.,** The influence of age and gender on the stereoselective metabolism and pharmacokinetics of mephobarbital in humans, *Clin. Pharmacol. Ther.,* 48, 633, 1990.
73. **Chandler, M. H. H., Scott, S. R., and Blouin, R. A.,** Age-associated stereoselective alterations in hexobarbital metabolism, *Clin. Pharmacol. Ther.,* 43, 436, 1988.
74. **Williams, K. M.,** Kinetics of misonidazole enantiomers, *Clin. Pharmacol. Ther.,* 36, 817, 1984.
75. **Eichelbaum, M., Ende, M., Remberg, G., Schomerus, M., and Dengler, H. J.,** The metabolism of D, L-[^{14}C] verapamil in man, *Drug Metab. Dispos.,* 7, 145, 1979.
76. **Eichelbaum, M.,** Pharmacokinetic and pharmacodynamic consequences of stereoselective drug metabolism in man, *Biochem. Pharmacol.,* 37, 93, 1988.
77. **O'Reilly, R. A.,** Ticrynafen-racemic warfarin interaction: hepatotoxic or stereoselective?, *Clin. Pharmacol. Ther.,* 32, 356, 1982.

78. **Nakamura, Y., Yamaguchi, T., Takahashi, S., Hashimoto, S., Iwatani, K., and Nakagawa, Y.,** Optical isomerization mechanism of R(–)-hydratropic acid derivatives, *J. Pharmacobiodyn,* 4, S-1, 1981.
79. **Rubin, A., Knadler, M. P., Ho, P. P. K., Bechtol, L. D., and Wolen, R. L.,** Stereoselective inversion of (R) -fenoprofen to (S) -fenoprofen in humans, *J. Pharm. Sci.,* 74, 82, 1985.
80. **Simmonds, R. G., Woodage, T. J., Duff, S. M., and Green, J. N.,** Stereospecific inversion of (R)- (–)-benoxaprofen in rat and man, *Eur. J. Drug Metab. Pharmacokinet.,* 5, 169, 1980.
81. **Jamali, F., Berry, B. W., Tehrani, M. R., and Russell, A. S.,** Stereoselective pharmacokinetics of flurbiprofen in humans and rats, *J. Pharm. Sci.,* 77, 666, 1988.
82. **Palatini, P., Montanari, G., Perosa, A., Forgione, A., Pedrazzini, S., and Furlanut, M.,** Stereospecific disposition of flunoxaprofen enantiomers in human beings, *Int. J. Clin. Pharmacol. Res.,* 8, 161, 1988.
83. **Foster, R. T. and Jamali, F.,** Stereoselective pharmacokinetics of ketoprofen in the rat, *Drug Metab. Dispos.,* 16, 623, 1988.
84. **Jamali, F., Singh, N. N., Pasutto, F. M., Russell, A. S., and Coutts, R. T.,** Pharmacokinetics of ibuprofen enantiomers in humans following oral administration of tablets with different absorption rates, *Pharm. Res.,* 5, 40, 1988.
85. **Hsyu, P. and Giacomini, K. M.,** Stereoselective renal clearance of pindolol in humans, *J. Clin. Invest.,* 76, 1720, 1985.
86. **Von Bahr, C., Hermansson, J., and Tawara, K.,** Plasma levels of (+)- and (–)-propranolol and 4-hydroxypropranolol after administration of racemic (I)-propranolol in man, *Br. J. Clin. Pharmacol.,* 14, 79, 1982.
87. **Paxton, J. W. and Norris, R. M.,** Propranolol disposition after acute myocardial infarction, *Clin. Pharmacol. Ther.,* 36, 337, 1984.
88. **Soons, P. A. and Breimer, D. D.,** Stereoselective pharmacokinetics of oral and intravenous nitrendipine in healthy male subjects, *Br. J. Clin. Pharmacol.,* 32, 11, 1991.
89. **Ariens, E. J., Wius, E. W., and Veringa, E. J.,** Stereoselectivity of bioactive xenobiotics. A pre-Pasteur attitude in medicinal chemistry, pharmacokinetics, and clinical pharmacology, *Biochem. Pharmacol.,* 37, 9, 1988.
90. **Ravis, W. R.,** *Stereoisomerism in Pharmaceuticals, Pharmacokinetics and Pharmacodynamics,* Technomic Publishing Lancaster, PA, 1990, chap. 4.
91. **Eichelbaum, M. and Somogyi, A.,** Inter- and intra-subject variation in the first-pass elimination of highly cleared drugs during chronic dosing, *Eur. J. Clin. Pharmacol.,* 26, 47, 1984.
92. **Evans, A. M., Nation, R. L., Sansom, L. N., Bochner, F., and Somogyi, A. A.,** Stereoselective drug disposition: potential for misinterpretation of drug disposition data, *Br. J. Clin. Pharmacol.,* 26, 771, 1988.
93. **Thomson, A. H., Murdoch, G., Pottage, A., Kelman, A. W., Whiting, B., and Hillis, W. S.,** The pharmacokinetics of R-and S-tocainide in patients with acute ventricular arrhythmias, *Br. J. Clin. Pharmacol.,* 21, 149, 1986.
94. **Vogelgesang, B., Echizen, H., Schmidt, E., and Eichelbaum, M.,** Stereoselective first-pass metabolism of highly cleared drugs: studies of the bioavailability of L- and D-verapamil examined with a stable isotope technique, *Br. J. Clin. Pharmacol.,* 18, 733, 1984.
95. **Sahajwalla, C. G., Longstreth, J., Karim, A., Purich, E. D., and Cabana, B. E.,** Consequences in pooling R- + S-verapamil in bioequivalence assessment, presented at ACCP 20th Annu. Meet., Atlanta, GA, October 1991.
96. **Jamali, F., Mehvar, R., Russell, A. S., Sattari, S., Yakimets, W. W., and Koo, J.,** Human pharmacokinetics of ibuprofen enantiomers following different doses and formulations: intestinal chiral inversion, *J. Pharm. Sci.,* 81, 221, 1992.

97. **Cox, S. R., Brown, M. A., Squires, D. J., Murrill, E. A., Lednicer, D., and Knuth, D. W.,** Comparative human study of ibuprofen enantiomer plasma concentrations produced by two commercially available ibuprofen tablets, *Biopharm. Drug Dispos.*, 9, 539, 1988.
98. **Walker, S. E. and Hardy, B. G.,** Alterations in apparent bioequivalency of ibuprofen based on isomer analysis, presented, ACCP 20th Annu. Meet., Atlanta, GA, October 1991.
99. **Hall, S. D., Rudy, A. C., and Brater, D. C.,** Bioavailability of ibuprofen enantiomers in humans, presented, ACCP 20th Annu. Meet., Atlanta, GA, October 1991.

Chapter 8

Animal Models and Their Role in Bioequivalence Studies

Wade J. Adams

CONTENTS

I. INTRODUCTION

The evaluation of the biopharmaceutical and pharmacokinetic characteristics of drug candidates is now recognized to be an essential aspect of drug development, rivaling in importance the pharmacological and toxicological evaluation of new drug entities. Indeed, bioavailability and pharmacokinetic studies in animal models are recognized to be of fundamental importance,[1-4] as are metabolism and disposition studies,[2,5-7] to the interpretation and rationalization of animal pharmacology and toxicology data and the extrapolation of these data to humans. Increasingly, *in vivo* bioavailability and pharmacokinetic studies are being conducted in animal models during lead selection, usually in rodents to conserve compound, to select from among multiple leads that have potent *in vitro* or *in vivo* activity in pharmacological screens. A major reason for conducting these *in vivo* studies is that the extent of absorption and presystemic metabolism (first-pass effect) of orally administered drugs cannot be predicted with certainty from the physicochemical and *in vitro* dissolution characteristics of drugs and drug formulations, and from *in vitro* metabolic studies. Although a number of *in vitro* and *in situ* preparations have found utility in screening for absorption of closely related structural analogs and for understanding the intimate details of absorption processes,[8] these preparations obviously do not take into account all of the absorption, distribution, metabolism, and excretion (ADME) processes of the physiologically intact animal.

0-8493-6930-4/94/$0.00+$.50

As drug development progresses for a compound that is intended to be administered by an extravascular route, *in vivo* biopharmaceutics and pharmacokinetic studies are frequently conducted in animal models to obtain basic information about the physicochemical and physiological factors affecting the rate and extent of absorption. These studies are done in a species that can accommodate a human-scale dosage formulation to evaluate the form of the drug that is most appropriate for development (e.g., a free base or a salt), whether micronization is necessary for drug candidates that have low aqueous solubilities under the physiological conditions encountered in the gastrointestinal (GI) tract, the effect of formulation excipients on oral bioavailability, and the effect of concomitant administration of food and fluids. An assessment of the exposure of animals to the intact compound, and metabolites when appropriate, is also made in conjunction with subchronic and chronic toxicity studies. Dose alone is clearly not a satisfactory index of exposure in toxicity studies, especially when comparing across species, since the same drug dose may result in very different levels of exposure to intact drug and metabolites; this is because of species-dependent drug absorption, distribution, metabolism, and elimination.[2,5-7] Thus, by the time that registration of a new drug entity occurs a considerable body of knowledge is frequently available concerning the ADME characteristics of the drug in several animal species as well as humans.

Common dosage formulations occasionally are administered to both animals and humans that provide insight into the suitability of an animal model, under a limited range of experimental conditions, for assessing the bioavailability/bioequivalence of new forms or dosage formulations of a drug prior to the conduct of definitive bioavailability studies in humans. Rarely, if ever, are these animal studies conducted with the aim of achieving high statistical power, as is the case with definitive human bioavailability/bioequivalence studies, but simply of providing assurance that the human study has a reasonable probability of success. Despite the numerous animal studies that may be conducted during the course of drug development, definitive bioavailability/bioequivalence studies in humans of the final formulation — manufactured under scaled-up conditions — are conducted before large-scale introduction of a new drug into patients; exceptions are a few special cases in which *in vivo* bioavailability data in humans are waived.[9-11] In addition, bioavailability studies of drug lots manufactured under extremes in manufacturing conditions are also necessary to set manufacturing and dissolution specifications for quality control release of drug lots. The conduct of bioavailability/bioequivalence studies in a limited number of healthy volunteers has not been a major concern for drugs with a demonstrated margin of safety. In certain circumstances, however, the conduct of bioequivalence studies in animal models is appealing, usually because of ethical considerations. A case in point are drugs for life-threatening diseases that cannot be tested in healthy patient populations because of safety concerns (e.g., the drug may be mutagenic). Frequently these drugs have low therapeutic ratios and are administered near the maximum tolerated dose (e.g., antineoplastic drugs). However, ethical questions are also raised when a drug formulation with unknown therapeutic value, because of its unknown bioavailability, is tested in patients who have life-threatening diseases when a formulation of known therapeutic value is available.

The purpose of the present chapter is to discuss the anatomy and physiology of animal models that can accommodate human-scale dosage formulations, to review published literature in which the same dosage formulations have been compared in humans and animals, and to discuss the role and limitations of animal models for the bioavailability and bioequivalence assessment of new human oral dosage formulations prior to their introduction into humans.

II. ANIMAL MODELS FOR BIOAVAILABILITY ASSESSMENT OF HUMAN ORAL DOSAGE FORMULATIONS

The anatomic and physiological features of the gastrointestinal tract vary greatly in different species[12-16] due to adaptations that have taken place because of differences in the dietary habits of higher animals. Animals are conventionally classified on the basis of their eating habits in nature, although their diets may be considerably different following domestication. In the carnivores and omnivores, digestion is mainly enzymatic with minimal digestion by microbial fermentation. In contrast, domesticated herbivores fall into one of two groups: (1) those with rumens (cow, sheep), in which extensive microbial fermentation of vegetable matter occurs in the forestomach of the gastrointestinal tract (reticulum, rumen, and omasum) prior to reaching the true stomach (abomasum); and (2) those with simple stomachs (horse), in which extensive microbial fermentation takes place in the large intestine (cecum and colon). Because there is no need for microbial fermentation in the carnivores, the gastrointestinal tract in the carnivore is much shorter and has a smaller relative capacity than in the herbivore.

The oral absorption of a solid drug dosage form is dependent on three major factors: the wetting and dissolution or release of the active drug, the residence time of the dosage form and the dissolved drug at the site of absorption, and the ability of the gastrointestinal mucosa to absorb the drug; all of these depend on the anatomy and physiology of the gastrointestinal tract.[12-16] The number of animal species that can be realistically used to investigate the biopharmaceutical and pharmacokinetic characteristics of human-scale dosage forms is limited by these same anatomic and physiological factors. These include the anatomic dimensions; the secretory levels of gastric, intestinal, and pancreatic juices and of bile; the presence of drug metabolizing enzymes and microorganisms; and the motility of the gastrointestinal tract. First and foremost, the digestive system in the animal model must be able to accommodate the human-scale dosage form without inducing abnormal physiological responses or traumatizing the mucosa. Ideally, the sizes of the stomach, small intestine, and large intestine in the animal model should be approximately proportional to those in humans so that the residence time of the lumenal contents in the animal are proportional to those in humans.

A. COMPARATIVE HUMAN AND ANIMAL GASTROINTESTINAL ANATOMY AND PHYSIOLOGY

1. Stomach

Comparison of the stomachs of man, dog, pig, horse, rat, cow, and llama (Figure 8–1) indicates that major differences exist in the structure and the function of the upper gastrointestinal tracts in these species.[15] Man, dog, pig, and horse have noncompartmentalized stomachs; the rat stomach is partially divided into two compartments; and the stomachs of the cow and llama are highly enlarged and compartmentalized. In ruminant herbivores the large forestomach constitutes a fermentation vessel, while in nonruminant herbivores the cecum and colon are large and provide a site for extensive microbial digestion. Thus, in ruminant herbivores enzymatic digestion occurs after microbial fermentation and the microbial bodies are themselves digested; whereas in simple herbivores fermentation takes place after enzymatic digestion, and only the fermentation products are available for digestion and absorption and not the bacterial bodies.[16] Because of the major differences in the upper gastrointestinal tract in ruminants as compared to man, even small ruminants such as sheep and goats are not considered suitable models for oral bioavailability and bioequivalence assessment of human dosage formulations. Furthermore, some herbivorous monkeys have compartmentalized stomachs[12] and, therefore, would not be considered suitable models.

Although rabbits have been used to a limited extent to study human-scale dosage formulations,[17-21] their size and the anatomic dimensions of their gastrointestinal tracts may be too small for them to be generally useful for this purpose.[12,22] Studies of enteric-coated barium sulfate tablets and granules indicated that stomach emptying is very prolonged in rabbits relative to humans, as is shown in Figure 8–2.[17] Furthermore, the cecum in the rabbit relative to that in humans is anatomically large compared to the rest of the gastrointestinal tract, and plays a much greater role in microbial metabolism than in humans. Finally, reingestion of the soft feces (coprophagia) is required in rabbits to

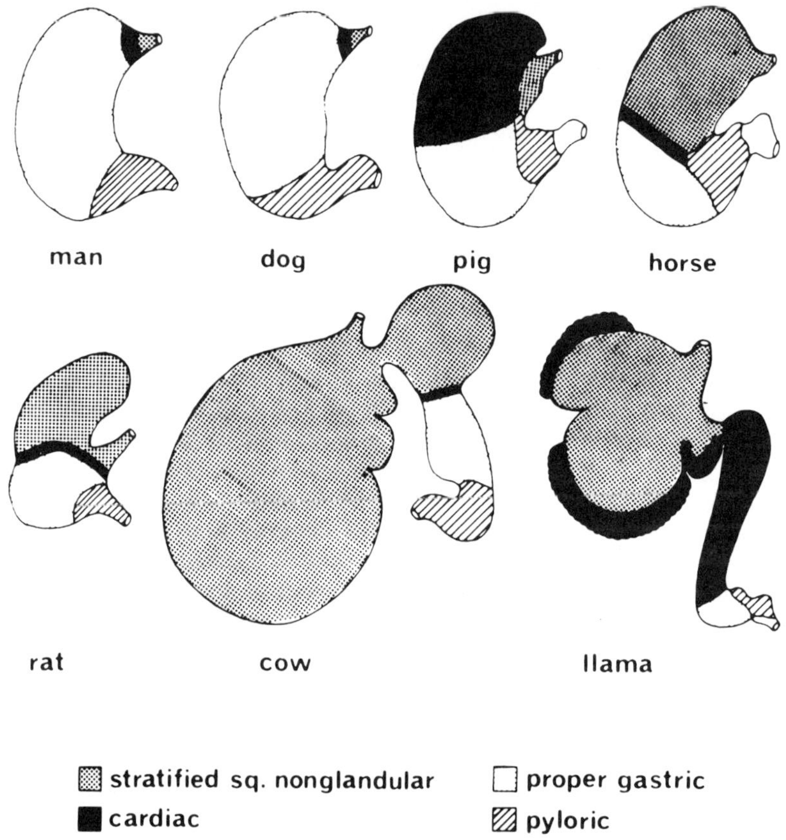

Figure 8–1 Comparison of the stomachs and the distribution of gastric mucosa in seven species. Stomachs are not drawn to scale (e.g., the capacity of the adult bovine stomach is approximately 70 times that of the adult human stomach). (From Argenzio, R. A., *Dukes' Physiology of Domestic Animals,* 10th ed., Comstock Publishing (Cornell University Press), Ithaca, NY, chap. 17. With permission.)

assure adequate nutritional status;[23] thus special precautions must be taken to assure fasted conditions in rabbit studies.[17-21] The use of stomach-emptying controlled rabbits appeared to be useful in assuring that the stomach was empty prior to the administration of griseofulvin tablets,[19] and a good rank order correlation was found in maximum plasma concentrations and areas under concentration-time curves between rabbits and humans for griseofulvin tablets having different dissolution rates. However, this technique does not appear to have gained acceptance, as other studies describing its use have not appeared; this is most likely because it is not a convenient approach to use. For these reasons the rabbit is not considered to be a very useful or generally applicable animal model for assessing the bioavailability or bioequivalence of human-scale dosage forms and will not be further considered here.

Humans, dogs, pigs, and rhesus monkeys all have simple stomachs that can readily accommodate a human-scale dosage formulation. Although the pig is classified as an omnivore, domesticated pigs are predominately herbivorous and a pouch or diverticulum is present at the top of their stomachs. The diverticulum probably serves as a site for limited microbial metabolism. As ruminants, pigs also have a projection from the pylorus called the torus pyloricus which is poorly developed in young animals.[24] Considerable differences exist in the composition of the epithelium lining the stomach of these species. Three types of mucosa are found — cardiac, proper gastric, and pyloric mucosa — as shown in Figure 8-1. Proper gastric mucosa makes up a large proportion of the human, dog, and rhesus monkey stomach; whereas cardiac mucosa makes up a much greater proportion of the pig stomach, and an additional small area of stratified squamous epithelium surrounds the gastroesophageal junction in the pig.[15] The stomach contains many gastric glands that empty their secretions onto the surface of the mucosa through small invaginations called gastric pits. The gastric glands located in the proper gastric mucosa of the stomach contain mucous neck cells that secrete a viscous, alkaline mucus; parietal or oxyntic cells that secrete hydrochloric acid; and zymogenic or chief cells that secrete pepsinogen, a precursor of the enzyme pepsin which is optimally active in cleaving peptidic bonds under acidic conditions.[25] The glands of the cardiac and pyloric regions of the stomach secrete mainly mucus; however, enteroendocrine cells are also present in the pyloric region that secrete the hormone gastrin. The mucus, which adheres to the stomach walls to a thickness of approximately 1 to 1.5 mm, protects the gastric mucosa and lubricates the walls of the stomach.

Comparative anatomic and physiological data for the stomachs of humans, dogs, pigs, and rhesus monkeys are tabulated in Table 8–1.[12] Gastric volumes vary considerably among these species; the rhesus monkey has the smallest volume (approximately one tenth that of humans) and pigs, the largest (approximately six times that of humans). Dogs have nearly the same gastric volume as humans. Since the stomachs of all four species have glandular mucosa that secrete mucus and gastric acid, their stomachs tend to have an acidic pH. Basal (unstimulated) gastric acid outputs typically range from 1 to 5 meq/h in humans, and with histamine or pentagastrin stimulation maximum outputs can reach 6 to 40 meq/h.[26] The ionic composition of the gastric secretions is dependent on the rate of secretion, with higher hydronium ion concentrations associated with higher secretory rates. The major anion present in gastric secretions is the chloride ion, independent of the rate of secretion. The basal rate of hydrochloric acid output varies diurnally in humans, with the highest output in the evening and the lowest in the morning.[26] Gastric acid output increases promptly after feeding in humans, dogs, pigs, and monkeys.[12]

Although the proper gastric mucosa regions of the stomach are of comparable size in dogs and humans (Figure 8–1), the basal output of gastric acid appears to be much higher in humans than dogs under fasting conditions. Investigations of gastric pH using the Heidelberg capsule technique indicate that the pH in young healthy human volunteers is significantly lower ($p < 0.05$) than in the dog (6.0 ± 0.14 vs. 7.3 ± 0.09),[27] with the gastric pH in some dogs indistinguishable from that of the small intestine.[12] Because of the high-fasting pH observed in some dogs, Dressman and Yamada[12] suggest screening the gastric pH of dogs prior to including them in absorption studies of pH-sensitive drugs and drug formulations. Peak gastric acid outputs appear to be higher in dogs than in humans,[12] however, which may explain why gastric pH changes very little after administration of food to beagle dogs.[28]

As previously noted, the stomach in the pig is approximately 6 times larger than that in humans. However, the parietal cell-containing proper gastric mucosa make up a smaller proportion of the stomach in pigs than humans (Figure 8–1). Under basal conditions, the volume of gastric acid secreted is comparable to that in humans (Table 8–1).[12] Confounding data exist in the literature concerning the fasting pH in the pig. In two different studies the fasted gastric pH was reported to be higher in the pig than in humans, with a pH of 3.75 to 4.00 found in one study[29] and a mean pH of 2.67 found 3 h postprandially in the other study.[30] However, a third study done in healthy young animals (4 or 8 weeks old) reported mean pH values of 1.6 to 1.8, very comparable to that in humans.[31] As in the case of dogs, postprandial acid output in the pig appears to be higher than that in humans.[12] The suitability of pigs for oral absorption studies is compromised by their susceptibility to gastric ulcers, with gastric ulcers reported in 5 to 50% of the domestic pig population.[32] Pigs used in the laboratory are frequently administered H_2-receptor blockers (e.g., cimetidine) because of their tendency to develop ulcers. Humans with gastric ulcers are reported to secrete less hydrochloric acid than normal individuals.[33]

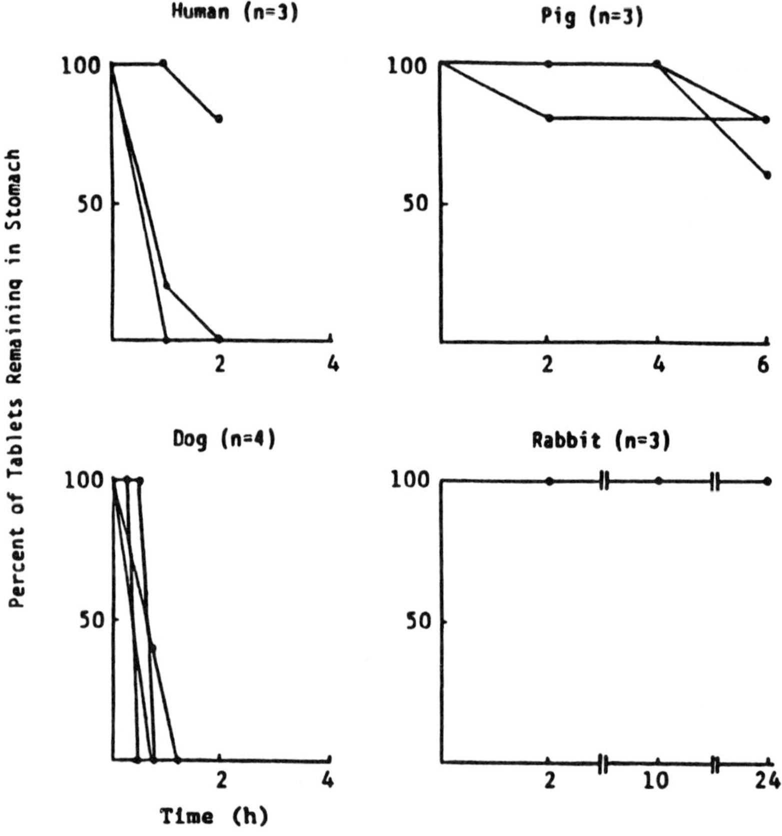

Figure 8–2 Gastric emptying of enteric-coated barium sulfate tablets — 11 mm in diameter (this page) — and barium sulfate granules — 1 mm in diameter (adjacent page) — in fasted humans, pigs, dogs, and rabbits. Five tablets were administered to all species except rabbits, which were administered two tablets. (Redrawn from Aoyagi, N., *Comparative Studies of Griseofulvin Bioavailability Among Man and Animals,* Kyoto University, Kyoto, Japan, 1986.)

Basal gastric acid output in monkeys is similar to that in humans when monkeys are allowed to range freely.[34] However, the gastric acid output of monkeys changes under restraint conditions. In Old World monkeys (e.g., rhesus and cynomolgus monkeys) gastric acid secretion very nearly stops under restraint conditions, with the gastric pH being neutral or slightly alkaline; whereas gastric acid secretion apparently increases in New World monkeys under restraint conditions.[12] The volume of gastric juice secreted and gastrointestinal motility also appear to be reduced in Old World monkeys under restraint conditions. The need to acclimatize animals prior to bioavailability and bioequivalence studies is recognized, but is particularly important in stress-sensitive species such as the monkey. These stress-induced changes in physiology make it particularly difficult to conduct bioavailability/bioequivalence studies in large monkeys since it is recommended that monkeys over 10 kg be restrained.[12]

2. Small Intestine

The presence of large valvelike circular folds (plicae circulares, valves of Kercking) and tiny fingerlike projections (villi) in the small intestine result in this region of the gastrointestinal tract having the largest absorptive surface area.[13,14] It has been estimated that these

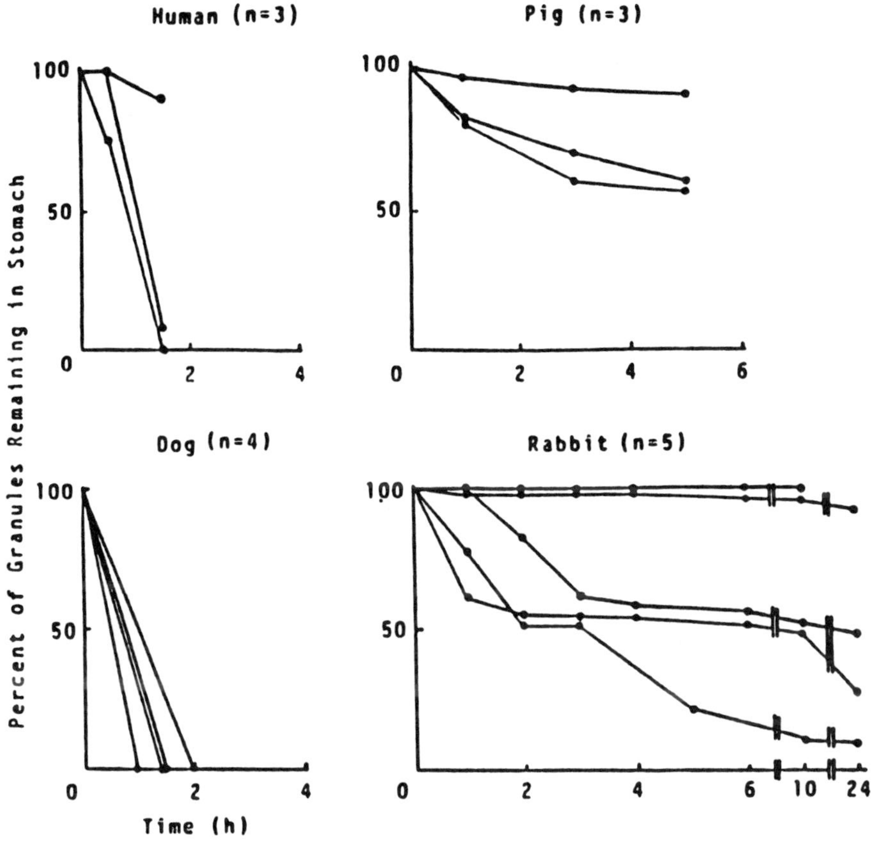

Figure 8–2 (continued)

morphological features of the small intestine increase its available surface area by as much as two million times relative to the surface area of a smooth tube.[35] Comparative anatomic and physiological data for the small intestine in humans, dogs, pigs, and rhesus monkeys are tabulated in Table 8–2.[12] The length of the intestine is highly dependent on intestinal tone, which is lost at death. In humans, the length of the intestine more than doubles at autopsy. Most of the data reported for animals were likely obtained at autopsy. The small intestine in dogs is about half as long as that in humans and has about the same lumenal dimensions. Thus, the intestinal transit time in the dog is expected to be approximately half that in humans. In a comparative study done in beagle dogs and humans, the mean residence time of a Heidelberg capsule in dogs was approximately 2 h as compared to approximately 4 h in humans.[36] The shorter intestinal transit time of dosage formulations in the dog results in a shorter contact time with the mucosa of the intestinal tract and may result in a substantial reduction in the extent of absorption of dosage forms having slow dissolution rates (e.g., poorly soluble drugs or sustained-release formulations). However, the shorter intestinal length in the dog may be compensated for to some extent by the longer and more slender villi in carnivores. In marked contrast to the dog, pigs have a small intestine that is approximately twice as long as that in humans, with the lumenal dimensions of the intestine being very comparable to those in humans. Since the villi in omnivores would be expected to be similar, the surface area for drug absorption is probably much greater in pigs than in humans.[12] Although the overall length of the small intestine in the rhesus monkey is unknown, the length of the duodenum is less than one fifth as long as that in humans. It therefore seems probable that the overall length of the small intestine is shorter than in

Table 8–1 **Comparison of anatomic and physiological data for the stomach of humans, dogs, pigs, and rhesus monkeys**

Parameter	Human	Dog	Pig	Monkey
Volume (l)	1–1.6	1	6–8	0.1
Gastric acid secretion				
Basal acid output				
Volume (ml/min)	1	0.3–1.5	1.05	[a]
Rate (meq/h)	2–5	0.1	5.6 (μg/h)	[a]
Postprandial acid output				
Rate (meq/h)	18–23	39	1.25 (μg/h)	
pH				
Fasted	1.7 (1.4–2.1)[b]	1.5 (Beagles)	2.7 3.75–4 (n = 20) 1.6–1.8 0.8–3.0[c]	
Fed				
During meal	5.0 (4.3–5.4)[b]	2.1 ± 0.1[d]	<2 (n = 1)	
Time to return to pH 3	56 ± 41 min[d]			

[a] Similar to humans unless stressed.
[b] Interquartile range.
[c] Range.
[d] Standard deviation.
From Dressman, J. B. and Yamada, K., *Pharmaceutical Bioequivalence,* Marcel Dekker, New York, 1991, chap. 9. With permission.

humans. The lumenal diameter of the intestine appears to be greater in the monkey and may, at least in part, compensate for its shorter length. However, the intestinal villi in the rhesus monkey are broad and leaf shaped compared to the filamentous villi in humans.[12] It seems probable, therefore, that the small intestine in rhesus monkeys has lower absorptive capacity than in humans.

Aggregated lymphatic nodules or Peyer's patches (tonsillae intestinales) are larger and more numerous in the distal ileum in humans and are occasionally seen in the jejunum.[13] Approximately one quarter of the intestinal mucosa in humans is lymphoid tissue made up of T (thymus-dependent) and B (bursa-dependent) cells.[33] As is the case with other lymphatic tissue, these patches atrophy with age. Immunoglobulins produced by this lymphoid tissue bind to antigens and prevent their absorption,[37] inhibit binding of bacteria to epithelial cells, and prevent bacterial colonization.[38,39] Deficiencies in immunoglobulin secretion may lead to inflammation. The distribution of Peyer's patches in monkeys is similar to that in man, whereas Peyer's patches are distributed throughout the intestine in dogs and pigs.[12]

The pancreatic juice secreted by humans, dogs, pigs, and monkeys contains both digestive enzymes and bicarbonate. The relative rates of secretion of gastric acid and bicarbonate determine the intestinal pH. Human intestinal juice has a pH that is slightly acidic (5.5 to 6.5). The duodenal pH is approximately 0.5 to 1.0 pH units higher in dogs and pigs than in humans, and may be comparable to humans or 0.5 to 2.5 pH units higher in monkeys. The higher pH of intestinal juice in the fasted dog compared to that in man is consistent with the lower basal gastric acid secretion rate and higher secretin-stimulated pancreatic bicarbonate secretion rate in dogs.[40] The pH of the intestinal contents tends to be lower in humans after ingestion of food by as much as 0.5 pH unit, whereas the pH of the intestinal juices in the dog is maintained at the fasted level after feeding. In those

Table 8–2 **Comparison of anatomic and physiological data for the small intestine of humans, dogs, pigs, and rhesus monkeys**

Parameter	Human	Dog	Pig	Monkey
Dimensions				
Length				
(Autopsy) (m)	7	4	15–20	5 cm[a]
(In vivo) (m)	3	1.5		
Duodenal diameter (m)	3–4	2–2.5	2.5–3.5	1.5–2
Villi				
Length	0.5–1.5		0.5–1	
Shape	Filamentous	Long, slender		Ridges, leaflike
Peyer's patches:				
location	Ileum	Duodenum, jejunum, ileum	Jejunum, ileum, colon	Ileum
Secretions				
Bile				
Major acid	Cholic	Cholic	Hyocholic	
Conc by gallbladder	×5	×8–10	×2	
Flow rate (l/day)	0.8–1	0.1–0.4		
Pancreatic juice flow rate (ml/min)	1	2–3	1	
Intestinal pH				
Fasted	6.1 [5.6–6.4]	6.5–7.5	7.2[a]	7.9; 5.5–6.0
Fed	5.4 [5.0–5.8]	6.5–6.9		

[a] Duodenum.

[b] Lower duodenum.

From Dressman, J. B. and Yamada, K., *Pharmaceutical Bioequivalence,* Marcel Dekker, New York, chap. 9. With permission.

cases where the pK_a of a poorly soluble drug falls in the range 5 to 8, there may be substantial differences in the rate and extent of absorption in dogs and humans.[27] Since secretin-stimulated pancreatic bicarbonate secretion is more variable in dogs than in humans,[40] it is expected that intestinal pH will be more variable and that absorption of poorly soluble drugs that have a pK_a in the range 5 to 8 will be more variable in dogs.

Humans, dogs, pigs, and rhesus monkeys all have a gallbladder from which bile is secreted into the duodenum.[13-16] Bile salts in humans and dogs are derived from cholic acid while those in pigs are derived from hyocholic acid. Pigs also produce a less concentrated bile than humans while dogs produce a bile that has a higher bile salt concentration. These differences in bile salt concentration and type of bile salt may result in differences in the solubilizing and wetting capacity of intestinal juices in these species, and may result in differences in the dissolution and absorption of poorly soluble drugs.

3. Large Intestine

Comparative anatomic and physiological data for the cecum and colon of humans, dogs, pigs, and rhesus monkeys are presented in Table 8–3.[12] The cecum and colon tend to be relatively large in herbivores, small in carnivores, and intermediate in size in omnivores like humans. The ascending colon, which comprises about 0.2 m of the 1 to 1.5-m length of the human colon, is thought to be the main location for absorption in the colonic region of the gastrointestinal tract. The overall length of the colon, including the ascending colon, is much longer in pigs than in humans while the colon is relatively short in dogs and rhesus monkeys. It should also be noted that the diameter of the colon in the dog is smaller than in humans. Thus, the transit times through the large intestine would be expected to be shorter for dogs and monkeys, particularly dogs. Humans, pigs, and monkeys have haustra,[13,14,16] morphological features caused by the puckering of the colon into pouches or sacculations. Although dogs do not have haustra, there is mass movement of the lumenal contents in the aborad direction in the dog similar to that in humans. The contents of the colon in dogs are apparently mixed in a manner similar to haustral shuttling in humans, pigs, and monkeys.

Since microbial metabolism occurs in both the cecum and colon, the extent of microbial metabolism would be expected to increase approximately in proportion with the dimensions of this region of the gastrointestinal tract. Significant production of volatile fatty acids from carbohydrates apparently occurs in pigs,[41,42] as well as the catabolism of amino acids and the synthesis of B vitamins;[32] and this occurs to a lesser extent in humans. Thus, the colon may play a greater role in the absorption and metabolism of drugs in pigs compared to humans even though both are omnivores.

4. Gastrointestinal Motility and Transit Times

The plexuses in the wall of the gastrointestinal tract function as a semiautonomous nervous system controlling motor and secretory activities.[14] Materials pass through the gastrointestinal tract because of rhythmic contractions along the gastrointestinal tract that originate in the pacemaker zone of the stomach. These contractions are relatively weak in the upper part of the stomach but become stronger in the pyloric region. In the fasted state the contractions are quiescent for 1 to 2 h followed by a short period (10 to 20 min) of intense contractions with concurrent relaxation of the pyloric sphincter. These strong contractions are strong enough to cause large pieces of food or nondisintegrating drug dosage forms to be expelled from the stomach.[12] This pattern of rhythmic activity is called the migrating myoelectric complex (MMC) and occurs every 75 to 90 min in humans. Plasma motilin concentrations have been shown to correlate with the MMC in dogs.[43,44] After ingestion of food, regular contractions occur with a frequency of about three per minute in humans. Because of the weakness of these contractions in the upper stomach, the contents of the stomach remain unmixed for a considerable period of time after ingestion of food. This results in a layering of the contents of the stomach by density.

Table 8–3 **Comparison of anatomic and physiological data for the cecum and colon of humans, dogs, pigs, and rhesus monkeys**

Parameter	Human	Dog	Pig	Monkey
Cecum				
Length (cm)	7	12–15	20–30	5–6
Diameter (cm)	6		8–10	
Volume (l)	ca. 1	0.25	1.5–2.2	
Colon				
Length, overall (m)	0.9–1.5	0.6–0.75	4–4.5	0.4–0.5
Length, asc. colon (cm)	20		Long, coiled	10
Diameter (cm)	6	Similar to SI	8–10	
Haustrae	Present	Absent	Present	Present
Microbial metabolism				
Colon	Volatile fatty acids Vitamins	Very minor	Volatile, fatty acids Vitamins	
pH	6 (Upper)			
Colon	7.5 (Lower)			

From Dressman, J. B. and Yamada, K., *Pharmaceutical Bioequivalence,* Marcel Dekker, New York, 1991, chap. 9. With permission.

Thus, fats form a layer at the top of the stomach and are emptied more slowly than more dense solids, while denser fluids that can flow around the solids are rapidly emptied into the duodenum.[33] The rate of gastric emptying is affected by the volume of material in the stomach, the volume and composition of the chyme entering the duodenum, and the relative hypertonicity or hypotonicity of the chyme and products of proteolytic digestion.[14] Both segmentation and peristalsis occur in the small intestine. Segmentation mixes the chyme thoroughly with intestinal, pancreatic, and biliary secretions and exposes the chyme to the intestinal mucosa. The frequency of the contractions in the small intestine are most rapid in the duodenum (11 to 12 cycles per minute in humans) and progressively decrease along the length of the intestine (about 6 to 7 cycles per minute at the terminus of the ileum in humans). The peristaltic waves of the small intestine are weak and travel only a short distance, resulting in the slow movement of the intestinal contents. The motility of the small intestine is increased by distension; by hypertonicity, hypotonicity, or excessive acidity; and selected products of digestion.[14] Movements of the large intestine are generally sluggish, and passage of materials through the colon may take 18 to 24 h in humans. Mixing by movements in the colon occurs with a lower frequency than in the small intestine. At infrequent intervals (3 to 4 times per day), strong contractions of large segments of the colon propel material along the colon. The strong contractions often occur following ingestion of food, indicating that stomach and duodenum activities influence colon motility.[14]

The basic gastrointestinal motility pattern and periodicity in dogs and monkeys appears to be the same as that described above for humans.[12] Emptying of radiopaque barium sulfate from the stomachs of humans and dogs was complete within about 2 h.[17] However, the emptying of food from the stomach has been reported to be slower in dogs than humans.[12] As noted previously, intestinal transit times in dogs are about half those in humans because of the shorter length of the intestine in dogs. Under fasting conditions pigs have the same motility pattern as humans, but after ingestion of food the pattern changes. Stomach emptying in the pig is bimodal, with about 30 to 40% of the contents emptied in 15 min, followed by a prolonged emptying about an hour later.[32] Food apparently remains in the stomach of the pig 24 h a day, since complete emptying of the stomach apparently never occurs.[12] Standard fasting periods used for humans, dogs, and monkeys are obviously not applicable to pigs. Furthermore, the basic differences in the stomach-emptying patterns between pigs and humans bring into question the applicability of the pig as an animal model for bioavailability or bioequivalence assessment of immediate-release dosage formulations.

B. GASTROINTESTINAL DRUG METABOLISM

A number of drugs are metabolized in the lumen or wall of the gastrointestinal tract, which can reduce bioavailability and introduce significant intra- and intersubject variability in systemic drug concentrations. Even the stomach mucosa contains metabolizing enzymes and appears to be the primary site of metabolism of ethanol.[45] L-dopa also appears to be metabolized by the gastric mucosa since its oral bioavailability is enhanced by metoclopramide, which increases gastric-emptying time; and is decreased by propantheline bromide, which decreases gastric-emptying time.[46,47] Lumenal enzymes in the proximal gastrointestinal tract principally originate from pancreatic secretions and desquamation. These enzymes appear to be involved in the hydrolysis of at least some esters (e.g., chloramphenicol[48]) and in the selective cleavage of amide bonds. The intestinal mucosal columnar epithelial cells are quantitatively the most important site of metabolism in the gastrointestinal tract and contain most of the drug-metabolizing enzymes normally found in the liver. The villous tips of these cells have been reported to have the highest enzyme activity, with enzymatic activity progressively decreasing toward the crypts of Lieberkühn.[49] In general, the metabolic activity of mucosal epithelial cells in the duodenum and jejunum is greater than for those in the ileum and colon.[50-53] In the mouse, however, metabolic activity is reported to be similar in the duodenum and the colon.[54] Phase I enzymes identified in the mucosal epithelial cells include monooxygenases (including the P-450 enzymes), alcohol dehydrogenase, monoamine oxidases, epoxide hydrolase, esterases, amidases, glucuronidases; and Phase II enzymes identified include glucuronyltransferases, sulfotransferases, *O*-methyltransferases and glutathione-SH transferases.[50,55-57] Phase I and II metabolic reactions in a number of animal species have been reported,[54] including the dog, pig, and monkey. The locations of the enzymes within the mucosal epithelial cells is shown schematically in Figure 8-3.[58] As with hepatocytes, Phase I enzymes in these cells can be induced or inhibited.[57] Generally, mucosal epithelial cells have lower enzymatic activity than hepatocytes, with the K_{max} similar but the V_{max} lower than for hepatocytes.[59] Because of the lower metabolizing capacity of these cells relative to hepatocytes and the fact that very high drug concentrations may exist in the lumen of the gastrointestinal tract after oral drug administration, the metabolism in the mucosal epithelial cells may become saturated.[60] The metabolic capacity of drug metabolizing enzymes and the extent of first-pass metabolism should be considered when selecting an animal model for oral bioavailability studies since a species having an extent of first-pass metabolism comparable to humans would be expected to have similar sensitivities to the rate of release of the drug from formulations. The absolute oral bioavailability of selected drugs in humans and animals has been reviewed.[61]

Microbial metabolism by gut flora is quantitatively less important than that occurring in mucosal epithelial cells for immediate-release formulations since most drug absorption occurs in the proximal intestine where the highest mucosal cell enzyme activity resides.[33] Interest in microbial metabolism has increased in recent years because of the proliferation of controlled-release formulations which release significant amounts of drug in the colon where bacterial levels are extremely high (10^{11} bacteria per gram).[58] About 60 different bacteria are present in the colon,[62] the composition of which is quite consistent among animal species and man.[58] An important metabolic role played by intestinal flora is in the enterohepatic recycling of drugs and endogenous compounds (e.g., cholesterol, bile salts) that are excreted in the bile as polar conjugates.[14] Hydrolysis of the polar drug conjugates

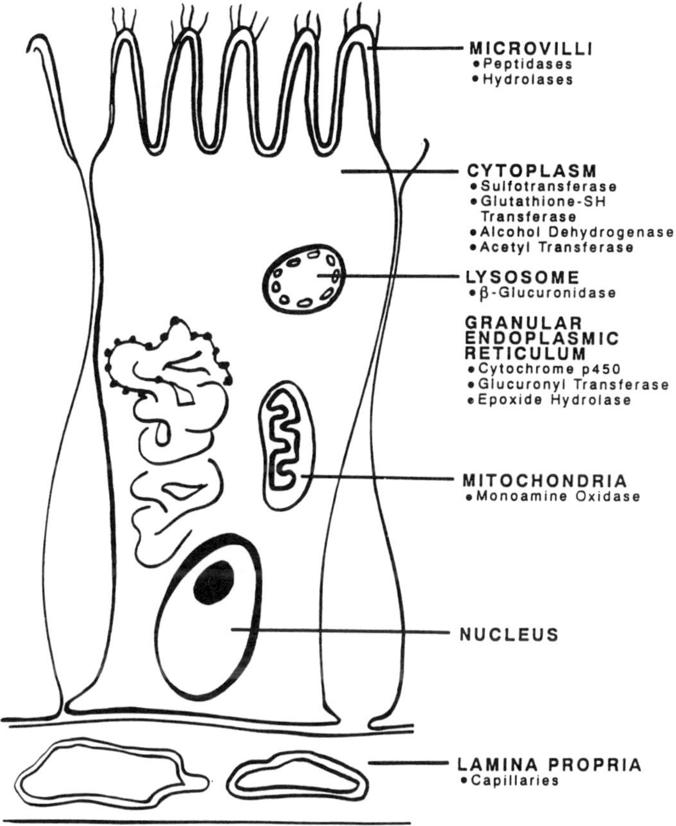

Figure 8–3 Schematic representation of a mucosal epithelial cell showing the location of enzymes within the cell. (Redrawn from Reference 58.)

to yield the intact drug are catalyzed by bacterial enzymes (e.g., β-glucuronidases, sulfatases). Whether enterohepatic recycling of drug conjugates occurs in humans should be a consideration when selecting an animal model for oral bioavailability or bioequivalence studies of human dosage formulations.

III. COMPARATIVE ANIMAL AND HUMAN ORAL BIOAVAILABILITY STUDIES

Although the results of a number of oral drug bioavailability studies in animal species have been reported in the literature, relatively few comparative human and animal studies have been reported in which the same dosage formulations were administered to both animals and man. Examination of the literature quickly reveals that the overwhelming number of published comparative human and animal oral bioavailability studies in which human dosage formulations were administered have been done in the dog. In fact, the only comparative oral bioavailability studies in humans and monkeys reported in the open literature were absolute oral bioavailability studies or radiolabel disposition studies. Although the absolute oral bioavailabilities of some drugs are comparable in monkeys and humans,[61] including some that are incompletely absorbed (e.g., nadolol, acyclovir, methyldopa, and menogaril),[63-66] the overall correlation in absolute oral bioavailability between humans and primates is low ($r^2 = 0.2$, $n = 7$).[61] Also, the overall correlation is less than the correlation between humans and dogs ($r^2 = 0.3$, $n = 36$), for which considerably more data are available.[61] It should be noted that the correlation in absolute oral bioavailability between humans and rodents ($r^2 = 0.4$, $n = 36$)[61] is actually higher than that between humans and dogs. Clearly, too little data are available to determine the general applicability of the monkey as a model for bioavailability/bioequivalence assessment in humans and will not be further considered.

The reasons for the larger number of comparative studies in dogs is likely related to more than anatomic and physiological considerations. Additional reasons for using dogs instead of monkeys or pigs for these studies are the ease of handling dogs and obtaining serial blood specimens or cumulative urine samples, their availability and low cost, and the fact that the dog is the nonrodent species most frequently used for subchronic and chronic toxicology studies. Monkeys by comparison are difficult and expensive to obtain, they require specialized housing and pose a health risk to laboratory personnel, and the ethics of using primates for laboratory studies may be a consideration. Although domestic pigs are readily available, they are not easy to handle, dose, and obtain blood and urine samples from because of their size and anatomy. Even miniature strains of pigs (e.g., Göttingen and Hanford minipigs, and Yucatan micropig) can be difficult to handle, and obtaining blood and urine samples from these animals can be technically challenging.

The use of animal models for oral bioavailability assessment has previously been reviewed,[12] and a joint Pharmaceutical Manufacturers Association/Federal Drug Administration (PMA/FDA) workshop was held on the use of animal models as substitutes for humans in oral bioavailability studies.[67] A compilation of case histories in which the dog was used as an animal model for oral bioavailability assessment of human dosage formulations has also appeared.[68-70] Most of the studies described in the above referenced compilation of case histories were done during preclinical phases of drug development that demonstrated the utility of the dog as an animal model for assessing bioavailability/bioequivalence prior to the conduct of definitive human studies, although several cases where the dog was not predictive were cited. In these case histories, the dog was used as an animal model to (1) select from among several ester prodrugs one for development,[68] (2) assess the extent of first-pass metabolism,[68] (3) evaluate the bioavailability of enteric-coated tablets,[68] (4) determine the importance of biliary excretion and the extent of enterohepatic recycling,[68] (5) evaluate multiple experimental dosage formulations prior to testing in humans,[68,69] (6) select an appropriate salt form of a basic drug for development,[69] (7) determine the effect of formulation excipients on oral bioavailability during formulation development,[69] and (8) determine the effect of micronization on oral bioavailability prior to the conduct of human studies.[68] Most of these studies were pilot studies that involved a limited number of animals and are typical of studies frequently done during the course of new drug development to provide guidance during the drug development process. Several specific examples from this compilation of studies in which dogs were used to assess oral bioavailability will be cited in greater detail below. However, the main focus of the remainder of this discussion will be devoted to comparative animal and human studies in which multiple commercial and/or experimental formulations were administered with the objective of obtaining high statistical power. In these studies, *in vitro* dissolution data were obtained for correlation with *in vivo* results; and in most studies, comparable numbers of animals and human volunteers were used (10 to 12 in most cases). A number of the drugs studied had low aqueous solubilities under the pH conditions encountered in the gastrointestinal tract, and several were extensively metabolized in the first pass in at least one of the species. Comparative data in two animal species were obtained for several drugs.

A. IMMEDIATE-RELEASE FORMULATIONS

1. Acidic Drugs

Three weakly acidic drugs with low aqueous solubilities at acidic pH — flufenamic acid,[71] nalidixic acid,[72,73] and indomethacin[74,75] — were investigated in comparative dog and human bioavailability studies designed to achieve high statistical power. Since the

pK_a of these compounds is in the range of 4 to 6, pH partition theory of gastrointestinal absorption[76] would predict that these compounds would dissolve mainly in the small intestine and then be absorbed. However, if the pH of the stomach is high because of low basal acid output, then significant dissolution might occur in the stomach.

The oral bioavailabilities of five commercially available formulations of flufenamic acid capsules were investigated in crossover design studies in humans (n = 15) and beagle dogs (n = 10) by monitoring intact drug concentrations in systemic circulation.[71] Mean maximum concentrations (C_{max}) of drug in humans (Figure 8–4) were about 2.5 times lower than mean C_{max} in dogs (Figure8–5). The mean time at which C_{max} was achieved (T_{max}) ranged from 1.5 to 2.42 h in humans and 1.5 to 2.25 h in dogs. Although the range of the mean T_{max} values were comparable in humans and dogs, the rank order of T_{max} for the treatments was different in the two species. There were no significant treatment differences in C_{max} or T_{max} in humans, but treatments D and E had significantly shorter T_{max} than treatment C in dogs. The extent of absorption of the formulations covered a very narrow and identical relative range in both humans (83.6 to 100%) and dogs (83.6 to 100%). Treatment A had the highest AUC in both humans and dogs, but the rank order of the bioavailability of the other treatments was different in humans and dogs. Statistically significant treatment differences ($p < 0.05$) in treatments A and B were found in humans and treatments A and D in dogs. It is not surprising given the small range in the extent of bioavailability of these formulations that the rank order correlations differ in humans and dogs. The fact that treatment A was highly bioavailable in both species was encouraging, but the fact that treatment D had a high bioavailability in humans but the lowest bioavailability in dogs led the authors to the conclusion that it would be difficult to predict the bioavailability of flufenamic acid capsules in humans from bioavailability tests in dogs.

The oral bioavailabilities of three commercial formulations and two experimental formulations of nalidixic acid tablets were investigated in Latin-square crossover design studies in humans (n = 13) and beagle dogs (n = 10) by monitoring intact drug concentrations in systemic circulation.[72,73] Mean C_{max} in humans were about 5 times lower than mean C_{max} in dogs. Major treatment differences in mean C_{max} and T_{max} were observed in both humans and dogs. Mean T_{max} ranged from 1.3 to 3.7 h in humans and 1.9 to 2.6 h in dogs. The narrower range in mean T_{max} in dogs relative to humans likely reflects the shorter gastrointestinal transit time in dogs. A good inverse correlation existed between the rate of absorption in humans and mean C_{max} and AUC in dogs. That is, short T_{max} in humans were associated with high C_{max} and AUC in dogs. In humans, significant differences ($p < 0.05$) were found in mean T_{max} for treatments A and B and treatments C, D, and E; however, no significant treatment differences in mean T_{max} were found in dogs. The correlation in mean C_{max} of the treatments between humans and dogs (Figure 8–6) was exceptionally good (r = 0.895), with the rank order of mean C_{max} for the treatments exactly the same in the two species. Although the correlation in the mean AUC of the treatments between humans and dogs was not as good as for mean C_{max}, treatment A was the most bioavailable and treatment E was the least bioavailable in both species. In humans, the mean AUC of treatments A and B were significantly greater than those of treatments D and E, but in dogs only treatments A and E were significantly different. These differences may, at least in part, be related to the fact that the range of treatment differences in mean AUC were greater in humans (59.4 to 100%) than in dogs (66.7 to 100%). Treatments that did not disintegrate and disperse well under mild *in vitro* dissolution conditions had higher relative bioavailabilities in dogs than in humans. This may be related to greater tablet dissolution of this acidic drug in the gastrointestinal tract of dogs, or perhaps to higher bile salt concentrations in dogs relative to humans. The dog appears to be a reasonably good screening model for assessing the rate of absorption of nalidixic acid tablets but not the extent of absorption. Thus, it does not appear that dogs can replace humans in definitive bioavailability/bioequivalence testing of nalidixic acid

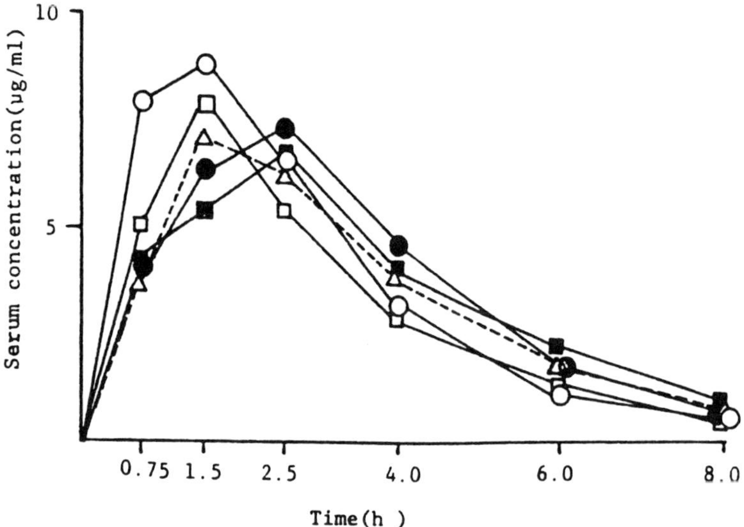

Figure 8–4 Mean serum concentrations of flufenamic acid in human volunteers after oral administration of five capsule formulations: (○) treatment A; (□) treatment B; (△) treatment C; (●) treatment D; and (■) treatment E. (Redrawn from Reference 71.)

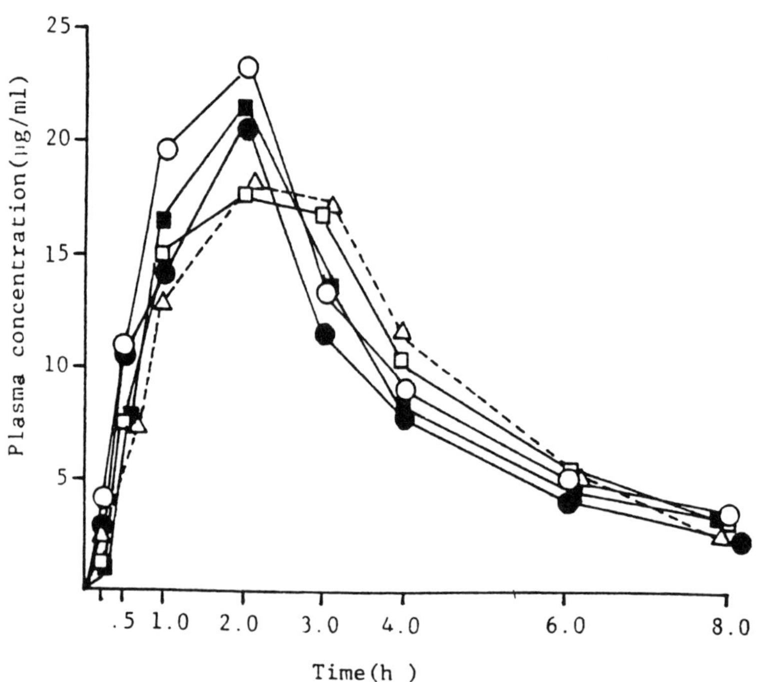

Figure 8–5 Mean plasma concentrations of flufenamic acid in beagle dogs after oral administration of five capsule formulations: (○) treatment A; (□) treatment B; (△) treatment C; (●) treatment D; and (■) treatment E. (Redrawn from Reference 71.)

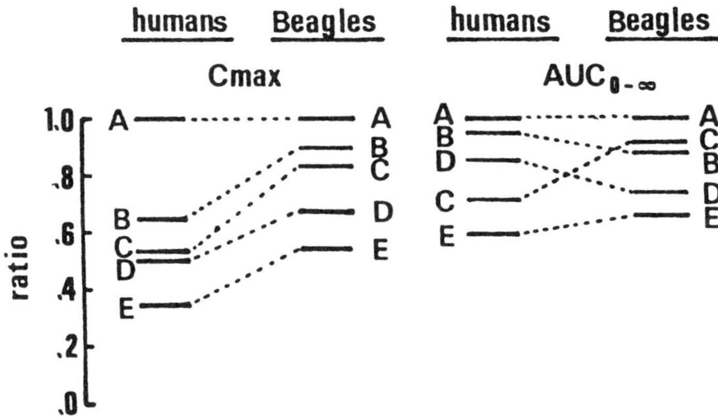

Figure 8–6 Comparison of the relative values of mean C_{max} and $AUC_{0-\infty}$ of four nalidixic acid tablet formulations in humans and beagle dogs (treatment A = 1.0). (Redrawn from Reference 73.)

tablets. The results of this study further suggest that the dog is not a good animal model for studying formulations that have prolonged release rates, probably because of the short intestinal transit time in the dog. Treatment of dogs with drugs to increase gastrointestinal transit times may be useful in studies of nalidixic acid.[47,77,78]

The oral bioavailabilities of two commercial formulations and three experimental formulations of indomethacin capsules were investigated in Latin-square crossover design studies in humans (n = 10) and beagle dogs (n = 10) by monitoring intact drug concentrations in systemic circulation.[74,75] Mean C_{max} in humans were about 2 times lower than mean C_{max} in dogs. The gastric acidities in the human volunteers were also estimated, with significant ($p < 0.05$) differences found in mean C_{max} and AUC in the high gastric acidity vs. low gastric acidity volunteers for some treatments. Major treatment differences in mean T_{max}, C_{max}, and AUC were observed in both humans and dogs. Mean T_{max} were shorter in dogs (range, 1.12 to 2.90 h) than in humans (1.0 to 5.0 h) for most of the treatments, with the notable exception of treatment A, which contained smaller particle size drug. The mean C_{max} of treatment A in humans was significantly higher than those of all the other treatments, while in dogs the mean C_{max} of treatment A was significantly greater than those of treatments D and E. The relative treatment differences in mean C_{max} and AUC for human volunteers with both high and low gastric acidities, and for dogs are shown in Figure 8–7. The relative differences in mean C_{max} between treatment A and the other treatments was greater for human volunteers having either high or low gastric acidities than for dogs. The correlation between mean C_{max} for humans and dogs was good, especially for the volunteers with high gastric acidities, but the correlation between mean AUC was very poor in humans and dogs. These results indicated that the dog may provide useful information about the rate of absorption of immediate-release indomethacin formulations, but is unlikely to provide useful information about the extent of absorption. These results also suggested that humans are more sensitive to changes in the particle size of the drug than are dogs.

Comparative oral bioavailability studies of potassium phosphanilate, a moderately acidic compound ($pK_a = 1.8$), were conducted in fasted dogs (n = 4) and humans (n = 10) by monitoring intact drug concentrations in systemic circulation.[69] No indication was given as to the design of the studies. The absolute oral bioavailability was 45% in the dog, and about 28% of the dose was excreted in the urine; whereas the oral bioavailability was very low in humans, and only 4% of the dose was excreted in the urine. Thus, the oral

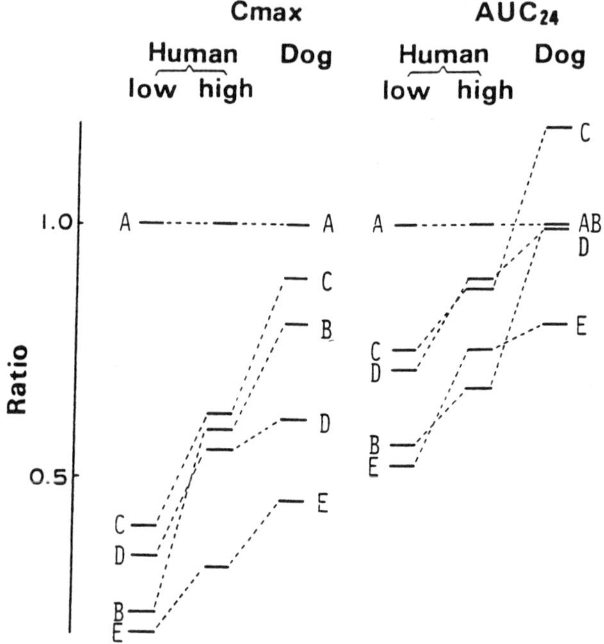

Figure 8–7 Comparison of relative values of mean C_{max} and $AUC_{0\text{-}24}$ of five indomethacin capsule formulations in humans having low and high gastric acidities and in beagle dogs (treatment A = 1.0). (Redrawn from Reference 75.)

bioavailability of potassium phosphanilate in dogs was not predictive of its oral bioavailability in humans because of major differences in the extent of first-pass metabolism in humans relative to dogs. The difference in first-pass metabolism may have been due to the fact that dogs, unlike most humans, are not good N-acetylators of aromatic amines.[69] This study demonstrates the importance of having comparative drug disposition data in animal models and humans prior to the selection of an animal model for bioavailability or bioequivalence assessment of human dosage formulations.

2. Basic Drugs

The oral bioavailability of poorly soluble, basic drugs are frequently dependent on the extent of dissolution of the drug in the stomach prior to its transfer to the small intestine. To increase the rate of dissolution, salts of the free base form of drugs are often used. Micronization may also prove beneficial. Studies of three basic drugs are reported here in which dogs were used to evaluate human dosage formulations that had different dissolution characteristics.[69,79-83]

Comparative oral bioavailability studies of experimental formulations of a basic quinazolinone drug (pK_a, conjugate acid = 2.4) were conducted in fasted beagle dogs (n = 12) in a randomized crossover design, and in fasted humans (n = 12) in a Latin-square design by monitoring intact drug concentrations in systemic circulation.[69] Treatments B, C, and D were administered to both dogs and humans. Treatment B had the lowest mean C_{max} and AUC in both dog and humans but the rank order in mean AUC for treatments C and D was different for dogs and humans (Table 8–4). Greater relative variabilities in C_{max} and AUC were observed for dogs than for humans. Absorption of all three formulations was considerably faster in humans than in dogs. Treatments A and D were subsequently selected for clinical studies. The investigators reported the dog to be useful in predicting the bioavailability tablet formulations and in the development of a dissolution procedure at an early stage of drug development.

Table 8–4 **Bioavailability[a] of free base and hydrochloride salt formulations of a basic quinazolinone in dogs[b] and humans[c]**

Species	Treatment	Dose	C_{max} (μg/ml)	T_{max} (h)	AUC (μg h/ml)
Human	A — Tablet, base	2 × 150 mg	2.7 ± 1.1	1.5	10.9 ± 2.1
Human	B — Tablet, base	1 × 300 mg	1.6 ± 0.7	1.5	6.8 ± 2.2
Dog		100 mg/kg	4.3 ± 1.7	2.4 ± 0.6	10.1 ± 5.4
Human	C — Capsule, salt	2 × 175 mg	3.1 ± 1.0	1.0	13.0 ± 2.8
Dog		100 mg/kg	7.9 ± 2.9	2.4 ± 1.0	19.4 ± 6.1
Human	D — Tablet, base	1 × 300 mg	3.1 ± 0.9	1.5	11.4 ± 2.9
Dog		100 mg/kg	9.2 ± 3.0	2.6 ± 0.8	23.4 ± 9.0

[a] All values expressed as mean ± standard deviation.

[b] Approximately 100 mg/kg administered, free base equivalents, as tablets or capsules to 12 dogs per dosage formulation.

[c] A 300-mg dose of each tablet or capsule formulation administered to 12 volunteers per dosage formulation.

From Smyth, R. D. et al., in *Animal Models for Oral Drug Delivery in Man,* American Pharmaceutical Association Academy of Pharmaceutical Sciences, Washington, D.C., 1983, chap. 4.

The oral bioavailabilities of two commercial capsule formulations of cinnarizine, selected from among 32 different formulations, that had extremes in *in vitro* dissolution were investigated in a randomized block design in humans (n = 12), and in a Latin-square crossover design in beagle dogs (n = 12) by monitoring intact drug concentrations in systemic circulation.[79,80] The gastric acidities of the human volunteers and dogs were also estimated because highly variable systemic concentrations of cinnarizine had been observed in humans that were highly correlated with the gastric pH of the volunteers. Mean T_{max} in dogs were considerably shorter than in humans having either high or low gastric acidities (Figure 8–8). Mean C_{max} in humans having high gastric acidities (pH < 3) were of comparable magnitude to mean C_{max} in dogs, and were 3 to 7 times greater than mean C_{max} in humans having low gastric acidities. Unlike humans, gastric pH did not affect the bioavailability of cinnarizine in dogs despite of the fact that the gastric pH in dogs, estimated 90 min after drug administration, ranged from 2 to nearly 9. Mean C_{max} and AUC were not significantly different ($p > 0.05$) for the two capsule formulations in humans having high gastric acidities and in dogs. However, these parameters were significantly different for the two cinnarizine formulations in humans having low gastric acidities. The reasons for the lack of correlation of gastric acidity and bioavailability in the dog are unclear. It is possible that the pH measurements taken 90 min after ingestion of the drug did not reflect the pH at the time of drug administration. Alternatively, the extent of dissolution of the drug may have been greater in the dog, possibly because of greater gastrointestinal motility or greater secretion of bile salts. Irrespective of the reasons for the apparent differences of gastric acidity on the bioavailability of cinnarizine in humans and dogs, the dog was not a suitable animal model for predicting the bioavailability of cinnarizine capsules in humans.

A third basic drug investigated in humans and dogs was diazepam (pK_a, conjugate base = 3.3), which has a pH-dependent *in vitro* dissolution rate that is especially slow in the pH range 3 to 7. The oral bioavailabilities of four commercial tablet formulations of diazepam were investigated in human volunteers (n = 12) and in beagle dogs (n = 12) using Latin-square study designs.[81-83] In addition to having low aqueous solubilities above pH 3, diazepam is extensively metabolized in the first pass to *N*-desmethyldiazepam in dogs, but not in humans. As a consequence, the bioavailabilities were determined in humans and dogs by monitoring systemic concentrations of intact drug and *N*-desmethyldiazepam,

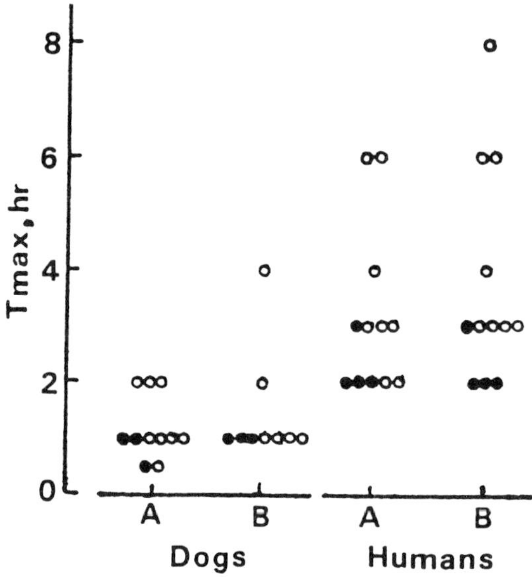

Figure 8–8 Comparison of T_{max} values for two cinnarizine capsule formulations in humans and beagle dogs having low (○) and high (●) gastric acidities. (Redrawn from Reference 80.)

respectively. The gastric acidities of the human volunteers were also estimated. When the data for all the human volunteers were analyzed together, independent of gastric pH, no significant differences in mean AUC were detected for any of the treatments (range of relative AUC, 90.8 to 100%); however, significant differences ($p < 0.05$) in mean C_{max} were detected for treatments A and B (range of relative C_{max}, 67 to 100%). In dogs the converse was true; there were significant differences in mean AUC (AUC for treatment A was significantly greater than that of all the other treatments), but there were no significant differences in mean C_{max} for any of the treatments. It should be noted, however, that treatment differences in dogs were small (Figure 8–9), and that the relative differences in mean AUC in dogs (82 to 100%) were less than the relative differences in mean C_{max} (77.4 to 100%). Although AUC in humans was independent of gastric pH for all of the treatments, C_{max} for all of the treatments were higher for volunteers with high gastric acidities (Figure 8–10). The three formulations having the slowest *in vitro* dissolution rates at pH 4.6 (treatments B, C, and D) had significantly higher ($p < 0.05$) C_{max} for volunteers with high gastric acidities. These data suggest that the extent of dissolution of treatments B, C, and D in humans was greater when gastric acidity was high, as had been observed for the weak base cinnarizine. Unlike cinnarizine, however, the extent of absorption of diazepam by humans was independent of gastric acidity. This difference in the bioavailability characteristics of the two drugs may be due to the relatively higher solubility and lower dose of diazepam. The shorter intestinal transit time in dogs relative to humans could account for the differences in extent of absorption seen in the dog. The fact remains, however, that treatment A was found superior to the other formulations in both dogs and humans for formulations having relatively small differences in bioavailability, despite the fact that there are large differences in the extent of first-pass metabolism in dogs relative to humans. Additional comparative oral bioavailability data for diazepam formulations having greater differences in the rate or extent of absorption would be useful in evaluating the utility of the dog as a model for bioavailability assessment of diazepam tablets in humans.

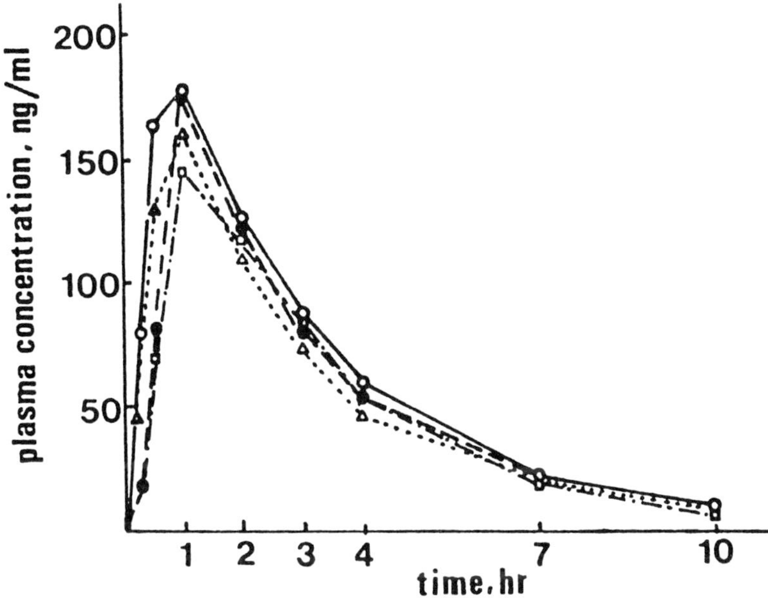

Figure 8–9 Mean plasma concentration-time profiles of *N*-desmethyldiazepam in beagle dogs after administration of four diazepam tablet formulations: (○) treatment A; (●) treatment B; (□) treatment C; and (△) treatment D. (Redrawn from Reference 83.)

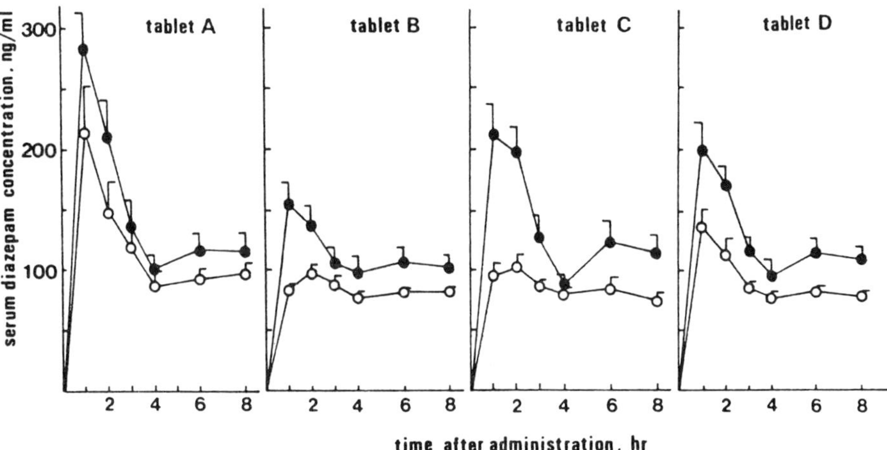

Figure 8–10 Mean serum concentration-time profiles of diazepam in humans having low (○) and high (●) gastric acidities after administration of four diazepam tablet formulations. Vertical bars represent standard errors. (Redrawn from Reference 82.)

3. Neutral Drugs

Cyclandelate is a low solubility drug (16.7 μg/ml) that is rapidly metabolized to mandelic acid. Approximately 50% of the mandelic acid is excreted by humans in the urine, but a part of the mandelic acid is further metabolized to phenylglyoxylic acid. The oral bioavailabilities of five commercial capsule formulations of cyclandelate were investigated in Latin-square crossover design studies in humans (n = 10) and in beagle dogs (n = 10) by monitoring the

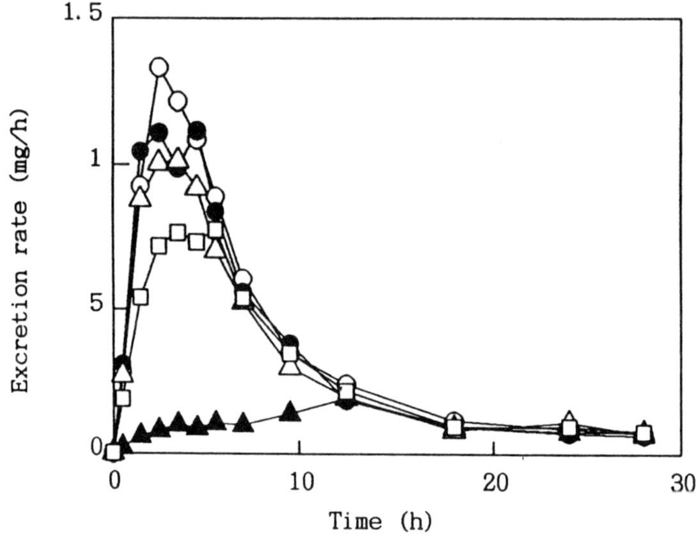

Figure 8–11 Mean excretion rate-time profiles of mandelic acid in humans after administration of five cyclandelate capsule formulations: (○) treatment A; (●) treatment B; (△) treatment C; (▲) treatment D; (□) treatment E. (Redrawn from Reference 84.)

rate of excretion of mandelic acid in the urine of humans (Figure 8–11),[84] and systemic concentrations of mandelic acid in dogs (Figure 8–12).[85] The tablets having the highest (treatment A) and lowest (treatment D) bioavailability in humans were also administered concomitantly with food in separate crossover design studies to the same human volunteers (n = 10), and six of the ten beagle dogs used in the previously described study. The formulation having the lowest extent of absorption in humans (36.3%) had the lowest bioavailability in dogs (70.3%). A significant correlation ($p < 0.05$) was found between the extent of absorption in humans and dogs. Food enhanced the bioavailability of cyclandelate from the formulations having the highest and lowest bioavailabilities, with both formulations bioequivalent in dogs after ingestion of food but not humans. Thus, the dog was not predictive of the bioavailability of cyclandelate in unfasted humans. Finally, the bioavailability in dogs was highly variable compared to the bioavailability in humans. Whether this was related to differences in absorption, differences in the extent of metabolism, or differences in clearance of mandelic acid by nonmetabolic processes cannot be determined. This study reflects the difficulty of using animal models to predict the bioavailability in humans of high clearance drugs.

Griseofulvin is a highly insoluble drug for which *in vivo* bioavailability in humans is improved by micronization. The oral bioavailability of four commercial tablet formulations were investigated in human volunteers (n = 12), in beagle dogs (n = 12), and in Göttingen minipigs (n = 7) using Latin-square study designs (humans, dogs) or a randomized block study design (minipigs).[86-88] Systemic concentrations of griseofulvin were monitored in humans (Figure 8–13) and minipigs (Figure 8–14). Systemic concentrations of 6-demethylgriseofulvin were monitored in the dog (Figure 8–15) because of extensive first-pass metabolism of the drug. The range of mean AUC values in humans was very narrow (91.6 to 100%); and, as a consequence, no significant treatment differences were found with the exception that C_{max} for treatment B was significantly greater than that of treatment C. In marked contrast to humans, a much wider range of relative AUC values were found in dogs (54.2 to 100%), with both mean C_{max} and AUC for treatment A significantly greater than those for treatments C and D. The range of relative bioavailabilities in Göttingen minipigs was intermediate those of humans and dogs (72.5 to 100%), with no significant

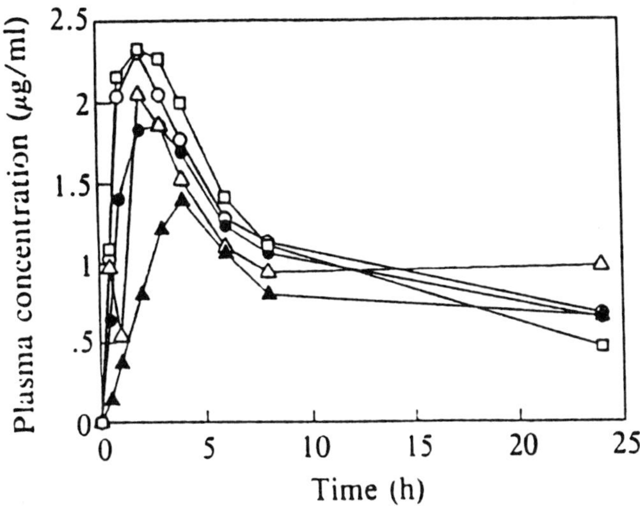

Figure 8–12 Mean plasma concentration-time profiles of mandelic acid in beagle dogs after administration of five cyclandelate capsule formulations: (○) treatment A; (●) treatment B; (△) treatment C; (▲) treatment D; (□) treatment E. (Redrawn from Reference 85.)

treatment differences found. The mean C_{max} and AUC of the treatments in pigs and humans were highly correlated. However, C_{max} and AUC were more variable in minipigs than in humans, indicating greater variability in absorption. Mean T_{max} for three of the four formulations were longer in minipigs than in humans. Delayed onset of absorption was observed in some minipigs, indicative of slow gastric emptying. Dogs were obviously much more sensitive to the dissolution characteristics of the formulations, possibly because of the shorter gastrointestinal residence time in dogs compared to humans and pigs. Additional comparative oral bioavailability data for griseofulvin formulations having greater differences in the extent of absorption would be useful in evaluating the utility of the dog as a model for bioavailability assessment of griseofulvin tablets in humans.

B. COATED TABLETS

Comparative oral bioavailability studies of five enteric-coated tablet formulations and a sugar-coated tablet formulation of pyridoxal phosphate were investigated in Latin-square crossover design studies in humans (n = 12) and beagle dogs (n = 12) by monitoring urinary excretion of 4-pyridoxic acid in humans[89] and systemic concentrations of pyridoxal in dogs.[90] Treatments A and B had significantly lower bioavailabilities than the other treatments in humans, and treatment B was significantly lower than the other treatments in dogs. Although the gastric emptying rates of enteric-coated tablets were faster in dogs than in humans, the rate and extent of absorption of pyridoxal phosphate were highly correlated in humans and dogs (Figure 8–16), suggesting that the beagle dog may be a suitable animal model for bioavailability assessment of enteric-coated tablets of pyridoxal phosphate.

The oral bioavailabilities of an enteric-coated tablet formulation and a granule formulation of aspirin were investigated in humans, in dogs, and in pigs by monitoring the urinary excretion rate of salicylic acid (humans) or systemic concentrations of salicylic acid (dogs, pigs).[17] Both the rate and extent of absorption of these formulations appeared to be highly correlated in humans and dogs (Figure 8–17), whereas the absorption of the enteric-coated tablet by pigs was delayed and was very low relative to the granule formulation. Furthermore, the salicylic acid concentrations in the pig were highly variable. These results suggest that the beagle dog has promise as an animal model for

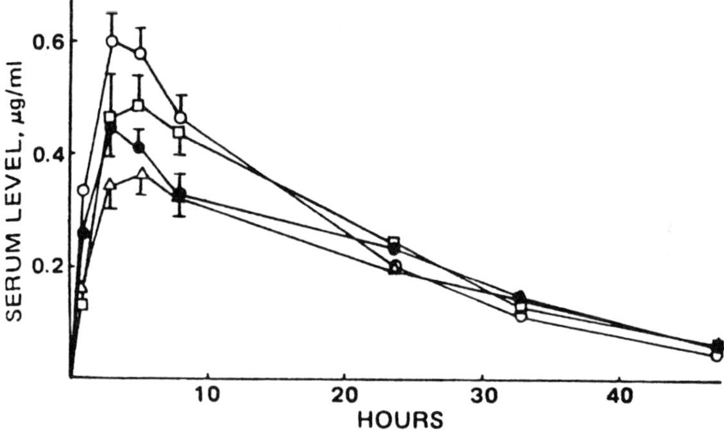

Figure 8–13 Mean plasma concentration-time profiles of griseofulvin in humans after administration of four griseofulvin capsule formulations: (●) treatment A; (○) treatment B; (△) treatment C; and (□) treatment D. Vertical bars represent standard errors. (Redrawn from Reference 86.)

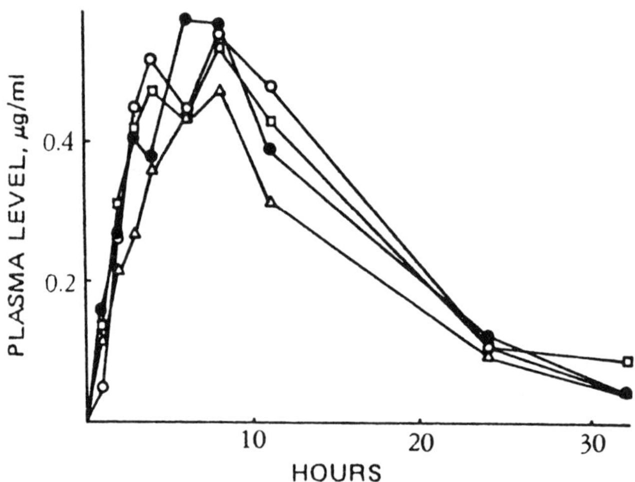

Figure 8–14 Mean plasma concentration-time profiles of griseofulvin in Göttingen minipigs after administration of four griseofulvin capsule formulations: (●) treatment A; (○) treatment B; (△) treatment C; and (□) treatment D. (Redrawn from Reference 88.)

bioavailability assessment of aspirin formulations, but the pig does not appear to be a suitable animal model.

Although metronidazole readily dissolves in aqueous solutions (solubility 11.6 mg/ml at pH 7) and is rapidly absorbed, the dissolution of some sugar-coated tablet formulations is very slow near neutral pH. The oral bioavailabilities of five commercial sugar-coated tablets of metronidazole were investigated in Latin-square design studies in humans (n = 10) and in beagle dogs (n = 11) by monitoring systemic drug concentrations.[91,92] The gastric acidities in the human volunteers and dogs were also estimated because of the effect of pH on the dissolution rates of these formulations. The authors stressed the importance of measuring the gastric pH in dogs at the time each treatment was administered because of large intradog

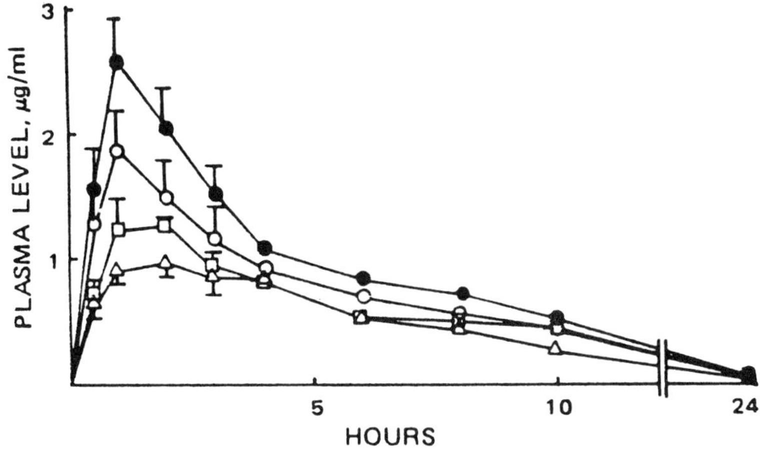

Figure 8–15 Mean plasma concentration-time profiles of griseofulvin in beagle dogs after administration of four griseofulvin capsule formulations: (●) treatment A; (○) treatment B; (△) treatment C; and (□) treatment D. Vertical bars represent standard errors. (Redrawn from Reference 87.)

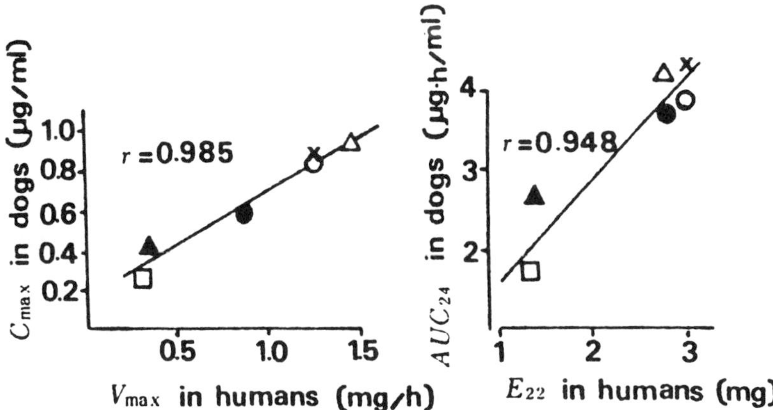

Figure 8–16 Comparison of the extent of absorption of six pyridoxal phosphate enteric-coated tablet formulations in humans and in beagle dogs: (▲) treatment A; (□) treatment B; (△) treatment C; (●) treatment D; (○) treatment E; and (×) treatment F. (Redrawn from Reference 90.)

variations in gastric pH. Gastric acidity in fasted humans remained relatively constant in comparison to that in dogs. Large gastric acidity-dependent differences in mean C_{max} and AUC were found for all but one of the formulations in both humans (Figure 8–18) and dogs (Figure 8–19). Mean C_{max} and AUC for humans and dogs classified as having low gastric acidities (pH > 3) were highly correlated (Figure 8–20). In contrast, these same parameters in humans and in dogs classified as having high gastric acidities (pH < 3) were not well correlated. These data suggest that the beagle dog may be a useful animal model for bioavailability tests of sugar-coated metronidazole tablets.

The bioavailabilities of enteric- or film-coated tablets of erythromycin were evaluated in a pilot dog study, and then in a human study.[69] No information was provided concerning the number of animals and human volunteers used in these studies. The dog was not

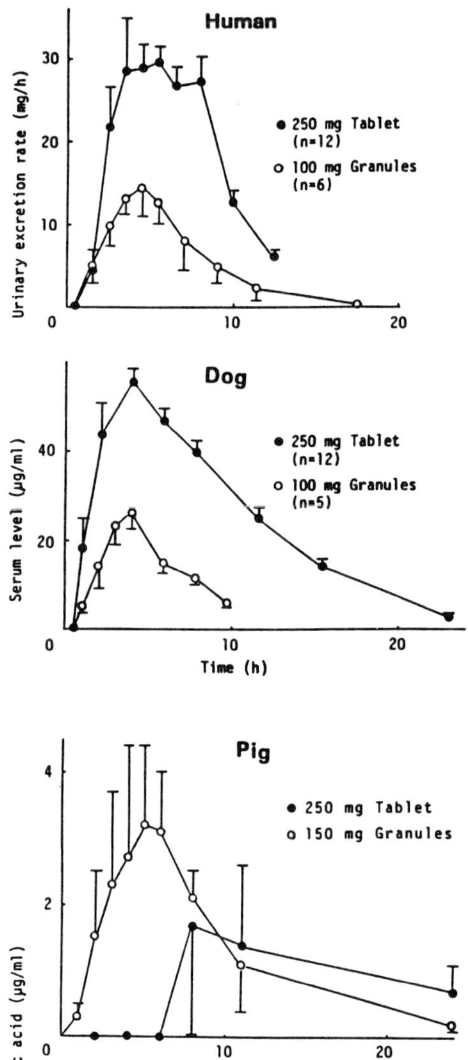

Figure 8–17 Mean salicylate levels, expressed as total salicylic acid urinary excretion rate or as serum concentrations, in fasted humans, in beagle dogs, and in pigs after administration of enteric-coated tablet (11 mm in diameter) or granule (1 mm in diameter) formulations of aspirin. (Redrawn from Reference 17.)

predictive of differences in the relative oral bioavailability of enteric-coated vs. film-coated tablets of acid-sensitive erythromycin in humans unless the dog was treated with a gastric secretagogue (histamine) to stimulate gastric acid secretion. This study demonstrates that administration of secretagogues to dogs to stimulate gastric secretion may be useful for the study of poorly soluble drugs that have pH-sensitive dissolution rates.

C. CONTROLLED-RELEASE FORMULATIONS

The oral bioavailabilities of solution and sustained-release tablet formulations of [^{14}C]aminorex were investigated in four or five human volunteers and two or three beagle dogs in parallel design studies by monitoring systemic concentrations of total radioactivity.[93] Complete absorption of [^{14}C]aminorex from the sustained-release formulation was

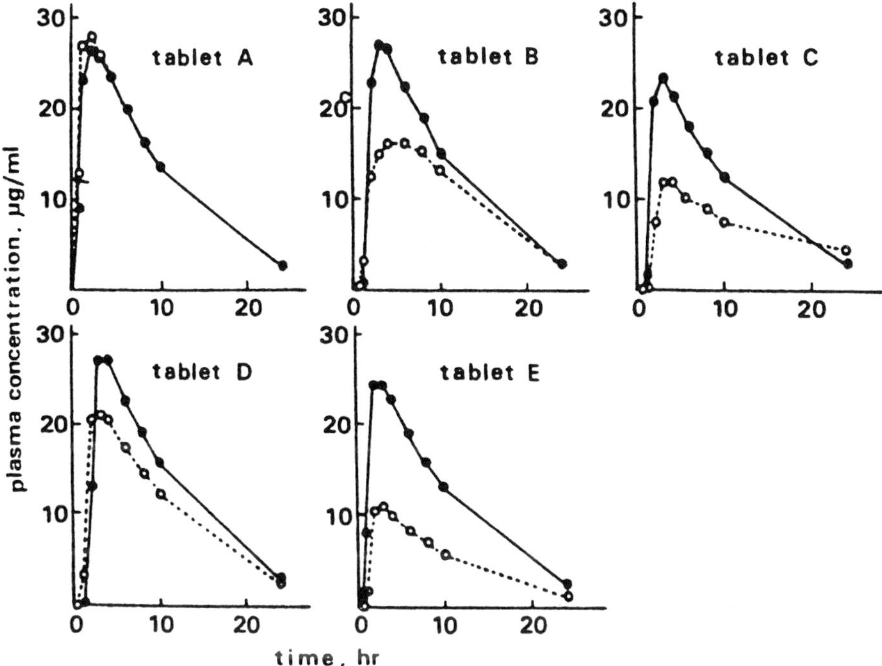

Figure 8–18 Mean serum concentration-time profiles of metronidazole in humans having low (○) and high (●) gastric acidities after administration of five sugar-coated tablet formulations of metronidazole. (Redrawn from Reference 91.)

found in humans relative to the solution formulation, whereas only 70 to 80% of the [^{14}C]aminorex was absorbed from the sustained-release formulation in the dog relative to the solution formulation (Figure 8–21). In a subsequent experiment with nondisintegrating sustained-release tablets in dogs, the nondisintegrating tablets were expelled in the feces in two of four dogs within 6 h and in the remaining two dogs within 8 to 12 h, demonstrating the short gastrointestinal transit time in the dog.

In an oral bioavailability study of sustained-release formulations of valproic acid,[94-96] two sustained-release formulations were compared to a standard immediate-release tablet formulation in humans (n = 6) and mongrel dogs (n = 5) by monitoring systemic concentrations of valproic acid (Figure 8–22). Although the bioavailabilities of the formulations had the same rank order in dogs and humans, the extent of absorption of the tablet having the slowest release rate was less than 50% compared to the immediate-release formulation in dogs and compared to the bioavailability of this formulation in humans.

Comparative oral bioavailability studies of sustained- and immediate-release formulations of acetaminophen were conducted in humans (n = 8) and dogs (n = 4) by monitoring systemic acetaminophen concentrations.[12] As in the previously cited comparisons of immediate- and sustained-release formulations, the extent of absorption for the sustained-release formulation of acetaminophen was substantially lower than that of the immediate-release formulation in the dog (57%), while absorption of the sustained-release formulation in humans was nearly complete (92%).

The results of comparative bioavailability studies of sustained-and immediate-release formulations of phenylpropanolamine in humans (n = 6) and dogs (n = 4) indicated that the extent of absorption of phenylpropanolamine from the sustained-release formulation

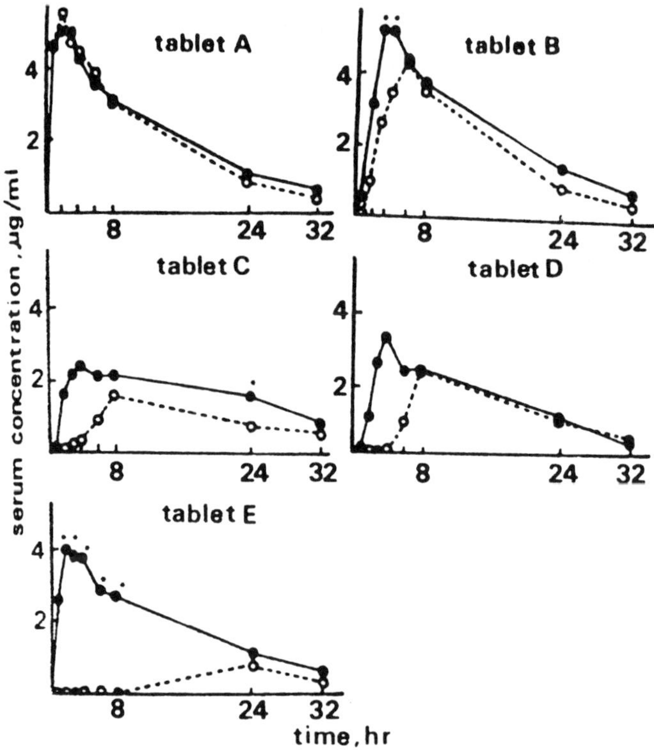

Figure 8–19 Mean plasma concentration-time profiles of metronidazole in beagle dogs having low (○) and high (●) gastric acidities after administration of five sugar-coated tablet formulations of metronidazole. (Redrawn from Reference 92.)

was nearly as high in dogs as in humans (Figure 8–23).[12] Drug absorption was also prolonged in the dog. A proposed explanation for the close agreement in the dog and human data for this drug is the fact that phenylpropanolamine is absorbed in the colon. Thus, the effective gastrointestinal residence time is longer for this compound which resulted in complete release of the drug from the formulation, even in the dog.

In an attempt to find an animal model that was predictive of food-induced changes in theophylline absorption from controlled-release formulations,[97-101] the effects of food on the absorption of controlled-release theophylline were investigated in Hormel-Hanford minipigs[102] (n = 5) and in beagle dog[103] (n = 4) in crossover design studies. The pharmacokinetics of orally administered theophylline were noticeably different in minipigs and humans,[98,99] although the absolute oral bioavailabilities under fasting conditions were quite comparable in minipigs and humans (81 vs. 71%). Furthermore, because of the high variability in the minipig data and the animal's intolerance to the high fat diet, it was difficult to accurately determine the food effect in the minipig. For these reasons, the minipig was judged not to be an ideal model to study the bioavailability of controlled-release formulations of theophylline. Although the absolute oral bioavailability of two different commercial theophylline products were only about 50% as bioavailable in dogs as in humans, the investigators found that the effects of food on the bioavailability of these formulations in dogs followed the same trend as had been reported in humans.[99] The investigators therefore concluded that the beagle dog, although not a perfect animal model for accurately predicting absolute oral bioavailability, appeared to be a good model

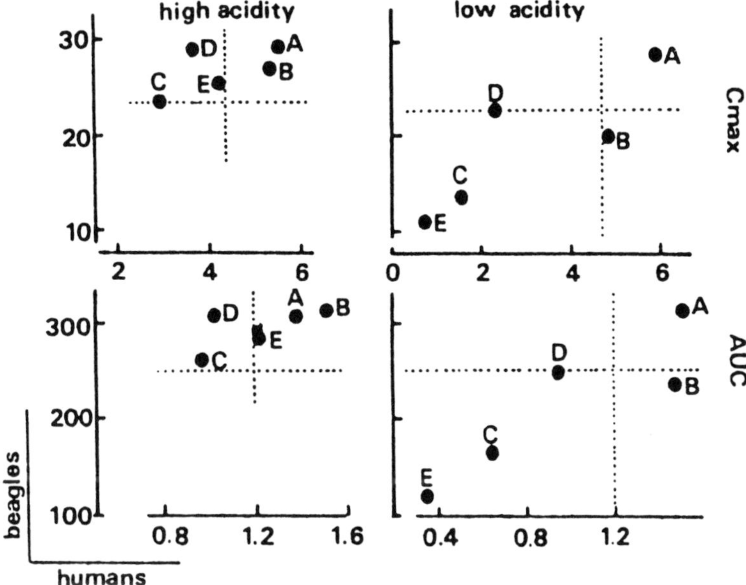

Figure 8–20 Comparison of mean C_{max} and $AUC_{0\text{-}24}$ of five sugar-coated metronidazole tablet formulations in humans and beagle dogs having high and low gastric acidities. Dotted lines represent 80% of the highest values of these parameters in each species. Correlation coefficients (r) for regression lines of the C_{max} and $AUC_{0\text{-}24}$ data were 0.843 and 0.650, respectively, for the high gastric acidity groups; and 0.856 and 0.899, respectively, for the low gastric acidity groups. (Redrawn from Reference 92.)

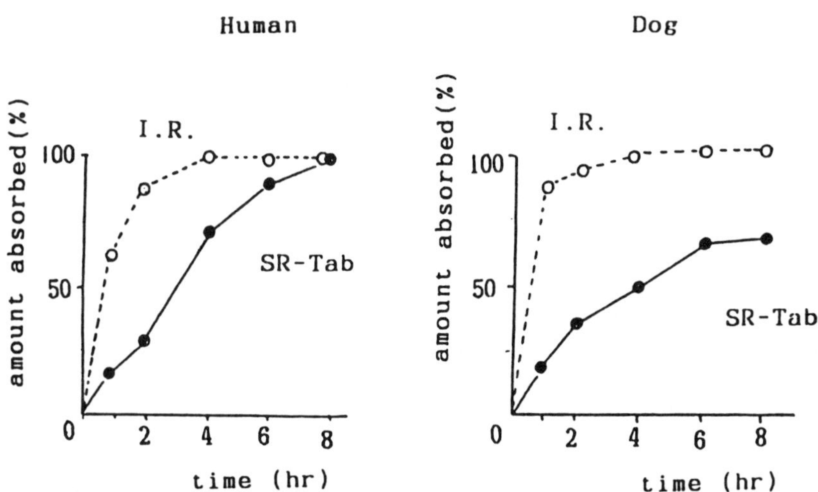

Figure 8–21 Cumulative percentage of aminorex absorbed by humans and beagle dogs after administration of immediate- (I.R.) and sustained-release tablet (SR-Tab) formulations of [^{14}C]aminorex. (Redrawn from Reference 93.)

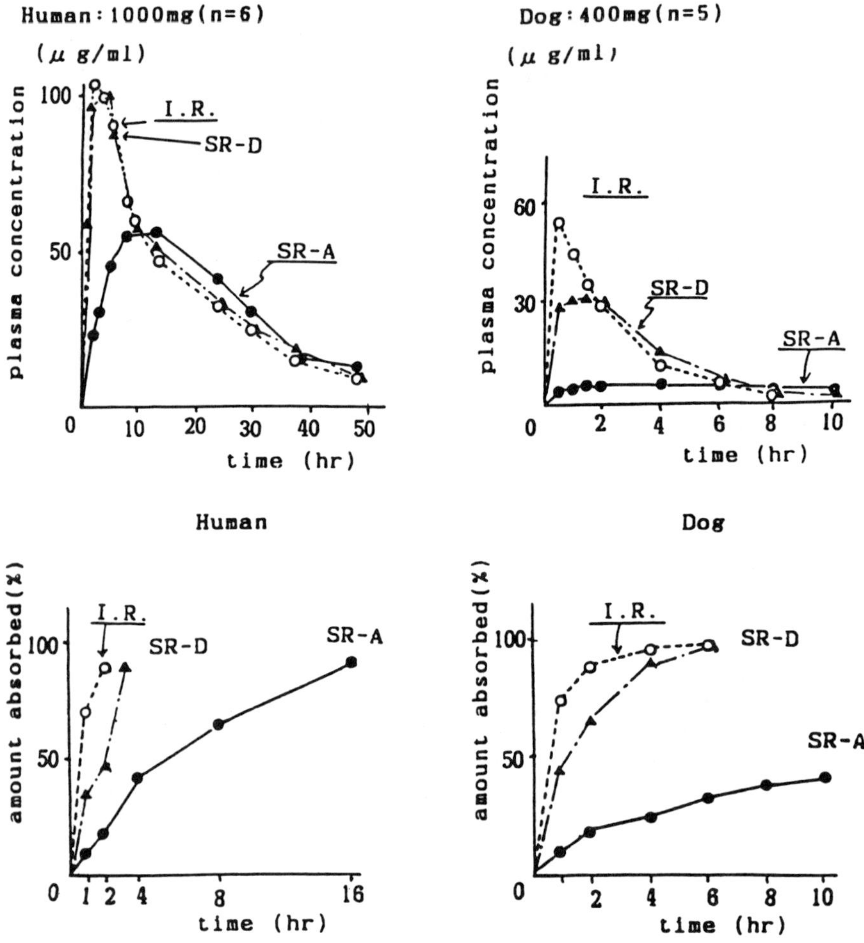

Figure 8–22 Mean plasma concentration-time profiles of valproic acid (top panels) and cumulative percentage of valproic acid absorbed (lower panels) in humans and in mongrel dogs after administration of immediate- (I.R.) and sustained-release (SR-A and SR-D) valproic acid formulations. (Redrawn from Reference 12.)

for predicting the effects of food on the relative bioavailability of controlled-release theophylline products in humans.

The low bioavailabilities of controlled-release formulations relative to immediate-release formulations of drugs in dogs that were cited here are consistent with the anatomically short gastrointestinal tract that results in a short intestinal residence time in dogs. Drugs that have low aqueous solubilities under the pH conditions encountered in the gastrointestinal tract frequently have low bioavailabilities in dogs relative to humans because of short intestinal residence times in dogs. Thus, increasing the gastrointestinal residence time in the dog may be beneficial in investigations of both controlled-release formulations and poorly soluble drugs. The results of several studies suggest that it may be possible to increase intestinal residence times significantly by administration of propantheline bromide,[47,77] loperamide hydrochloride,[104] or atropine sulfate[78] to control intestinal transit times. In gastrointestinal physiology-regulated dogs, a combined treatment of intramuscular pentagastrin and intravenous atropine sulfate was used to achieve a gastric pH of approximately 2 and a small intestinal transit time of 4 h. The absorption

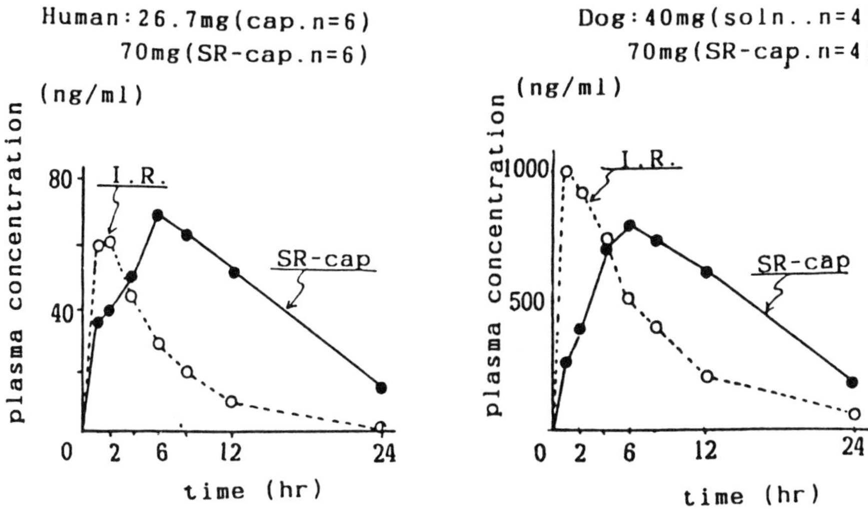

Figure 8–23 Mean systemic concentration-time profiles of phenylpropanolamine in humans and dogs after administration of immediate-(I.R.) and sustained-release (SR-cap) phenylpropanolamine capsule formulations. (Redrawn from Reference 12.)

profiles of sustained-release diclofenac sodium in these dogs were bimodal[78] (Figure 8-24), just as reported for sustained-release diclofenac sodium in normal human volunteers.[105] In marked contrast, the absorption profiles of sustained-release diclofenac sodium in nonregulated dogs were comparable to the absorption profiles of immediate-release diclofenac sodium,[78] except absorption was slower (Figure 8–25).

IV. CONCLUSIONS

The number of animal species that can realistically be used to investigate the biopharmaceutical and pharmacokinetic characteristics of human dosage formulations is limited. First and foremost, the digestive system in the animal model must be able to accommodate human-scale dosage formulations. Ideally, the sizes of the stomach, small intestine, and large intestine in the animal model should be approximately proportion proportional to those in humans so that the residence time of the lumenal contents in the animal are proportional to those in humans. Because of major differences in the gastrointestinal tracts of ruminants as compared to man, even small ruminants such as sheep and goats are not considered suitable models for oral bioavailability and bioequivalence assessment of human dosage formulations. Although rabbits have been used to a limited extent to study human dosage formulations, the anatomic dimensions of their gastrointestinal tracts and the fact that stomach emptying is very prolonged in rabbits relative to humans does not make them generally useful for this purpose.

Dogs, pigs, and rhesus monkeys all have simple stomachs that can readily accommodate a human-scale dosage formulation. Gastric volumes vary considerably among these species. Dogs have nearly the same gastric volume as humans; rhesus monkeys have about one tenth the gastric volume as humans; and pigs have a gastric volume that is approximately 6 times that of humans. The stomachs of these species have glandular mucosa that secrete mucus and gastric acid as in humans. The basal output of gastric acid appears to be much higher in humans than in dogs under fasting conditions, while pigs and monkeys have gastric acid outputs that are similar to humans. However, gastric acid output in monkeys is very sensitive to restraint conditions. The small intestine in dogs is

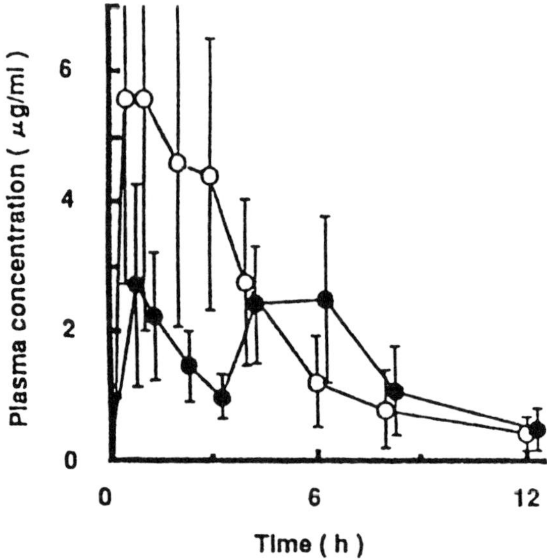

Figure 8–24 Mean plasma concentration-time profiles of diclofenac in gastrointestinal physiology-regulated beagle dogs after administration of immediate- (○) and sustained-release (●) diclofenac sodium formulations. Vertical bars represent standard deviations. (Redrawn from Reference 78.)

about one half as long as that in humans and has about the same lumenal dimensions. Thus, the intestinal transit time in the dog is expected to be approximately one half that in humans, and may result in a substantial reduction in the extent of absorption of dosage forms having slow dissolution rates (e.g., poorly soluble drugs or controlled-release dosage formulations). For formulations with rapid dissolution rates, the shorter intestinal length in the dog may be compensated for to some extent by the longer and more slender villi in the carnivore. In marked contrast to the dog, pigs have a small intestine that is approximately twice as long as that in humans and lumenal dimensions that are comparable to those in humans. Basic differences in the stomach-emptying patterns between pigs and humans (food apparently remains in the stomach of the pig 24 h a day) bring into question the applicability of the pig as an animal model for bioavailability or bioequivalence assessment of immediate-release dosage formulations. The overall length of the small intestine in monkeys appears to be shorter than in humans, but the lumenal diameter appears to be greater and may compensate to some extent for its shorter length. However, the intestinal villi in rhesus monkeys are broad and leaf shaped compared to the filamentous villi in humans. It seems probable, therefore, that the small intestine in rhesus monkeys has lower absorptive capacity than in humans. Thus from an anatomic and physiological perspective, there is no one animal species that can be predicted *a priori* to be the most suitable animal model for evaluation of human dosage formulations.

The conduct of bioavailability studies in animal models unquestionably provides valuable information about the biopharmaceutical and pharmacokinetic characteristics of new drugs during their development. Although little may be known during the early phases of drug development about the suitability of an animal model for bioavailability and bioequivalence assessment of human dosage formulations, a body of knowledge that is accumulated as data from multiple species becomes available from pharmacokinetics, bioavailability, and dose proportionality studies; toxicokinetics studies; and absorption, distribution, metabolism, and excretion studies. Common dosage formulations are occasionally administered to animal models and humans in biopharmaceutical studies that provide insight into the suitability of an

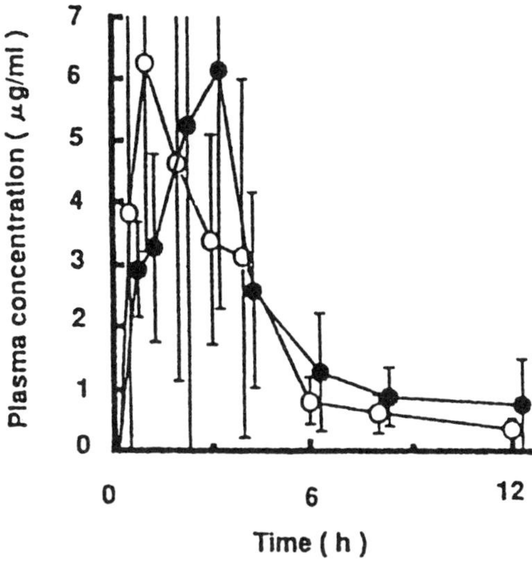

Figure 8–25 Mean plasma concentration-time profiles of diclofenac in nonregulated beagle dogs after administration of immediate-(○) and sustained-release (●) diclofenac sodium formulations. Vertical bars represent standard deviations. (Redrawn from Reference 78.)

animal model, under a limited range of experimental conditions, for assessment of the bioavailability or bioequivalence of human dosage formulations prior to the conduct of definitive bioavailability studies in humans. Rarely, if ever, are these animal studies conducted with the aim of achieving high statistical power, but of simply providing assurance that the human study has a reasonable probability of success. Despite the numerous animal studies that may be conducted during the course of new drug development, definitive bioavailability and/or bioequivalence studies in humans of the final formulation are conducted before large-scale introduction of a new drug into patients; exceptions are a few special cases in which *in vivo* bioavailability data in humans are waived.

Review of data available in the open literature from a number of comparative animal and human bioavailability studies in which common dosage formulations were administered confirmed that the *a priori* substitution of animal models for humans in definitive bioavailability studies is not warranted because no animal species was generally able to predict the bioavailability/bioequivalence of formulations in humans. Most of the comparative studies were done in dogs, but several studies were done in pigs. Too little comparative data were available to determine the general applicability of monkeys as a model for bioavailability/bioequivalence assessment in humans. Studies of both immediate-release and controlled-release formulations were reported. Relative to humans, dogs underestimated the bioavailability of controlled-release formulations compared to immediate-release formulations, except for a drug that is absorbed in the colon as well as the small intestine (phenylpropanolamine). It was suggested that administration of poorly soluble drugs or controlled-release formulations of drugs to dogs that have been pretreated with agents that increase gastric acidity or intestinal residence time may result in better correlation of dog and human bioavailability data. In some cases the dog was found useful for providing a preliminary assessment of the bioavailability of immediate-release dosage formulations, under a limited range of test conditions, prior to the conduct of definitive studies in humans. Pigs were not found to be very useful in reported studies because of slow stomach-emptying of drugs and high variability in drug absorption. These studies clearly demonstrated that the utility of an animal model must be verified by human studies of each drug and for each biopharmaceutical test condition.

Just as comparative metabolism and disposition studies are recognized to be of fundamental importance to the interpretation and rationalization of animal pharmacology and toxicology data and the extrapolation of these data to humans, it must be recognized that comparative pharmacokinetics and biopharmaceutical studies are of fundamental importance to the verification of an animal model in each biopharmaceutical test condition. Thus, considerable comparative information is needed before the predictive value of animal biopharmaceutical studies can be assessed. Based on available data, the anatomy and physiology of any one animal model simply does not appear to reflect that in humans closely enough to allow definitive oral bioequivalence decisions to be made with a high level of confidence. Consequently, definitive bioavailability/bioequivalence studies should be conducted in a limited number of closely monitored patients or normal volunteers to assure against exposure of patients to subtherapeutic or toxic levels of a drug.

REFERENCES

1. **Clark, B. and Smith, D. A.,** Pharmacokinetics and toxicity testing, *CRC Crit. Rev. Toxicol.,* 12, 343, 1984.
2. **Zbinden, G.,** Biopharmaceutical studies, a key to better toxicology, *Xenobiotica,* 18, 9, 1988.
3. **Adams, W. J.,** The metabolic background, in *Human Drug Evaluation,* O'Grady, J. and Linet, O. I., Eds., Macmillan Press, London, 1991, chap. 3.
4. **Peck, C. C., Barr, W. H., Benet, L. Z., Collins, J., Desjardins, R. E., Furst, D. E., Harter, J. G., Levy, G., Ludden, T., Rodman, J. H., Sanathanan, L., Schentag, J. J., Shah, V. P., Sheiner, L. B., Skelly, J. P., Stanski, D. R., Temple, R. J., Viswanathan, C. T., Weissinger, J., and Yacobi, A.,** Opportunities for integration of pharmacokinetics, pharmacodynamics, toxicokinetics in rational drug development, *Pharm. Res.,* 9, 826, 1992.
5. **Glocklin, V. C.,** General considerations for studies of the metabolism of drugs and other chemicals, *Drug Metab. Rev.,* 13, 929, 1982.
6. **Zbinden, G.,** Metabolic studies in chemical safety studies, in *Foreign Compound Metabolism,* Caldwell, J. and Paulson, G. D., Eds., Taylor & Francis, Philadelphia, 1984, 203.
7. **Smith, R. L.,** The role of metabolism and disposition studies in the safety assessment of pharmaceuticals, *Xenobiotica,* 18, 89, 1988.
8. **Stavchansky, S. A. and McGinity, J. W.,** Bioavailability in tablet technology, in *Pharmaceutical Dosage Forms,* Vol. 2, 2nd ed., Lieberman, H. A., Lachman, L., and Schwartz, J. B., Eds., Marcel Dekker, New York, 1990, chap. 6.
9. Food and Drug Administration, Bioequivalence requirements and *in vivo* bioavailability procedures, *Fed. Regist.,* 42, 1624, 1977.
10. Criteria for Waiver of Evidence of *in vivo* Bioavailability, 21 Code of Federal Regulations, 320.22.
11. Drug Price Competition and Patent Term Restoration Act of 1984, Public Law 98–417, 98 Stat. 1585, September 24, 1984.
12. **Dressman, J. B. and Yamada, K.,** Animal models for oral drug absorption, in *Pharmaceutical Bioequivalence,* Welling, P. G., Tse, F. L. S., and Dighe, S. V., Eds., Marcel Dekker, New York, 1991, chap. 9.
13. **Clemente, C. D.,** Ed., *Gray's Anatomy,* 30th Am. ed., Lea & Febiger, Philadelphia, 1985, chap. 16.
14. **Spence, A. P. and Mason, E. B.,** *Human Anatomy and Physiology,* 3rd ed., Benjamin/Cummings Publishing, Menlo Park, CA, 1987, chap. 23.

15. **Argenzio, R. A.,** Secretory functions of the gastrointestinal tract, in *Dukes' Physiology of Domestic Animals,* 10th ed., Swenson, M. J., Ed., Comstock Publishing (Cornell University Press), Ithaca, NY, 1984, chap. 17.
16. **Argenzio, R. A.,** Introduction to gastrointestinal function, in *Dukes' Physiology of Domestic Animals,* 10th ed., Swenson, M. J., Ed., Comstock Publishing (Cornell University Press), Ithaca, NY, 1984, chap. 15.
17. **Aoyagi, N.,** *Comparative Studies of Griseofulvin Bioavailability Among Man and Animals,* Kyoto University, Kyoto, Japan, 1986.
18. **Maeda, T., Takenaka, H., Yamahira, Y., and Noguchi, T.,** Use of rabbits for GI drug absorption studies, *J. Pharm. Sci.,* 66, 69, 1977.
19. **Maeda, T., Takenaka, H., Yamahira, Y., and Noguchi, T.,** Use of rabbits for GI drug absorption studies: relationship between dissolution rate and bioavailability of griseofulvin tablets, *J. Pharm. Sci.,* 68, 1286, 1979.
20. **Aoyagi, N., Ogata, H., Kaniwa, N., and Eima, A.,** Bioavailability of griseofulvin plain tablets in stomach-emptying controlled rabbits and the correlation with bioavailability in humans, *J. Pharm. Dyn.,* 7, 630, 1984.
21. **Venho, V. M. K. and Eriksson, H.,** The rabbit: an animal model for comparative bioavailability studies of drugs, *Int. J. Pharm.,* 30, 91, 1986.
22. **Chiou, W. L., Riegelman, S., and Amberg, J. R.,** Complications in using rabbits for the study of oral drug absorption, *Chem. Pharm. Bull.,* 17, 2173, 1969.
23. **Okerman, L.** (R. Sundahl, Transl.), *Diseases of Domestic Rabbits,* Blackwell Scientific, Oxford, 1988.
24. **Shively, M. J.,** *Veterinary Anatomy; Basic, Comparative, and Clinical,* Texas A&M University Press, College Station, TX, 1984.
25. **Allen, G.,** Specific cleavage of the protein, in *Laboratory Techniques in Biochemistry and Molecular Biology-Sequencing of Proteins and Peptides,* Vol. 9, 2nd ed., Burdon, R. H. and van Knippenberg, P. H., Elsevier, Amsterdam, 1989, chap. 3.
26. **Kutchai, H. C.,** Gastrointestinal secretions, in *Physiology,* 2nd ed., Berne, R. M. and Levy, M. N., Eds., C. V. Mosby, St. Louis, MO, 1988, 682.
27. **Lui, C. Y., Amidon, G. L., Berardi, R. R., Fleisher, D., Youngberg, C., and Dressman, J. B.,** Comparison of gastrointestinal pH in dogs and humans: implications on the use of the beagle dog as a model for oral absorption in humans, *J. Pharm. Sci.,* 75, 271, 1986.
28. **Youngberg, C. A., Wlodyga, J., Schmaltz, S., and Dressman, J. B.,** Radiotelemetric determination of gastrointestinal pH in four healthy beagles, *Am. J. Vet. Res.,* 46, 1516, 1985.
29. **Huber, W. G. and Wallin, R. F.,** Gastric secretion and ulcer formation in the pig, in *Swine in Biomedical Research,* Tumbleson, M. E., Ed., Plenum Press, New York, 1966, 21.
30. **Maner, J. H., Pond, W. G., Loosli, J. K., and Lowley, R. S.,** Effect of isolated soybean protein and casein on the gastric pH and rate of passage of food residues in baby pigs, *J. Anim. Sci.,* 21, 49, 1962.
31. **Altman, P. L.** (Comp.), Blood and other body fluids, *FASEB,* Washington, D.C., 1961.
32. **Pond, W. G. and Houpt, K. A.,** *Biology of the Pig,* Comstock Publishing (Cornell University Press), Ithaca, NY, 1978.
33. **Selen, A.,** Factors influencing bioavailability and bioequivalence, in *Pharmaceutical Bioequivalence,* Welling, P. G., Tse, F. L. S., and Dighe, S. V., Eds., Marcel Dekker, New York, 1991, chap. 5.
34. **Lapin, B. A. and Cherkovich, G. M.,** Biological normals — GI juice and motility, in *Pathology of Simian Primates, Part I,* Fiennes, R. N., Ed., S. Karger, Basel, 1972, 127.
35. **Wilson, T. H.,** *Intestinal Absorption,* W. B. Saunders, Philadelphia, 1962.

36. **Dressman, J.,** Comparison of canine and human gastrointestinal physiology, *Pharm. Res.,* 3, 123, 1986.
37. **Kagnoff, M. F.,** Immunology of the digestive system, in *Physiology of the Gastrointestinal Tract,* Johnson, L. R., Ed., Raven Press, New York, 1981, 1699.
38. **Walker, W. A., Wu, M., and Bloch, K. J.,** Stimulation by immune complex of mucus release from goblet cells of the rat small intestine, *Science,* 197, 370, 1977.
39. **Fubara, E. S. and Freter, R.,** Protection against enteric bacterial infection by secretory IgA antibodies, *J. Immunol.,* 111, 395, 1973.
40. **Anderson, N. V.,** *Veterinary Gastroenterology,* Lea & Febiger, Philadelphia, 1980, 247.
41. **Argenzio, R. A. and Southworth, M.,** Sites of organic acid production and absorption in gastrointestinal tract of the pig, *Am. J. Physiol.,* 228, 454, 1975.
42. **Clemens, E. T., Stevens, C. E., and Southworth, M.,** Sites of organic acid production and pattern of digesta movement in the gastrointestinal tract of swine, *J. Nutr.,* 105, 759, 1975.
43. **Itoh, Z. and Sekiguchi, T.,** Interdigestive motor activity in health and disease, *Scand. J. Gastroenterol.,* Suppl. 82, 121, 1983.
44. **Phillips, S. F. and Devroede, G. J.,** Functions of the large intestine, in *International Review of Physiology,* Vol. 19, *Gastrointestinal Physiology III,* Crane, R. K., Ed., University Park Press, Baltimore, 1979, 236.
45. **Caballeria, J., Baraona, E., Rodamilans, M., and Lieber, C. S.,** Effects of cimetidine on gastric alcohol dehydrogenase and blood alcohol levels, *Gastroenterology,* 96, 388, 1989.
46. **Mearrik, P. T., Wade, D. N., Birkett, D. J., and Morris, J.,** Metoclopramide, gastric emptying and L-dopa absorption, *Aust. N.Z. J. Med.,* 4, 144, 1974.
47. **Sandler, M., Ruthven, R. J., Goodwin, B. L., Hunter, K. R., and Stern, G. M.,** Variation of levodopa metabolism with gastrointestinal absorption site, *Lancet,* 1, 238, 1974.
48. **Glazko, A. J., Dill, W. A., Kazenko, L. M., Wolf, L. M., and Carnes, H. E.,** Physical factors affecting the rate of absorption of chloramphenicol esters, *Antibiot. Chemother.,* 8, 517, 1958.
49. **Pestalozzi, D. M., Buhler, R., von Wartburg, J. P., and Hess, M.,** Immunohistochemical localization of alcohol dehydrogenase in the human gastrointestinal tract, *Gastroenterology,* 85, 1011, 1983.
50. **Hartiala, K.,** Metabolism of hormones, drugs and other substances by the gut, *Physiol. Rev.,* 53, 496, 1973.
51. **Boström, H., Brömster, D., Nordenstam, H., and Wengle, B.,** The occurrence of phenol and steroid sulphokinases in the human gastrointestinal tract, *Scand. J. Gastroenterol.,* 3, 369, 1968.
52. **Traber, P. G., Chianale, J., Florence, R., Kim, K., Wojcik, E., and Gumucio, J. J.,** Expression of cytochrome P450b and P450e genes in small intestine mucosa of rats following treatment with phenobarbital, polyhalogenated biphenyls, and organochlorine pesticides, *J. Biol. Chem.,* 263, 9449, 1988.
53. **Russel, R. I., MacAllister, R., and Campbell, R.,** Relationship of β-gluronidase activity in gastric juice to the histology of the gastric mucosa, *Gastroenterology,* 58, 352, 1970.
54. **Ilett, K. F., Tee, L. B. G., Reeves, P. T., and Minchin, R. F.,** Metabolism of drugs and other xenobiotics in the gut lumen and wall, *Pharmacol. Ther.,* 46, 67, 1990.
55. **Hartiala, K.,** Metabolism of foreign compounds in the gastrointestinal tract, in *Handbook of Physiology,* American Physiology Society, 1977, sect. 9, 375.
56. **Caldwell, J.,** The metabolism of drugs by the gastrointestinal tract, in *Pre-systemic Drug Elimination,* George, C. F., Ed., Butterworths, London, 1981, chap. 2.
57. **Hänninen, O.,** Mucosal biotransformation of toxins in the gut, in Receptors and Other Targets for Toxic Substances, *Arch. Toxicol.,* Suppl. 8, 83, 1985.

58. **Barr, W. H.,** The Role of intestinal metabolism in bioavailability, in *Pharmaceutical Bioequivalence,* Welling, P. G., Tse, F. L. S., and Dighe, S. V., Eds., Marcel Dekker, New York, 1991, chap. 6.
59. **Shirkey, R. S., Chakraborty, J., and Bridges, J. W.,** Comparison of drug metabolizing ability of rat intestinal mucosal microsomes with that of liver, *Biochem. Pharmacol.,* 28, 2835, 1979.
60. **Barr, W. H., Aceto, T., Chung, M., and Shukur, M.,** Dose dependent drug metabolism during the absorptive phase, *Rev. Can. Biol.,* Suppl. 32, 31, 1973.
61. **Sietsema, W. K.,** The absolute oral bioavailability of selected drugs, *Int. J. Clin. Pharmacol. Ther. Toxicol.,* 27, 179, 1989.
62. **Donaldson, R. M.,** Normal bacterial populations of the intestine and their relation to intestinal function, *N. Engl. J. Med.,* 270, 938, 1967.
63. **Dreyfus, J., Shaw, J. M., and Ross, J. J.,** Absorption of the β-adrenergic-blocking agent, nadolol, by mice, rats, hamsters, rabbits, dogs, monkeys, and man: an unusual species difference, *Xenobiotica,* 8, 503, 1979.
64. **de Miranda, P., Krasny, H. C., Page, D. A., and Elion, G. B.,** The disposition of acyclovir in different species, *J. Pharm. Exp. Ther.,* 219, 309, 1981.
65. **Kwan, K. C.,** Merck & Co., presented at the PMA/FDA Workshop on the Use of Animals as Substitutes for Humans in Oral Bioavailability Studies, Washington, D.C., June 28–29, 1989.
66. **Adams, W. J.,** The Upjohn Co., presented at the PMA/FDA Workshop on the Use of Animals as Substitutes for Humans in Oral Bioavailability Studies, Washington, D.C., June 28–29, 1989.
67. PMA/FDA Workshop on the Use of Animals as Substitutes for Humans in Oral Bioavailability Studies, Washington, D.C., June 28–29, 1989.
68. **Crouthamel, W. and Bekersky, I.,** Preclinical evaluation of new drug candidates and drug delivery systems in the dog, in *Animal Models for Oral Drug Delivery in Man,* Crouthamel, W. and Sarapu, A. C., Eds., American Pharmaceutical Association Academy of Pharmaceutical Sciences, Washington, D.C., 1983, chap. 3.
69. **Smyth, R. D., Dandekar, K. A., Lee, F. H., DeLong, A. F., and Polk, A.,** Use of the dog in bioavailability and bioequivalence testing, in *Animal Models for Oral Drug Delivery in Man,* Crouthamel, W. and Sarapu, A. C., Eds., American Pharmaceutical Association Academy of Pharmaceutical Sciences, Washington, D.C., 1983, chap. 4.
70. **Sarapu, A. C. and Bibart, C. H.,** Drug product formulation and manufacturing process studies utilizing the beagle dog as a model for *in vivo* drug release, in *Animal Models for Oral Drug Delivery in Man,* Crouthamel, W. and Sarapu, A. C., Eds., American Pharmaceutical Association Academy of Pharmaceutical Sciences, Washington, D.C., 1983, chap. 5.
71. **Kaniwa, N., Ogata, H., Aoyagi, N., Shibazaki, T., Ejima, A., Watanabe, Y., Motohashi, K., Sasahara, K., Nakajima, E., Morioka, T., and Nitanai, T.,** The bioavailability of flufenamic acid and its dissolution rate from capsules, *Int. J. Clin. Pharmacol. Ther. Toxicol.,* 21, 56, 1983.
72. **Ogata, H., Aoyagi, N., Kaniwa, N., Shibazaki, T., Ejima, A., Takasugi, N., Mafune, E., Hayashi, T., and Suwa, K.,** Bioavailability of nalidixic acid from uncoated tablets in humans. I. Correlation with dissolution rates of the tablets, *Int. J. Clin. Pharmacol. Ther. Toxicol.,* 22, 175, 1984.
73. **Ogata, H., Aoyagi, N., Kaniwa, N., Shibazaki, T., Ejima, A., Takasugi, N., Mafune, E., Hayashi, T., and Suwa, K.,** Bioavailability of nalidixic acid from uncoated tablets in humans. II. Bioavailability in beagles and its correlation with bioavailability in humans and *in vitro* dissolution rates, *Int. J. Clin. Pharmacol. Ther. Toxicol.,* 22, 240, 1984.

74. **Aoyagi, N., Ogata, H., Kaniwa, N., and Ejima, A.,** Bioavailability of indomethacin capsules in humans. I. Bioavailability and effects of gastric acidity, *Int. J. Clin. Pharmacol. Ther. Toxicol.,* 23, 469, 1985.
75. **Aoyagi, N., Ogata, H., Kaniwa, N., Ejima, A., Nakata, H., Tsutsumi, J., and Fujita, T.,** Bioavailability of indomethacin capsules in humans. III. Correlation with bioavailability in beagle dogs, *Int. J. Clin. Pharmacol. Ther. Toxicol.,* 23, 578, 1985.
76. **Shore, P. A., Brodie, B. B., and Hogben, C. A. M.,** The gastric secretion of drugs: a pH partition hypothesis, *J. Pharmacol. Exp. Ther.,* 119, 361, 1957.
77. **Kimura, Y., Goto, N., Yoshimura, N., Kitazawa, H., Sugiyama, M., Okamura, K., and Satake, K.,** *Yakuzaigaku,* 48, 313, 1988.
78. **Sagara, K., Nagamatsu, Y., Yamada, I., Kawada, M., Mizuta, H., and Ogawa, K.,** Bioavailability study of commercial sustained-release preparations of diclofenac sodium in gastrointestinal physiology regulated-dogs, *Chem. Pharm. Bull.,* 40, 3303, 1992.
79. **Ogata, H., Aoyagi, N., Kaniwa, N., Ejima, A., Sekine, N., Kitamura, M., and Inoue, Y.,** Gastric acidity dependent bioavailability of cinnarizine from two commercial capsules in healthy volunteers, *Int. J. Pharm.,* 29, 113, 1986.
80. **Ogata, H., Aoyagi, N., Kaniwa, N., Ejima, A., Kitaura, T., Ohki, T., and Kitamura, M.,** Evaluation of beagle dogs as an animal model for bioavailability testing of cinnarizine capsules, *Int. J. Pharm.,* 29, 121, 1986.
81. **Ogata, H., Aoyagi, N., Kaniwa, N., Koibuchi, M., Shibazaki, T., Ejima, A., Tsuji, T., and Kawazu, Y.,** The bioavailability of diazepam from uncoated tablets in humans. I. Correlation with the dissolution rates of the tablets, *Int. J. Clin. Pharmacol. Ther. Toxicol.,* 20, 159, 1982.
82. **Ogata, H., Aoyagi, N., Kaniwa, N., Koibuchi, M., Shibazaki, T., and Ejima, A.,** The bioavailability of diazepam from uncoated tablets in humans. II. Effect of gastric fluid acidity, *Int. J. Clin. Pharmacol. Ther. Toxicol.,* 20, 166, 1982.
83. **Ogata, H., Aoyagi, N., Kaniwa, N., Koibuchi, M., Shibazaki, T., Ejima, A., Shimamoto, T., Yashiki, T., Ogawa, Y., Uda, Y., and Nishida, Y.,** Correlation of the bioavailability of diazepam from tablets in beagle dogs with its dissolution rate and bioavailability in humans, *Int. J. Clin. Pharmacol. Ther. Toxicol.,* 20, 576, 1982.
84. **Kaniwa, N., Ogata, H., Aoyagi, N., Ejima, A., Takahashi, T., Uezono, Y., and Imazato, Y.,** Effect of food on the bioavailability of cyclandelate from commercial capsules, *Clin. Pharmacol. Ther.,* 33, 641, 1991.
85. **Kaniwa, N., Ogata, H., Aoyagi, N., Ejima, A., Takahashi, T., Uezono, Y., and Imazato, Y.,** Bioavailability of cyclandelate from capsules in beagle dogs and dissolution rate: correlations with bioavailability in humans, *J. Pharmacobio.-Dyn.,* 14, 152, 1991.
86. **Aoyagi, N., Ogata, H., Kaniwa, N., Koibuchi, M., Shibazaki, T., and Ejima, A.,** Bioavailability of griseofulvin from tablets in humans and the correlation with its dissolution rate, *J. Pharm. Sci.,* 71, 1165, 1982.
87. **Aoyagi, N., Ogata, H., Kaniwa, N., Koibuchi, M., Shibazaki, T., Ejima, A., Tamaki, N., Kamimura, H., Katougi, Y., and Omi, Y.,** Bioavailability of griseofulvin from tablets in beagle dogs and correlation with dissolution rate and bioavailability in humans, *J. Pharm. Sci.,* 71, 1169, 1982.
88. **Aoyagi, N., Ogata, H., Kaniwa, N., Koibuchi, M., Ejima, A., Yasuda, Y., and Tanioka, Y.,** Bioavailability of griseofulvin from plain tablets in Göttingen minipigs and the correlation with bioavailability in humans, *J. Pharm. Dyn.,* 7, 7, 1984.
89. **Kaniwa, N., Ogata, H., Aoyagi, N., Koibuchi, M., Shibazaki, T., Ejima, A., Takanashi, S., Kamiyama, H., Suzuki, H., Hinohara, Y., Nakano, H., Okazaki, A., Fujikura, T., Igusa, K., and Bessho, S.,** Bioavailability of pyridoxal phosphate from enteric-coated tablets. I. Apparent critical dissolution pH and bioavailability of commercial products in humans, *Chem. Pharm. Bull.,* 33, 4045, 1985.

90. **Kaniwa, N., Ogata, H., Aoyagi, N., Koibuchi, M., Shibazaki, T., Ejima, A., Takanashi, S., Kamiyama, H., Suzuki, H., Hinohara, Y., Nakano, H., Okazaki, A., Fujikura, T., Igusa, K., and Bessho, S.,** Bioavailability of pyridoxal phosphate from enteric-coated tablets. III. Correlations between bioavailability in humans and beagle dogs and between bioavailability in humans and *in vitro* dissolution rates, *Chem. Pharm. Bull.,* 33, 3906, 1985.
91. **Ogata, H., Aoyagi, N., Kaniwa, N., Shibazaki, T., Ejima, A., Takasugi, N., Ogura, T., Tomita, K., Inoue, S., and Zaizen, M.,** Bioavailability of metronidazole from sugar-coated tablets in humans. I. Effect of gastric acidity and correlation with *in vitro* dissolution rate, *Int. J. Pharm.,* 23, 277, 1985.
92. **Ogata, H., Aoyagi, N., Kaniwa, N., Shibazaki, T., Ejima, A., Takasugi, N., Ogura, T., Tomita, K., Inoue, S., and Zaizen, M.,** Bioavailability of metronidazole from sugar-coated tablets in humans. II. Evaluation of beagle dogs as an animal model, *Int. J. Pharm.,* 23, 289, 1985.
93. **Cressman, W. A. and Sumner, D.,** The dog as a quantitative model for evaluation of nondisintegrating sustained-release tablets, *J. Pharm. Sci.,* 60, 132, 1971.
94. **Bialer, M., Friedman, M., and Dubrovsky, J.,** Effect of sustained release on the pharmacokinetics of valproic acid in the dog, *Int. J. Pharm.,* 20, 53, 1984.
95. **Bialer, M., Friedman, M., and Dubrovsky, J.,** Comparative pharmacokinetic analysis of a novel sustained release dosage form of valproic acid in dogs, *Biopharm. Drug Dispos.,* 5, 1, 1984.
96. **Bialer, M., Friedman, M., and Dubrovsky, J.,** Pharmacokinetic evaluation of novel sustained-release dosage forms of valproic acid in humans, *Biopharm. Drug Dispos.,* 6, 401, 1985.
97. **Leeds, N. H., Gal, P., Purohit, A. A., and Walter, J. B.,** Effect of food on the bioavailability and pattern of release of a sustained-release theophylline tablet, *J. Clin. Pharmacol.,* 22, 196, 1982.
98. **Weinberger, M.,** Theophylline QID, TID, BID and now QD?, *Pharmacotherapy,* 4, 181, 1984.
99. **Hendeles, L., Weinberger, M., Milavetz, G., Hill, M., III, and Vaughn, L.,** Food-induced "dose-dumping" from a once-a-day theophylline product as a cause of theophylline toxicity, *Chest,* 87, 758, 1985.
100. **Karim, A., Burns, T., Wearly, L., Streicher, J., and Palmer, M.,** Food-induced changes in theophylline absorption from controlled-release formulations. I. Substantial increased and decreased absorption with Uniphyl tablets and Theo-Dur Sprinkle, *Clin. Pharmacol. Ther.,* 38, 77, 1985.
101. **Karim, A., Burns, T., Janky, D., and Hurwitz, A.,** Food-induced changes in theophylline absorption from controlled-release formulations. II. Importance of meal composition and dosing time relative to meal intake in assessing changes in absorption, *Clin. Pharmacol. Ther.,* 38, 642, 1985.
102. **Shiu, G. K., Sager, A. O., Velagapudi, R. B., Prasad, V. K., and Skelly, J. P.,** The effect of food on the absorption of controlled-release theophylline in mini-swine, *Pharm. Res.,* 5, 48, 1988.
103. **Shiu, G. K., LeMarchand, A., Sager, A. O., Velagapudi, R. B., and Skelly, J. P.,** The beagle dog as an animal model for a bioavailability study of controlled-release theophylline under the influence of food, *Pharm. Res.,* 6, 1039, 1989.
104. **Van Wyk, M., Dormehl, I. C., Sommers, D. K., and Maree, M.,** *Med. Sci. Res.,* 16, 575, 1988.
105. **Tsunoo, M., Yoshimura, K., Maruyama, Y., Takahashi, M., Oikawa, T., Iwasa, A., Nishimura, T., Inoue, M., Kokita, T., and Numata, H.,** Basic and clinical studies on sustained release preparation of diclofenac sodium. Pharmacokinetics of diclofenac and its metabolites by single administration and consecutive administration of sustained release capsules of diclofenac sodium (SR-318), *Prog. Med.,* 9 (Suppl.) 2, 877, 1989.

Commentary I

Issues in Bioequivalence: An Industrial Scientist's Perspective

Prem K. Narang

CONTENTS

I. INTRODUCTION

Under the Drug Price Competition and Patent Term Restoration Act of 1984, the Food and Drug Administration (FDA) is authorized to approve generic copies of pioneer drug products. Before the passage of the law, manufacturers of generic versions of pioneer drugs approved after 1962 had to submit clinical studies to demonstrate the safety and effectiveness of their products. The 1984 law permits the FDA to approve a generic drug without clinical evidence if the drug is shown to be "bioequivalent" to the innovator's product.

Bioequivalence (BE) testing is based on the assumption that the circulating systemic drug level is predictive of drug clinical effect. Thus, if two different preparations of the same active ingredient produce similar drug concentrations in blood, it is assumed that the two preparations will be therapeutically equivalent and thus interchangeable. The typical crossover design of an *in vivo* BE study is not always satisfactory for the approval of new formulations/generic copies. As every drug has individual physicochemical, biopharmaceutical, and kinetic profiles, to ensure that a new formulation may be interchanged with an already marketed formulation, a number of basic issues pertaining to active drug moieties need to be addressed prior to developing designs for an *in vivo* BE study. Before a study is planned/designed, these issues that this book addresses must be considered for meeting the primary objective and/or gaining additional scientific knowledge to make concise BE decisions.

II. ANALYTICAL ASPECTS

The primary purpose of the analytical method is to provide a best possible unbiased estimate of the analyte concentration in the biological matrix. Before one has to deal with the missing or spurious data from a study, it is imperative that the bioanalytical method development and validation be robust, with performance characteristics that match its

0-8493-6930-4/94/$0.00+$.50

intended use. One of the most crucial facets of bioanalytics in BE testing is establishing *interday precision estimates* and documenting sufficient stability information to support the study sample collection, shipment, and handling. Extensive use of quality controls (QCs) is highly recommended. Criteria for data acceptance, rejection, and reassay must be defined *a priori;* and standard *GLP* (good laboratory practice) should be strictly implemented, followed, and enforced. There is minimal debate on general principles governing this issue and what impact they may have on kinetics and PK/PD correlations. From an industrial perspective, the apparent precision one is able to achieve depends not only on good analytical technique but also on the range of concentration being measured, e.g., microgram (μg) or picogram (pg) per milliliter (ml). Realistically, for methodologies where one is near the limit of quantitation, regulatory prudence requires that not only the degree of difficulty of the assay, analyte stability, and interferences from endogenous compounds, metabolites, and degradation products be taken into consideration, but also reasonable accommodation should be made in light of the drug pharmacology. Drugs exhibiting a wide therapeutic window should pose less of a concern than those with narrow indices.

III. *IN VITRO* AND *IN VIVO* CORRELATIONS

Application of *in vitro* dissolution data as a surrogate measure of BE occurs both during pre- and post-NDA approval. Sometimes these dissolution profiles may be the only measures of performance available during development that link *in vivo* bioequivalence (BE) between the test formulation (new or those tested in Phase III studies) and the production batches. *In vivo* BE studies postapproval are required if there is a change in the manufacturing site for a controlled-release formulation or a major change in the composition of the drug product. For other minor changes in process, *in vitro* dissolution in most physiologically representative fluids/methodology is regarded sufficient for documenting BE. Even with suitable dissolution methodology and profiles, a question remains about its ability to predict *in vivo* performance. Suffice it to say, there is considerable debate and controversy on this issue.[3]

Dissolution testing is useful in the early product development and for quality assurance of the processes and product batches postmarketing. *In vitro/in vivo* correlations should be explored over a specified range of variables using dissolution rate or fraction released vs. absorption rate profile as assessed by deconvolution or statistical moment theory. It has been proposed that depending on the level of correlation found, guidelines can be established when an *in vivo* assessment would be required.[4] Literature is replete with examples of attempts at establishing predictive *in vitro/in vivo* correlations; however, most of these have been less than successful/fruitful. Continuously changing environment of the GI tract with respect to enzyme activity, pH, motility, gastric emptying, and presence of varying amounts of endogenous and exogenous substances influence dissolution from a formulation which is difficult to duplicate *in vitro*. How these factors influence availability of drug *in vivo* depends not only on the physiology, but also on the drug, dosage form, dose, and target patient characteristics. Drug-drug interactions, food and age effects, and underlying disease in the target population can also have an unpredictable effect on the rate and extent of absorption. Given the past success, *in vitro/in vivo* correlations cannot be recommended as surrogates for BE testing in man. I believe that, like any other model which has not been tested or validated over another experimental frame, good correlation does not always guarantee predictability or a similar outcome with another batch or another formulation of the same drug. Model robustness must be treated as a critical issue. Therefore, these explorations can only be considered interesting research exercises.

IV. SINGLE VS. MULTIPLE DOSE

When single-dose studies suffice for demonstrating BE and when multiple-dose studies are warranted are very important design issues. To some extent, these issues are primarily governed by drug kinetics and extent of variability. When intrasubject variance is smaller than the intersubject variance and the drug exhibits linear kinetics (good predictability of steady state from single doses), crossover designs where each subject serves as his/her own control result in a more powerful study to discriminate formulation differences. In such situations, data from single or multiple doses are equally adequate, and single-dose studies should suffice. However, to demonstrate BE for highly variable drugs displaying large first-pass metabolism and saturable/nonlinear kinetics in the therapeutic range and >30 to 40% intrasubject variability measured by the residual coefficient of variation, preference of data following multiple doses is certainly justified. Although more appealing, the requirement for multiple-dose studies with such drugs is primarily to detect input rate differences. Drugs for which the rate of absorption is important (e.g., analgesics, hypnotics, and anesthetics) or those in whom the absorption rate has been modified or controlled relative to the conventional immediate-release dosage form, multiple-dose studies are warranted. However, when there is no direct relationship of response with the drug input rate and prolonged dosing is necessary before an effect is elicited, cost-benefit justification for multiple-dose studies should be assessed on a case-by-case basis.

V. ACTIVE METABOLITES/CHIRALITY

An issue that has gained prominence in the last few years is the role of active metabolites and stereoisomers. Inability to measure the parent drug or its highly variable dispositional characteristics, and/or a firm establishment of the activity of its metabolite strongly advocates the use of metabolite data in BE assessment. Both the area under the plasma metabolite concentration vs. time curve and the metabolite mean residence time are reasonable estimators of the rate and the extent of absorption. This is especially true for drugs with low renal clearance compared to total clearance. Metabolite mean residence times may, in fact, be more sensitive to changes in the first-pass metabolism. One of the caveats in relying on the metabolite data is a lack of knowledge on the dispositional properties of the metabolite which may be required for unambiguous interpretation. The availability of even this information does not guarantee a successful outcome. It is interesting to keep in perspective that what we may refer to as the major metabolite may often not be, unless significant up-front metabolite isolation and identification work has been completed in man to identify this major metabolite. Quantitation of the measurable metabolite does not preclude the possibility that nonquantifiable metabolites do not possess higher affinity for the receptors that elicit the response of interest. Therefore, extensively metabolized drugs require that a more cautious approach be taken in selecting what metabolite to use in BE assessment. From a regulatory perspective, it seems reasonable that the confidence limits for the metabolite data, for demonstrating BE, should be somewhat relaxed compared to those for the parent drug analysis.

The impact of stereoisomeric composition of some widely prescribed drugs possessing an asymmetric carbon (chiral) center has recently been realized, not only in development but also in regulation and therapeutics. The surfacing of this issue has been spurred on by the realization that the pharmacodynamics (toxicity, efficacy) of the individual enantiomers often differ due to their unique pharmacological disposition, e.g., absorption, distribution, metabolism, and excretion.[1] It is well known that the (–) enantiomer of pentobarbital is more sedating while the (+) enantiomer is a central nervous system stimulant,[2] and that the primary metabolic route for the S(–)-enantiomer of warfarin is oxidation to form 7-hydroxywarfarin, while it is only a minor metabolic path for the R(+)

form. The availability of various chiral stationary phases and possibility for enantioselective separation (not always easy and robust due to column characteristics) has further fueled the debate as to what should be quantitated during BE testing. On the surface, it seems rational to apply stereospecific methodologies to quantitate not only the two antipodes but also their active metabolites. However, these approaches have a tendency to add substantially to the cost, and appear unjustified when dosing decisions are strictly based on the dose of the drug rather than systemic concentrations of the drug and/or its active metabolite. Further complications can arise for drugs with prochiral centers, e.g., phenytoin, which form chiral metabolites.

Before reasonable solutions to the role of stereoselectivity and active metabolites can be found, one must resist putting the cart in front of the horse. The relative impact of metabolite potency relative to the parent, the validity of the model used to assess activity and especially its capability to forecast human response, the fraction of the dose converted to metabolite, and the relative contribution of the parent and metabolite to pharmacological response must be reasonably well delineated before taking the arduous task of quantitating all that is feasible. A thorough understanding of the systemic clearance of the active epimer is extremely crucial in establishing adequate study designs, however. It may be of assistance if concentration-response relationships have been previously established.

VI. PHARMACODYNAMICS

BE between two formulations is demonstrated by a similarity in kinetic profiles of the active ingredient or therapeutic moieties, especially in the rate and extent of absorption. Similar plasma concentrations are then assumed to elicit similar pharmacological response. Although ultimate proof of the efficacy of a drug (formulation) resides in a controlled, randomized trial, such trials are not needed for demonstrating BE. However, the role of pharmacodynamics in BE is a rapidly evolving arena. Measurement and application of dynamic concepts is probably the most acceptable way to obtain indirect evidence of the systemic availability of a test formulation, when specific chemical or sometimes less specific bioassays are not available. Such approaches are gaining popularity for drugs used orally or topically that are not systemically absorbed. A major criticism of the application of the dynamic concepts is a lack of belief or data supporting a relationship between the dynamic end point (surrogate marker) and the true therapeutic effect, e.g., survival or response rate. This is especially true if the relationship with surrogate end point is weak. Implementation of these concepts in a reasonable number of patients from the target population showing altered responses due to underlying disease, compared to volunteers, can require extensive standardization of the population selection criteria. The confounding role of concomitant medications on our ability to estimate formulation differences in a clinical setting makes this approach less robust. Therefore, dynamic end points should be used only when no other alternatives exist for demonstrating equivalence. However, dynamic measures can assist in establishing drug concentration based standards, e.g., estimates of EC_{50}, E_{max}, etc. Several modeling approaches are covered in this book. Because modeling is a subjective art, this author's contention is that some specific guidelines be set for acceptance and rejection of what one would consider a validated, predictive model — especially predictive.

VII. POSSIBLE ROLE OF ANIMAL MODELS

The role of animals in understanding toxicology during new drug development has been invaluable. It is unclear as to what impact these assessments have had in determining or predicting "human risk". Several discussions recently have indicated that without successful demonstration of a similarity between the animal species and man, extrapolations from them may be meaningless. However, when it comes to assessing BE, it seems prudent to consider animal testing. If our primary goal is to assess differences between two formulations, it is not necessary that all human *in vivo* conditions (e.g., the GI tract, hepatic metabolism) be mimicked. Use of animals in some sense could be considered a similar extension of *in vitro* dissolution to *in vivo* performance. As long as the dispositional characteristics of the drug have been delineated in the animal species of choice and man, and the doses to be tested are in the apparent linear dispositional range, a demonstration of species similarity between the animal and man should not be a question/or warranted. Therefore, animal models could serve as an adequate surrogate (alternative) to support dissolution data and to establish BE. Several studies assessing BE using animal models have been performed but have only achieved mixed results. However, for drugs known to possess carcinogenic or serious toxicity potential in healthy volunteers, e.g., oncologics, the use of animals for BE should be promoted. At least on a scientific basis it seems rational, that if animal models can be used in screening of various formulations during the product development phase, why their use is not more prevalent/acceptable for assessing BE.

VIII. STATISTICAL CONSIDERATIONS

Based on the initial FDA criteria,[5] bioequivalency could be claimed when the null hypothesis of similarity of means for the rate and extent of absorption (typically C_{max} and AUC) could not be rejected at a 95% significance level employing a sufficient sample size to detect a 20% difference. This ±20% limit is arbitrary and subjective. The initial 1977 regulations contained no criteria concerning variability, and were expanded by the introduction of the so-called 75/75 rule which required the bioavailability (BA) estimator or the test to be within 75% of the reference formulation in at least 75% of the sample subjects. This rule fell out of favor and was abandoned because of heavy criticism of its poor statistical properties. The null hypothesis-power rule approach allows the use of a minimum sample size that would produce 80% power; a larger sample, however, increased the risk of detecting an unimportant difference. The negative aspects of this approach have been overcome by the two one-sided *t*-test procedure developed by Schuirmann.[7] This is currently the standard test for BE. It is apparent that when variability in the rate and extent measures is small, sample sizes for BE studies are reasonable; however, as the coefficients of variation in each subject bioavailability parameter estimator increases, the sample sizes become prohibitive.

Although not discussed here in depth, there are several other issues that pertain to the analysis of BE data. Logarithmic transformation of the C_{max} and AUC data, to achieve homoscedasticity in within-treatment variances seems well justified. The identification, use (or misuse), and removal of outliers is very critical in BE assessment. Unless there is an experimental reason for removing an outlier, or if objective statistical tests mandate its removal, no datum should be considered an outlier. Either way, I believe that data with and without inclusion of this outlier(s) should be presented. Sequence and period effects are sometimes detected in analysis of variance (ANOVA) of standard, two treatment-two period designs. Although statistical significance may be reached, these effects alone should not invalidate the BE study. Investigation of the sequence/period effects should be pursued in order to learn as much as possible about the dosage form, drug, physiological system, or their interactions.

A. VARIABILITY: INTRA- AND INTERSUBJECT

The problem with accepting ±20% difference in average extent of absorption of the two formulations is the inability of this estimate to accommodate intra- and intersubject variability. BE determinations are based on means and do not adequately characterize different types of variation that can occur both within a given individual as well as among different individuals. For example, a subject may handle a single formulation differently at different times (intrasubject variability). In addition, the way in which a formulation is handled by one subject is not necessarily predictive of how a different subject will respond to that same formulation (intersubject variability). This becomes especially important for drugs with "narrow therapeutic indices", where there is heightened sensitivity in clinicians who believe that special precautions need to be taken as relatively small changes in systemic concentrations can lead to marked changes in response (efficacy/toxicity).

It is important to remember that the decision making for establishing BE criteria should not be simply based on the concept of narrow or broad therapeutic indices, but on an understanding of intrapatient variability, e.g., variation in subjects taking the same dosage form on repeated administrations. Estimates of intrasubject variability ought to be required information for all approved dosage forms: both for innovator and generic products. The magnitude of this variability for a particular dosage form must be considered in light of the kinetic-dynamic relationship of drug concentration to response before decisions regarding BE criteria can be devised and established.

IX. CONCLUSIONS

In conclusion, Benet[8] has recently proposed some of the following interesting alternatives for refining the current BE guidelines, specifically for drugs with narrow therapeutic indices. The principle, though scientifically sound, has yet to be tested. Only application and the robustness of this methodology in addressing some of the concerns mentioned above will attest to its merits.

1. Innovator manufactures should be required to provide both inter- and intrasubject variability measures of extent and rate of availability for each marketed dosage form, and this should be included in the pharmacokinetic section of the package insert.
2. BE studies for new products (comparison of proposed marketed formulation with the formulation used in Phase III studies or for the approval of a generic equivalent product) should always be conducted utilizing a replicate design. That is, as a minimum, each subject would receive each dosage form at least twice. Comparisons of intrasubject variability should be included in the BE acceptance criteria.
3. Finally, Bayesian statistical approaches should be developed for use to evaluate formulation changes for approved products. Our present requirement of a full bioequivalency study for each significant manufacturing change encourages bad science and bad drug development.

The present BE requirements seem unrealistic at times, and prevent improvements in previously approved substandard formulations. Benet[8] has argued for defining a new set of BA/BE criteria by defining explicitly what we need to know, rather than what may be useful. This distinction holds primarily for measures of bioavailability. An estimate of the measure of bioavailability is only needed when alternate dosage forms of the drug are marketed, and when one attempts to maintain systemic concentrations by adjusting the dose based on differences in bioavailability from commercially available dosage forms.

Finally, the process of drug development has traditionally focused on the safety and efficacy of the new drug per regulatory directives. Drug development/approvals are based on achieving statistical significance for one of the primary efficacy variables by testing population locators, e.g., means or medians, between the treatment and the placebo (or active control) arms of a randomized study. Postapproval, however, physicians intend to dose patients on an individual basis, but use a fixed (approved) dose. In order to be competitive, the industry has often sacrificed an understanding of the basic clinical pharmacology: an assessment of dose (concentration) response for some time. A lack of understanding and integration of kinetic principles in early development has led to dosing paradigms that employ fixed doses, and dose modifications based only on purported dose-effect relationships. In such a competitive scenario, adequate resources are needed to support kinetic/dynamic programs that isolate the important issues discussed above, so as to develop adequate designs for the conduct of BE studies pre- or post-NDA approval.

The challenge to those involved with the process of drug development and regulation is to find scientifically sound alternatives that incorporate an understanding of basic science, and allow for an enhancement in scientific efficiency without sacrificing the commercial competitiveness needed for business, and certainly without compromising the patient care.

The commentary presented above reflects the author's personal perspective, and in no way reflects the views/beliefs or opinions that may be held by Adria Laboratories.

REFERENCES

1. **Wainer, I. W. and Drayer, D. E., Eds.,** *Drug Stereochemistry, Analytical Methods and Pharmacology,* Marcel Dekker, New York, 1988.
2. **Drayer, D. E.,** Pharmacokinetic and pharmacodynamic differences between drug enantiomers in humans: an overview, *Clin. Pharmacol. Ther.,* 40, 125, 1986.
3. PMA Comments on USP Stimuli to the Revision Process, *In vitro/in vivo* correlation from extended release oral dosage forms, December 1988.
4. **Leeson, L. J.,** *In vitro-in vivo* correlations for oral extended release dosage forms, Int'l Open Conference on Dissolution, Bioavailability and Bioequivalence, 1992.
5. *Federal Register,* 42, 1648, 1977.
6. *Federal Register,* 43, 6965, 1978.
7. **Schuirmann, D. J.,** A comparison of the two one-sided tests procedure and the power approach for assessing the equivalence of average bioavailability, *J. Pharmacokinet. Biopharm.,* 15, 657, 1987.
8. **Benet, L. Z.,** Definitions and difficulties in acceptance criteria, in Proceedings of Bio '92, Blume, H. H. and Midha, K. K., Eds., in press.

Commentary II

Progress in Harmonization of Bioavailability and Bioequivalence Standards

Iain J. McGilveray

Any account of a current state of policies based on science will be selective and biased by the observer's background. However, there is no doubt that the modern era of bioavailability and bioequivalence began in 1945 when Oser et al.[1] published an article on nutrition in an engineering journal, which defined the concept of physiological availability. The advance in trace analytical techniques in the 1960s, in particular, provided methods sensitive enough to permit urine and subsequently blood (plasma) concentrations of administered drug (or metabolites) to be measured; this, in turn, allowed comparison of formulations in volunteers. The early papers from such groups as Chapman, Campbell, and Morrison in Ottawa; Levy and Nelson in Buffalo; and Wagner in Michigan were reviewed by Wagner.[2] These investigations demonstrated clearly that major differences in bioavailability can occur and be detected among different formulations of the same drug (chemical entity).

Following compulsory licensing legislation in 1969, which facilitated entry of generic drugs to the Canadian market, the Drugs Directorate of the Canadian Federal Department of Health and Welfare began to use bioequivalence as a drug approval measure in the 1970s.[3] Along with other information, the Canadian program was examined by the U.S. Food and Drug Administration (FDA); this was the first regulatory agency to enact regulations for bioequivalence, which were published in the *Federal Register* in 1977.[4] These were landmark regulations and globally the definitions have been used in many jurisdictions. The application of the regulations was enlarged in the Drug Price and Competition Act to encompass post-1962 approved drugs. Following the bioequivalence hearing of 1986, various amendments to the 1977 regulations were adopted.[5]

During the 1980s a number of European regulatory agencies published guidances;[6,7,8] and, in fact, the European Economic Community issued a directive[9] concerning bioavailability. However, it was in 1989 in Toronto, that a major effort was made toward harmonization of bioavailability/bioequivalence requirements with the conference Bio International '89 (Bio '89). The timing of this conference convening as the United States generics scandal[10] broke, was coincidental; however, a number of issues were discussed, and it was obvious that specific topics would generate other conferences. The genesis of the December 1990 Bioanalytical Conference at Crystal City arose from discussion of that topic at Bio '89. The report[11] from the meeting has assisted pharmaceutical manufacturers, contractors, and regulatory reviewers internationally in dealing with analytical aspects of NDAs or ANDAs.

The Bio International '89 conference developed consensus reports for three topics: rate of absorption in bioequivalence determinations, design and assessment of equivalence of highly variable drugs, and statistical analysis of bioequivalence data.[12] The first two topics remain to be resolved but there has been much progress in statistical analysis.

A conference in Barcelona in 1991[13] provided a further opportunity for regulatory agencies to discuss harmonization; to provide general definitions, statistical design, validation, and quality assurance advice; and to indicate under what circumstances bioavailability/bioequivalence studies would or would not be needed. For example, a drug product offering a different strength or strengths than originally approved might be

0-8493-6930-4/94/$0.00+$.50

exempt from bioequivalence study, based on manufacturing and control information with dissolution data, if the formulation was proportional to the existing strength which already exhibited acceptable bioequivalence. This conference provided the basis for the European "note for guidance" on bioavailability[14] produced by the Working Party on Efficacy reporting to the European Commission (EC).

The second Bio International conference held in Germany in 1992 (Bio '92) provided conference statements[15] on highly variable drugs, the importance of metabolites in bioequivalence, and the determination of food effects. The latter topic provided a useful decision tree for consideration of pilot study information to intensively pursue food effects in drug formulation development. Although there was general guidance on use of metabolite information, it was left for case-by-case decision. Again there was no agreement on highly variable drugs, but various research ideas arose from this session that are expected to provide information in the near future. It appears that, in many cases, steady-state studies of highly variable drugs (if ethically allowed) can be used to diminish variability. Also, a replicate design, in which each subject receives two separate doses of reference and perhaps the test product as well, will allow estimation of the intrasubject variation. There have also been many conferences on modified-release formulations, including two with senior FDA authors of reports[16,17] and a more recent Stockholm conference that influenced the EC notes for guidance.[18,19] There are many areas of agreement regarding the bioavailability/bioequivalence of modified-release dosage forms. However, a major unresolved problem is to define criteria governing differences in the shape of plasma/serum concentration curves between products. Peak concentration (C_{max}), trough concentration (C_{min}), and some measure of fluctuation are not sufficient to assure "superimposition" of profiles; this is a particular concern when the relationship of pharmacokinetics to pharmacodynamics is ill-defined.

The FDA Office of Generic Drugs, guided in part by its Generic Drugs Advisory Committee, over the past 3 years has examined many of the problem issues of bioequivalence and initiated research to examine them. As well as focusing on equivalence concerns such as change of formulation and interlot consistency, committee discussions have been concerned with establishing bioequivalence of topical and other nonoral administrations.

Currently major areas of agreement exist between regulatory agencies (EC and other European jurisdictions, Australia, and Japan) in the conduct and design of bioequivalence studies, biological fluid analysis procedures and quality aspects, and most bioequivalence metrics and their statistical evaluation. For conventional, immediate-release oral formulations area under the curve (AUC) following a single dose is accepted as the measure of extent of absorption. Whereas AUC can often be reliably extrapolated to infinity, problems such as enterohepatic recycling can confound the estimate; thus generally the AUC to the last quantifiable concentration (AUC_t) is applied. Also, the rule that AUC_t should be at least 80% of the AUC infinity estimate is widely accepted. Exceptions would be for drugs of long half-lives when plasma concentrations would have to be followed for weeks. (The Canadian approach calls for following AUC to 72 h). A consensus has also been reached on statistical treatment of AUC and on logarithmic transformation of concentration data.[20] The two one-sided test of Schuirmann[21] used by the FDA and the 90% confidence interval provide the same decision rule for the AUC parameter. For the log transform, comparison of test and reference equivalency is declared the 90% confidence interval and is between 80 and 125%.

Estimation of rate of absorption indicators for bioequivalence is under intensive review, but currently C_{max} remains the metric used by all agencies. However, there is not general agreement on the statistical treatment for this variable. Although the FDA requires the same confidence interval as for AUC (90%, range 80 to 125%), the European, Canadian, and Australian approach is more flexible. Guidelines from these agencies suggest that when the rate is known to be more critical, as with an oral analgesic, then

C_{max} should have a stated confidence interval. There is no doubt that better estimators of rate will emerge from new work. While various pharmacokinetic models do not have general application, the use of partial areas (AUC) may have application.[22] The time to attain peak (T_{max}) has been found to be one of the more variable functions. However, most jurisdictions reserve its use for situations like the analgesics, but statistical treatment has still to be determined. The EC note for guidance[14] indicates use of nonparametric procedures.

For many drug products there is some harmonization of requirements. With the drugs (and formulations) termed "complicated" in the Canadian guideline[23] and Expert Advisory Committee report,[24] the authorities find more divergence of opinion. Interestingly, despite a hiatus since 1989, the FDA has begun to revise some guidances on individual drugs. A recent Canadian report[24] attempted to define groups of drugs (complicated) and provide guidance for difficult cases: narrow therapeutic range, nonlinear kinetics, highly toxic, etc. Difference in regulatory approaches can be expected for such products compared with products with a large therapeutic index because of the greater risk associated with interchangeability of these products. The perception of risk may also differ because the risk: benefit ratio is difficult to quantify precisely. However, discussions should aim at developing criteria to obtain standards for regulating the bioequivalence of such products.

Areas of disagreement remain with modified-release dosage forms, e.g., whether clinical studies will be needed when changing from conventional (such as four times a day to once a day) definition of profile and how to deal with enteric-coated products. Harmonization also has not yet been achieved in dealing with products for which plasma concentration data cannot be measured or is confounded in some way, as with albuterol metered-dose inhalers (from which perhaps 10% is absorbed from the airway and 90% in the gastrointestinal tract and plasma concentrations from the two routes cannot be differentiated), topical drugs, and highly toxic drugs that cannot be given to healthy volunteers. Also under discussion are decision criteria for reassessment of products which have been involved in formulation or processing changes, including new strengths with different ingredient proportion, changes of site of manufacture, apparatus, source of raw material, and major or minor variations in formulation. An area of concern is the use of dissolution when no association with *in vivo* metrics has been shown. Some of the above topics have been addressed in other workshops.

A major problem in harmonization of bioequivalence is the reference formulation. Virtually all jurisdictions demand that generic products be compared with innovator or certainly a product approved for marketing based on a full NDA or equivalent. For many drugs, the innovator manufacturer differs among countries; and even with the same international innovator, there can be intentional differences between formulas of the same proprietary "named" product in different countries and further different portfolios of strengths. Decision rules for mutual acceptance of reference products could allow acceptance of studies among countries and conserve precious human, clinical, and analytical resources.

REFERENCES

1. **Oser, B. L., Melnick, P., and Hochberg M.,** Physiological availability of the vitamins study of methods for determining availability in pharmaceutical products, *Ind. Eng. Chem. Anal. Educ.,* 17, 401, 1945.
2. **Wagner, J. G.,** *Biopharmaceutics and Relevant Pharmacokinetics,* Drug Intelligence Publications, Hamilton, IL, 1971, 82.
3. **McGilveray, I. J.,** Bioequivalence: a Canadian regulatory perspective, in *Pharmaceutical Bioequivalence,* Welling, P. G., Tse, F. L. S., and Dighe, S. V., Eds., Marcel Dekker, New York, 1991, 381.

4. Food and Drug Administration, Bioequivalence requirements and *in vivo* bioavailability procedures, *Fed. Regist.,* 42, 1624, 1977.
5. Food and Drug Administration, Abbreviated new drug regulations, finale rule, *Fed. Regist.* 57, 17950, 1992.
6. Medicines Act: Notes on Applications for Product Licenses, Annex II to MAL 2, Department of Health and Social Security, London, 1983.
7. Recommendation: Study of Bioavailability and Bioequivalence, Committee for Evaluation of Medicines, Rijswijk, The Netherlands, 1985 (revised 1987).
8. Nordic Guideline, Bioavailability Studies in Man, NLN Publication No. 18, Nordic Council on Medicines, Uppsala, Sweden, 1987.
9. **Rauws, A. G.,** Bioequivalence: a European Community regulatory perspective, in *Pharmaceutical Bioequivalence,* Welling, P. G., Tse, F. L. S., and Dighe, S. V., Eds., Marcel Dekker, New York, 1991, 419.
10. **Parker, R. E., Martinez, D. R., and Covington, T. R.,** Drug product selection. I. History and legal overview, *Am. Pharm.,* NS31, 524, 1991.
11. **Shah, V. P., Midha, K. K., Dighe, S. V., McGilveray, I. J., Skelly, J. P., Yacobi, A., Layloff, T., Viswanathan, C. J., Cook, C. E., McDowall, R. D., Pittman, K. A., and Spector, S.,** Conference report, analytical methods validation: bioavailability, bioequivalence and pharmacokinetic studies, *Pharm. Res.,* 9, 588, 1992.
12. **McGilveray, I. J.,** Consensus report on Bio International '89: issues in the evaluation of bioavailability, *Pharm. Res.,* 8, 136, 1991.
13. **Cartwright, A. C.,** International Harmonization and Consensus DIA Meeting on bioavailability and bioequivalence testing requirements and standards, *Drug Inform. J.,* 25, 471, 1991.
14. Commission of the European Communities, Committee on Proprietary Medicinal Products (CPMP) Working Party on Efficacy, Note for Guidance, Investigation of Bioavailability and Bioequivalence, December 1991.
15. **Blume, H. and Midha, K. K.,** Conference Report: Bio International '92, Conference on Bioequivalence and Pharmacokinetic Studies, *Pharm. Res.,* 10, 1806, 1993.
16. **Skelly, J. P., Barr, W. H., Benet, L. Z., Doluision, J. T., Goldberg, A. H., Levy, G., Lowenthal, D. T., Robinson, J. R., Shah, V. P., Temple, R. J., and Yacobi, A.,** Report of the Workshop on Controlled-Release Dosage Forms: issues and controversies, *Pharm. Res.,* 4, 75, 1987.
17. **Skelly, J. P., Amidon, G. L., Barr, W. H., Benet, L. Z., Carter, J. E., Robinson, J. R., Shah, V. P., and Yacobi, A.,** Workshop report: *in vitro* and *in vivo* testing and correlation for oral controlled/modified-release dosage forms, *Pharm. Res.,* 7, 975, 1990.
18. Commission of the European Communities, CPMP, Ad hoc Working Party on Efficacy and Medicinal Products, Note for Guidance: Clinical Testing of Prolonged-Action Forms with special Reference to Extended-Release Forms, 1991.
19. Commission of the European Committees, CPMP Working Party on Quality of Medicinal Products, Note for Guidance Quality of Prolonged-Release Oral Solid Dosage Forms, 1992.
20. **Midha, K. K., Ormsby, E. D., Hubbard, J. W., McKay, G., Hawes, E. M., Gavalas, L., and McGilveray, I. J.,** Logarithmic transformation in bioequivalence: application with two-formulations of perphenazine, *J. Pharm. Sci.,* 82, 138, 1993.
21. **Schuirmann, D. J.,** A comparison of the two one-sided tests procedure and the power approach for assessing the equivalence of average bioavailability, *J. Pharmacokinet. Biopharm.,* 15, 657, 1987.
22. **Mei-Ling, Chen,** An alternative approach for assessment of rate of absorption in bioavailability studies, *Pharm. Res.,* 9, 1380, 1992.

23. Health and Welfare Canada, Drugs Directorate Guidelines: Conduct and Analysis of Bioavailability and Bioequivalence Studies. Part A. Oral Dosage Formulations Used for Systemic Effects, The Government Publishing Centre, Supply and Services Canada, Ottawa, 1992.
24. Drugs Directorate, Health Protection Branch, Health and Welfare Canada, Expert Advisory Committee on Bioavailability, Report on Bioavailability of Oral Formulations of Drugs Used for Systemic Effects. Report C. Report on Bioavailability of Oral Dosage Formulations, Not in Modified-Release Form, of Drugs Used for Systemic Effects, Having Complicated or Variable Pharmacokinetics, December 1992.

INDEX

A

B

C

H

I

K

L

M

Q

R

S

T

U

V

W

Z

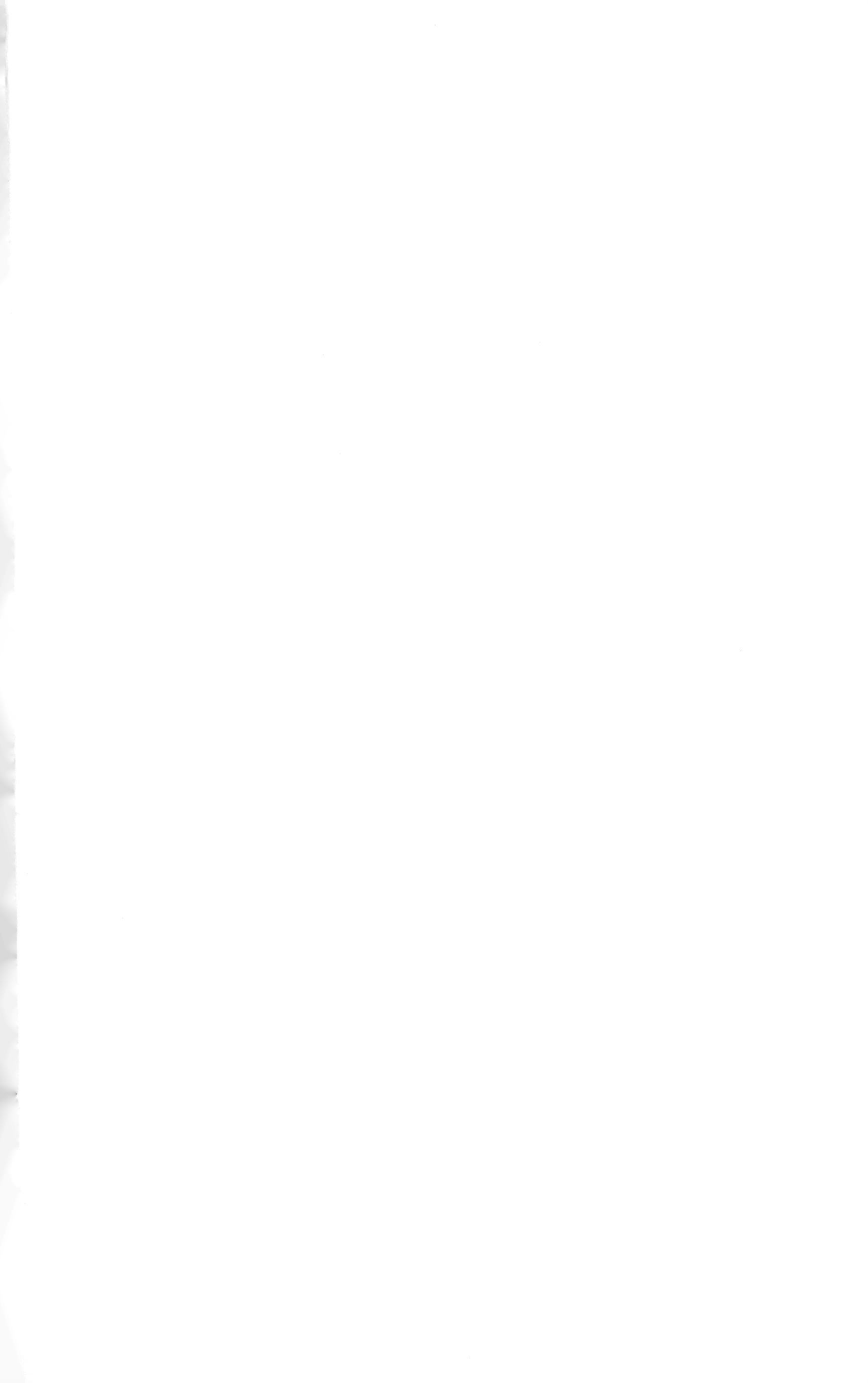